Epidemic Disease and Human Understanding

Epidemic Disease and Human Understanding

A Historical Analysis of Scientific and Other Writings

CHARLES DE PAOLO

McFarland & Company, Inc., Publishers
Jefferson, North Carolina, and London

LIBRARY OF CONGRESS CATALOGING-IN-PUBLICATION DATA DATA

De Paolo, Charles, 1950–
    Epidemic disease and human understanding : a historical
analysis of scientific and other writings / Charles De Paolo.
        p.   cm.
    Includes bibliographical references and index.

    ISBN-13: 978-0-7864-2506-8
    softcover : 50# alkaline paper ∞

    1. Epidemics— History. 2. Epidemiology— History. I. Title.
[DNLM: 1. Disease Outbreaks— history. 2. Epidemiology—
history. 3. Attitude to Health. WA 11.1 D422e 2006]
RA649.D47 2006
614.4 — dc22   2006000198
                                                      (DNLM)101264802

British Library cataloguing data are available

On the cover: Photomicrograph of *Yersinia pestis* bacteria, the infectious
agent of bubonic plague *(Public Health Image Library)*

Manufactured in the United States of America

McFarland & Company, Inc., Publishers
  Box 611, Jefferson, North Carolina 28640
    www.mcfarlandpub.com

To Andrea, Victoria, and Patrick

Contents

Contents

Acknowledgments

I would like to thank my colleagues at Borough of Manhattan Community College for encouraging and supporting my work. I am especially indebted to Antonio Pérez, Sadie Bragg, Michael Gillespie, Daisy Alverio, John Montanez, Erwin Wong, Robert Zweig, Frank Elmi, and Phil Eggers. I am grateful, as well, to the College for awarding me a Faculty Development Grant and to the Professional Staff Congress of the City University of New York, for offering me release time to pursue research. Medical professionals and literature scholars outside the College community offered invaluable advice and encouragement: Alan Greenberg, M.D., M.P.H., Mary Ann Chiasson, Dr. P.H., Carol McGuirk, and John S. Partington.

Permission to use material from the following sources is gratefully acknowledged: the Hench-Reed Collection of The Health Services Library of the University of Virginia. The Yellow Fever / Walter Reed Commission Exhibit and the Hench-Reed Collection can be accessed at the website of the University of Virginia Health Sciences Library: www.med.virginia.edu; a translation of Pasteur's "The Anthrax Vaccination: Reply of M. Pasteur to a paper of M. Koch," by David and Evelyn Cohen; papers by Pasteur, Koch, Lister, and Jenner can be accessed at their website: http://www.founersofscience.net/p'sReply.htm; and *Milestones in Microbiology: 1546 to 1940*, edited and translated by Thomas D. Brock, published by the American Society for Microbiology, Washington, D.C.

Abbreviations

CDC	Centers for Disease Control and Prevention
KJV	King James Version of the Bible
LD	Legionnaires' Disease
OED	Oxford English Dictionary (1st ed., 1933)
WHO	World Health Organization

Introduction

For more than three millennia of recorded history in the West, human beings have struggled to understand the meaning of the *epidemic* (Greek, *epi + demos,* "among the people"), a familiar word referring to the rapid spread of contagious disease (*Random House,* 444). Before we can survey how human beings have reacted to epidemic disease and the manner in which they have communicated these reactions, we need to have a firm understanding of what an *epidemic* is and of how it differs from related terms.

An etymological survey of the terms *epidemic, pandemic, endemic,* and *outbreak* will help us to understand their respective developments. Samuel Johnson, in his *Dictionary of the English Language* (1755), defines epidemic as a disease that "falls at once upon great numbers of people, as a plague" (p. 243). The mid-eighteenth century meaning of epidemic, of which Johnson's definition is representative, ascribes to it two distinguishing traits: sudden appearance and rapid spread.

From an etymological perspective, we find that the word *pandemic,* a Greek compound of *pan-* ("common") and of *demos-* ("people"), developed from the epidemic idea over centuries. In 1799, according to Hooper's *Medical Dictionary,* for example, the words epidemic and pandemic were used interchangably (*OED* XII: 417; "pandemic"), and, as late as 1853, were synonyms, as we find in Dunglison's *Medical Lexicon* (*OED* XII: 417; "pandemic"). But, by 1876, a standard text, Wagner's *General Pathology,* includes an important distinction: "an epidemic exists in one community only, *but in its greater extension, over a whole land, it is called a pandemic*" (*OED* XII: 417; "pandemic"; italics added). A *Times* article of September 2, 1892 makes it unequivocally clear that a pandemic, unlike an epidemic, is marked by geographical extensiveness and that it strikes many more people as a result; hence, the author writes that, in 1892, "[they were] face to face with a pandemic outbreak of cholera similar to those which fell upon Europe in 1830, 1847, 1853, 1866" (*OED* XII: 417; "pandemic").

In modern terminology, epidemic and pandemic are distinct but

1

closely-related terms. In *The Oxford English Dictionary*, an epidemic is a contagious malady "prevalent among a community or people at a special time and produced by some special causes not generally present in the affected locality" (*OED* IV: 239; "epidemic"). Read in conjunction with earlier definitions, the modern denotation of epidemic involves the *eruption* of a *non-indigenous* disease that affects a *limited* region and population (italics added). The *OED* distinguishes between the two terms explicitly: whereas a pandemic is "prevalent over the whole of a country or continent, or over the whole world," it differs from *epidemic*, which "may connote limitation to a smaller area" (*OED* XII: 417; "pandemic"). Thus, epidemic and pandemic diseases are virulent, non-indigenous, and eruptive, but they differ from one another in terms of physical extensiveness. The use of the optative mood in the phrase *may connote* in the *OED* suggests that the question of geographical borders demarcating an epidemic from a pandemic is not as clear as one would hope; for instance, a pandemic, usually thought of as a global phenomenon, can be used to describe a disease prevalent in a single country or in a single continent. For our purposes, however, the epidemiological realities these terms represent are differentiated from each other in terms of degree: in our experience, pandemics are intercontinental and involve more than one country.

Two related terms to appear in the course of our discussion also need to be clarified: they are *endemic* and *outbreak*. Deriving from the Greek *endemos*, which means "of or belonging to a state or people," endemicity refers to a disease "[h]abitually prevalent in a certain country, and due to permanent local causes" (*OED* IV: 159; "endemic"). As early as the seventeenth century, the distinction between endemic and epidemic had been recognized. Dr. Johnson (citing the English physician, William Harvey [1578–1657]) writes that an endemic disease proceeds "from some cause peculiar to the country where it reigns" (p. 237); that is, its source is not a foreign element introduced into the local ecology, the opposite being true for an epidemic.

The word *outbreak*, understood as an "eruption," has been used since the seventeenth century to describe emotional behavior and creativity; in 1806, it was even employed to convey how igneous rocks can burst from below the surface, and the word has since been included in the lexicon of geology. As far as disease is concerned, one of the term's initial applications has been traced to an 1879 publication of *St. George's Hospital*, in which reference is made to two "diphtheritic outbreaks" (*OED* XI: 248; "outbreak"). Robert De Salle and Marla Jo Brickman have recently defined the term aptly as "a suddenly occurring and explosively rapid increase in the incidence of an infectious disease in a population" (113). Once again, we are concerned with matters of degree: an outbreak involves an especially virulent infection, possibly the flashpoint or flashpoints of an epidemic.

More specific terms have a place in this study, so I would like to define them briefly in the course of previewing the content of the book. To make sense of the mysterious nature of epidemic disease, the writers of antiquity subsumed the experience under religious, mythological, or philosophical paradigms. One of the earliest ways of comprehending the disorientating effects of an outbreak, then, was to ascribe it to supernatural or cosmic powers, and I call this interpretation *pre-conceptuality*. A dogmatic rather than naturalistic view, *pre-conceptuality* (which is the focus of Part I) was manifested in Greco-Roman ascriptions of disease to mythic demi-gods, in Judeo-Christian assimilations of disease into sacred theodicy, and in philosophical speculations on the origin and cause of illness. In each case, the cause of the disease was *pre*conceived, that is, formulated in terms of received doctrines and of intellectual assumptions about nature.

In certain instances, ancient and classical writers found it difficult to explain the course of a disease dogmatically. If the faithful, for example, were not immune to an illness that was decimating their persecutors, then the dogmatic rationale had to be revised to render the inconsistency intelligible. Thus, one could say that the suffering of the steadfast elect was intended to inspire conversions. Or one could say that disease, along with other natural catastrophes, fulfilled the prophecies of sacred literature, such as those in *The Revelation of St. John the Divine*. If we look at the period of the Black Death for an example, we find writers such as the Franciscan Jean de Roquetaillade (c. 1310–c.1365) avowing that, in 1348–49, the end of the world was surely imminent (McGinn 174–75). For some chroniclers of the period, the plague which had come to Europe from the mysterious Orient was undeniably a punishment from God (Ziegler 16). Before the seventeenth century, then, many looked to the heavens or to philosophy for comfort in times of plague.

Gradually, the epidemic experience came to be interpreted as a natural phenomenon rather than as an instrument of divine purpose. The transition from an emphasis on received doctrine to one on direct experience is the focus of Part II. As early as the sixth century A.D., historians had begun to perceive epidemic disease, not as the fulfillment of divine aims or as the effect of cosmic perturbations, but as an *anomaly*—an occurrence deviating from preconceived expectation (*Random House* 55). Since the epidemic anomaly is such a useful index in the development of Western biomedical thought, I will briefly define the origin and modern understandings of the term.

In the seventeenth century, two diametrically opposed meanings circulated. On the one hand, Sir Thomas Browne (1605–1682), English physician and religious thinker, wrote, in 1646, that an *anomaly* was a radical imperfection and a divergence from the natural order whereas, to a contemporary of Browne, a natural anomaly evidenced the plenitude of divine creation (*OED* I: 346; "anomaly"). For modern philosophers and historians of science, anomalies have been perceived not so much as reflections of divine workmanship but as fresh insights into natural reality. In the first place, according to several contemporary writers, the ability to identify an anomaly in an experiment presupposes that the investigator is trained in the discipline and, in the light of this training, knows what to expect and what is out of the ordinary (Beveridge 102, 96–105; Medawar 734–35). An anomaly cannot be ignored since it may lead to new knowledge. And, if that knowledge is valid, it may, in turn, have the capacity to redefine established scientific paradigms (Kuhn [1970], 52–3). The writers of antiquity, on the other hand, struggled to make sense of horrible epidemics in the context of what they believed to be true about creation.

In Western history, early epidemiological thought did not suddenly supplant pre-conceptuality. As I show in Part II. The Observational Modality, these perspectives developed concurrently and, in places, overlapped with one another. Pre-conceptual epidemiology survives today; in its worst, exclusionary form, it has appeared as a fearful, ignorant, and anti-scientific response to disease. The beginning of an objective way of looking at pestilence, surprisingly, dates as far back as the fifth century B.C. in Greece. I use the modern phrase *eyewitness report* to describe the heritage of objective description, from which modern biomedical discourse derives. The eyewitness account, to which I refer, can be composed of first- or of secondhand sources, or it can be a combination of the two. Thucydides' description of the plague of Athens in 430 B.C. is a seminal example of the firsthand form, while Giovanni Boccaccio's plague description in *The Decameron* is possibly an amalgam of first- and of secondhand material.

The systematic examination of biomedical phenomena that I call the *investigative modality* emerged from eyewitness reports and developed gradually from the seventeenth century to the present. How this method developed is the focus of Part III. Eschewing dogmatic interpretations, certain observers speculated on anomalous aspects of pestilence and were particularly interested in causes, in clinical symptoms, and in the disorienting effects of epidemic disease. Girolamo Fracastoro (1478–1553), Nathaniel Hodges (1629–1688), and others arrived at common sense solutions in regard to the control of illnesses. Representative of this transitional phase in the development of epidemiological thought is the testimony of Dr. Hodges, written during the frightful plague epidemic of 1664–1665. As a critical historian, he condemned heterodox medicine, untested drugs, and criminal activity, while advocating reasonable adjustments of the quarantine system to control the spread of the disease. His overriding concern was for the suffering populous. Though Hodges labored under the misconception that the disease was atmospheric in origin, he still resisted superstitious and untrustworthy remedies, and his work adumbrated more critical forms of documentary discourse.

Equipped with the compound microscope (invented in 1609), seventeenth-century investigators, such as Athanasius Kircher (1602–1680), Anton van Leeuwenhoek (1632–1723), and Robert Hooke (1635–1703), contemplated the nature of invisible organisms and their relationship to disease (Winslow 144–60; Summers, "Microbiology"). The *investigative modality* arose from the pioneering work of seventeenth-century inventors and naturalists. As explained in chapters 8 and 9, investigation (as I see it) comprises three interactive phases: the *inferential* (logical assumptions made about disease causation); the *etiological* (the rigorous testing of these assumptions); and the *synergistic* (the interdisciplinary treatment, control, and prevention of outbreaks).

The greatest accomplishments in epidemiology began with tentative assumptions, with inferences subjected to rigorous, experimental trials. To illustrate how assumptions of this kind stimulated research, I discuss in Chapter 8 the early histories of smallpox, of puerperal fever, and of cholera. Pre-experimental ideas, the most important links in the chain of discovery, often amounted to little more than anecdotes, intuitions, and guesses. Yet progress against epidemic disease would have been impossible had it not been for intelligent guesswork. Those who inferred ideas from the smallpox experience, for instance, provided a bridge between folkloric medicine and the praxis of immunization. A critical juncture in the inferential history of variola, historians point out, occurred in ancient India and China, where it had become a commonplace observation that pockmarked survivors of the disease rarely experienced severe recurrences (Tucker 15, 17; I. and J. Glynn 6–9); the crucial assumption was that the matter of infection somehow protected against a second attack. The French philosopher, historian, and dramatist Voltaire (1694–1778) was one of the first Europeans to infer as much in 1733, citing the inoculative practices of the Turks. Thomas Dimsdale (1712–1800), the personal physician to Catherine the Great of Russia (1729–1796), inoculated the Empress in October 1768, and the record of her treatment stands as one of the first official documents in this line of inquiry. Similarly, Edward Jenner's (1749–1823) work on vaccination as a safer alternative to variolation was stimulated, during his early years, by the local belief in Gloucestershire that contracting cowpox brought immunity to smallpox.

A simple observation among rural folk, therefore, was behind the practice of vaccination in Britain.

The campaign against puerperal or childbed fever, the second example of inferentiality I present, also underscores the importance to scientific research of assumptions based on probability. Oliver Wendell Holmes (1809–1894), in his 1843 survey of childbed-fever research, compiled the experiences and assumptions of physicians who believed that the disease was contagious. On the basis of circumstantial evidence and of anecdotes, he surmised that medical practitioners unknowingly carried the infectious agent on their bodies and that antiseptic precautions were imperative. The high incidence of puerperal fever in a clinic where obstetricians regularly performed autopsies prompted the physician Ignaz Semmelweis (1818–1865) to conclude that practitioners carried the disease from the autopsy room to parturient women, a view contrary to the opinions of many contemporary doctors. Semmelweis (and later Louis Pasteur [1822–1895]) moved from inference to praxis and recorded the results of using simple hygienic procedures as a way of lowering the morbidity rate. Dr. John Snow (1813–1858), whose work on cholera is the third prominent example of inferentiality to be discussed, linked an 1855 cholera outbreak in London to a public water source. Visual inspection of water samples, residential interviews, along with medical and geographical assessments, provided circumstantial evidence to warrant the incapacitation of the Broad Street pump.

A branch of medicine concerned with disease causation, *etiology* (from the Greek word *aitiologia*: "determining the cause of something") relies upon inference (*OED* I: 149; "aetiology"). Robert Koch (1843–1910), German bacteriologist, physician, and 1905 Nobel Prize recipient, demonstrated that the organism *Bacillus anthracis* caused anthrax. Emerging from an inferential context, his work depended on the theories of Casimir Davaine (1812–1882), of Ferdinand Cohn (1828–1898), and of others who had initially inferred that blood-borne particles in sheep were related to anthrax disease (Lord 1). Through the study of the life-cycle of the organism, both *in vitro* and *in vivo*, Koch was able to prove that the bacillus caused the disease. In 1882, he distilled a methodology from his anthrax work, a series of postulates that, if systematically adhered to, could establish causation between suspect bacteria and disease. Once Koch had established the etiology or cause of anthrax, he was able to articulate his "perfect proof," a five-part process involving: (1) the isolation of foreign substances from diseased tissue so as to differentiate between the pathogen and its possible by-products (e.g., toxins); (2) the culturing of the suspected pathogen outside of its host; (3) the introduction of the culture into uninfected laboratory animals; (4) the identification of the microbial extract as the probable cause of disease in laboratory animals; and (5), through tissue and blood analysis, the identification of the pathogen found in laboratory animals with the one that had afflicted the original animal naturally. In addition, Koch learned that, for some diseases, the inoculation of a small quantity of diseased blood into healthy animals induced the illness.

Louis Pasteur, French chemist and bacteriologist, ingeniously applied immunization methods that Jenner had used against smallpox to the creation of an anthrax vaccine for veterinary use. The conquest of anthrax, a collaborative achievement, involved an accumulation of precedents, of inferences, of complex etiological experimentation, and, finally, of interventions (in the use of vaccine). Benefiting from the works of Jenner and Koch, Pasteur and his medical advisors contributed to the campaign against puerperal fever by demonstrating the importance of clinical observations and record-keeping, of laboratory assays, and of autopsies. Pasteur's rabies vaccine depended on the achievements of Friedrich Johannes Löffler, of Paul F. Frosch, and of others who inferred that filterable pathogens were responsible for foot-and-mouth disease. Jenner's method led Pasteur to assume that inoculation with graduated strengths of virulent material directly affected the immunological response. Throughout the rabies experimentation, Pasteur surmounted barriers inferentially, but he encountered a difficult problem: though the vaccine was successful with dogs, he could not be sure if it benefited man since human experimentation, using volunteers in a laboratory setting, was impossible. When the opportunity materialized for human experimentation, however, Pasteur went to work and achieved positive results.

In the late nineteenth century, a pattern of intellectual discovery, similar to that identified for anthrax, can be traced for bubonic plague. In his 1894 field work, the bacteriologist Alexandre Yersin (1863–1943) inferred that rat epizootics, the mass dying-off of rodents with plague, were connected to outbreaks of the disease, not only because the rodent plague or epizootic suspiciously preceded human ones, but also because there was a considerable body of anecdotal opinion and of popular belief to that effect among the people of Canton Province, China. On the basis of this idea, and concurrently with the Japanese microbiologist, Shibasaburo Kitasato (1852–1931), Yersin formulated the hypothesis that animals were intermediaries in the cycle of human disease. His on-site laboratory work on transmission raised the possibility that insect vectors were involved, and he made a substantive contribution when he speculated that plague inoculum had immunizing potential. Neither Yersin nor Kitasato, however, contributed to the etiological understanding of plague.

Paul-Louis Simond (1858–1947) proved experimentally, in 1898, that bubonic plague could be contracted without one having had close contact with a sick person. Once again, etiology depended on inference. Simond not only profited from the popular belief in Yunnan, China, that ratfall signaled an imminent outbreak, but he also made a startling assumption: flea bites in anatomical proximity to plague-infected lymph nodes indicated that insects transmitted the pathogen through blood-feeding.

Inferences punctuate the early history of typhus research. During the time between the outdoor preparation of typhus patients and their admission to the hospital, Dr. Charles Nicolle (1866–1936) noticed an anomaly: hospital personnel were especially susceptible to the disease during this period. From observations, he inferred that close physical contact rather than atmospheric pathogens was responsible for the transmission of the malady. He later hypothesized that the body louse transmitted the disease from patient to worker: the louse attached itself to the skin rather than to discarded clothing, and soap and water caused it to abandon patients for new hosts, often the hospital personnel who disrobed and bathed the sick.

To exemplify the development of etiological thought into a interdisciplinary, synergistic approach, I discuss the discovery and treatment of Legionellosis, a disease caused by a ubiquitous, aquatic microbe. The campaign against this disease began, in 1977, when doctors encountered patients stricken with an unknown pneumonia. Its diagnosis and treatment, which profited from the recollection of personal experiences and from archived specimens, depended on teamwork involving pulmonologists, entomologists, molecular biologists, geneticists, technicians, and many others.

In Part IV, I consider the ways in which epidemic disease has been treated in contexts other than the laboratory or clinic. In the modern eyewitness report, in fiction, and with figurative language, writers have described the human experience with pestilence in various ways. I begin, in Chapter 10, with descriptions of extensive disease and the means by which debilitation was managed. Captivity narratives, three of which I survey in this chapter, recount extreme ordeals and, therefore, are the most impressive discourses of survival. I present the personal narratives of a prisoner of war, of a traveler to a leper colony, and of a concentration camp prisoner. John McElroy (1846–1929), a Federal prisoner of war at Andersonville, Georgia, wrote a riveting account of his internment in 1864 and of the degree to which prisoners suffered from parasitic and infectious diseases in a camp lacking adequate housing, medicine, food, water, or clean clothing. The results were catastrophic, one-third of the prisoners dying in a matter of weeks from typhus, from dysentery, and from other disorders.

Andersonville contrasts sharply with life in Molokai, Hawaii, where, according to Jack London's (1876–1916) 1906 travelogue, the government had established a humane leper colony. Contrary to expectations, London found that the disease was being efficiently managed on Molokai, due to adequate nutritional and medical support. Though both Andersonville in 1864 and Molokai in 1906 were closed communities, in the former, overseers were contemptuous of human life while, in the latter, life was valued and nurtured.

A third variant of the captivity narrative is based upon experiences in the German concentration camp at Auschwitz in 1945. The narrative of Primo Levi (1919–1987), an Italian chemist and prisoner assigned to the labor detail, conflates features of McElroy's Andersonville and of London's Molokai. Levi experiences horrors on par with Andersonville but survived through ingenuity, and through cooperation with fellow prisoners. He and his companions acquired enough material and food to create a refuge in a clinic. Up to the moment of their liberation, Levi's refuge fostered hope in the future. The keys to their survival were inventiveness, good fortune, sufficient food, medicine, and electrical power (produced by a battery).

Along with historiography, the investigative report, and the autobiographical account, imaginative writing belongs to the heritage of epidemic discourse. I use the term *extrapolation* to describe a successful formula for the writing of epidemiological fiction or drama. By fictional extrapolation, I do not mean to estimate statistically the value of a variable beyond its observed range (*OED* IV: 473; "extrapolation"; *Random House* 469); rather, I am concerned with the degree to which epidemic worlds in fiction conform to historical and biomedical facts. I focus, specifically, on fictional environments afflicted by the bubonic plague.

History and fiction interpenetrate each other in Sinclair Lewis' (1885–1951) *Arrowsmith*. The early history of bacteriophage, a naturally-occurring, viral antagonist of bacteria, is the experimental context of the novel. Its discoverers initially encountered this biological anomaly in cultures of pathogenic bacteria. From the visual inspection of bacterial colonies, the scientists Hankin, Twort, and d'Hérelle independently inferred that an invisible agent, either microbe or enzyme, could destroy certain species of bacteria. Their experimentation was limited, since they were actually studying a virus which (unknown at the time) could only be seen through an electron microscope (invented independently, in 1932, by Ernst Ruska and Rheinhold Ruedenberg). Lewis' protagonist is portrayed as a contemporary of Dr. Felix d'Hérelle and (like Dr. Twort) as the unacknowledged codiscoverer of phage in 1917. Like d'Hérelle, Arrowsmith tries but fails to conduct definitive vaccine research during a plague outbreak. Just as d'Hérelle's failure in this pursuit was attributed to misguided altruism and to faulty research methods, Arrowsmith fails to test the discovery exhaustively and does not strictly adhere to scientific procedures; in part, his failure to prove the phage a viable therapy against plague is due to ignorant, obstructive authorities who interfere with his fieldwork on the fictitious Caribbean island of St. Hubert.

A second work to be discussed is Albert Camus' *The Plague* (1947), a fictive documentary written from the viewpoint of the protagonist, Dr. Bernard Rieux. Despite steadfast medical and civil efforts to stem the pestilence, the medical establishment of Oran, Algeria, achieves little beyond palliative measures as the disease runs its natural course. Whereas Arrowsmith experiences some success with phage vaccine, Rieux is woefully underequipped and technologically disadvantaged, so much so that he appears as effective in his endeavors as a fourteenth-century physician in opposing the Black Death.

The obstructionism of St. Hubert and the unpreparedness of the Oranais' medical establishment are major themes in *The Black Death* (1976), by Gwyneth Cravens and John S. Marr, M.D. To prevent the disease from spreading exponentially in New York City, the epidemiologist David Hart, M.D., initiates an aggressive public-health campaign. Unforeseen factors, similar to those on St. Hubert and in Oran, complicate the campaign. Budget cuts, bureaucratic red tape, untrained personnel, and ignorance subvert Dr. Hart's emergency program to stop the disease from gaining momentum. The plot is entirely plausible: plague is unknowingly transported by a female traveler who was infected in New Mexico where it is endemic to species of ground squirrel (its fleas transmit the blood-borne infection to other mammals). From the outset, Hart's work is hampered. Without a team and a network in place, and when the doctor is sickened himself, the disease spreads as predicted, especially when aerosolized and inhaled like the common cold. Barely avoiding mass fumigation at the hands of a desperate government, the survivors of the plague escape through tunnels from Manhattan into Queens.

The common theme of these novels, especially relevant to post–911 America, is that preparedness is essential if an outbreak is to be curtailed. Like the disasters on St. Hubert and in Oran, the pestilence in New York City runs its deadly course and eventually subsides, modern biotechnology, in the final analysis, having little impact on its ebb and flow.

In Chapter 12, about figurative language in epidemiologic discourse, I discuss the need in biomedical discourse of language that is exact and unambiguous. Figurative language (e.g., metaphor and personification), I emphasize, should not be used if it interferes with the comprehension of biomedical realities. To test the informational accuracy and value of figurative constructs, one needs to compare them not to popular culture or politics but to the biomedical information they purport to communicate. Whereas pre-conceptual writers, such as Procopius of Caesarea (6th century A.D.), personified plague because no other means of conveying its ubiquity, destructive power, and imperviousness was available, writers from the later nineteenth century to the present have experimented with rhetorical constructs, often leading to confusion. Ferdinand Cohn's general portrayal of bacteria and Hans Zinsser's personification of typhus, for instance, exemplify the injudicious use of figurative tropes. Contemporary writers, such as Laurie Garrett and Robert De Salle, with varying degrees of success, experiment with personification and analogy. Although Joshua Lederberg's 1998 essay on the history of infectious disease up to the present exhibits figurative language that distorts scientific fact, he revised its content meritoriously in the essay "Infectious History" (2000). The obvious rhetorical difference between the two essays is the elimination of figurative language from the variant of 2000.

The cognitive and technological phases of epidemiological thought that I trace over millennia are replicated in specific campaigns and over brief periods of time. In Chapter 13, I demonstrate how the cognitive progression from inference to synergy informs the campaign against yellow fever, 1881 to 1908. A selection of primary texts reveals the sequential workings of three modalities: the inferential-hypothetical, the investigative (etiological, autobiographical, and preventive), and the extrapolative (the dramatic).

The Cuban physician, Carlos Juan Finlay (1833–1911), hypothesized, in 1881, that a species of mosquito, rather than contaminated atmosphere, transmitted yellow fever. He attained limited experimental support for his hypothesis; nevertheless, Finlay's thinking motivated Walter C. Reed, M.D. (1851–1902) and his team to conduct large-scale human experiments on mosquito-borne contagion. One volunteer, John J. Moran, describes in his memoirs that the experiment, commencing on November 20, 1900, involved his exposure to fifteen infected mosquitoes. Whereas other participants who were exposed to yellow fever secretions on infected clothing and bedding did not contract the disease, Moran became ill after enduring repeated bites, but he survived. Thanks to the courage of Moran and others, Finlay's hypothesis was borne out, as Walter Reed established the etiology of the disease. Reed's colleague, William Crawford Gorgas, M.D. (1854–1920), stamped out mosquito breeding grounds in Cuba (in the preventive phase of the campaign), once it was understood that certain species of the insect transmitted the virus to and between human beings. Through a rigorous, threefold strategy — the treatment of breeding sites, the use of fumigation to kill infected female mosquitoes, and, ironically, the isolation of infected patients from non-infected mosquitoes (which ingested infected human blood and transmitted the virus to healthy persons), Gorgas et al. suppressed the disease. In 1905, he successfully brought this new knowledge to bear on the yellow fever epidemic in the Panama Canal Zone. The extrapolative aspect of the series, however, is a disappointment. Sidney Coe Howard's famous drama, *Yellow Jack: A History* (1933), seriously distorts the events and motives of the characters. Whereas extrapolative writing ideally aims to recreate epidemic events in accordance with biographical and epidemiologic realities, the drama in question misrepresents intellectual, personal, and ethical aspects of the story.

As I survey human responses to epidemic disease, I relate three subgenres of epidemiological writing to one another: the encyclopedia, the intellectual history, and the biographical collection. In this survey, I have chosen primary texts reflecting the historical unity of epidemiological thought over three millennia. Because my scope is broad, this study differs significantly from works devoted to the comprehensive history of a single epidemic disease. The histories of the influenza pandemic of 1918, of anthrax, and of smallpox exemplify the latter. Thus, for a comprehensive historical understanding of the influenza epidemic of 1918, Alfred W. Crosby's *America's Forgotten Pandemic: The Influenza of 1918* (1989), Gina Kolata's *Flu: The Story of the Great Influenza Pandemic of 1918 and the Search for the Virus That Caused It* (1999), and John M. Barry's *The Great Influenza: The Epic Story of the Deadliest Plague in History* (2004) are required readings; for anthrax, one will benefit greatly from Richard M. Swiderski's *Anthrax: A History* (2004); and for smallpox, three recent books are especially useful: Jonathan B. Tucker's *Scourge: The Once and Future Threat of Smallpox* (2001), Richard Preston's *The Demon in the Freezer: A True Story* (2002), and Ian and Jenifer Glynn's *The Life and Death of Smallpox* (2004). Unlike historiographers who are concerned with a single disease, I focus on interpretations of, and reactions to, a number of epidemic diseases as they are expressed in selected primary texts. To position this study in the scholarly corpus, I compare it closely to related generic forms mentioned above.

Encyclopedias on world epidemics are essential on every level of study in the field. Two texts, in particular — the *Encyclopedia of Plague and Pestilence from Ancient Times to the Present* (1995, revised 2001), edited by George Childs Kohn et al., and Mary Ellen Snodgrass' *World Epidemics: A Cultural Chronology of Disease from Prehistory to the Era of SARS* (2003) — convey the chronological, topical, cultural, and geographical breadth of the subject.

Kohn's book contains cross-referenced information, organized under three categories: pathology, chronology, and geography. Each entry provides important facts regarding the time and place of specific outbreaks, possible reasons for occurrences and dissemination, whom the epidemic mainly affected, and what the most significant outcomes of these events were. Overall, Kohn et al. discuss forty-eight diseases in twenty geographical locations (i.e., continents, regions, and nations).

Mary Ellen Snodgrass, in her impressive, chronological digest of world epidemics, presents readers with "a panoramic overview of patterns in human behavior" (p. 6). Epidemic diseases have extreme consequences, destroying social, political, and cultural structures, debasing or ennobling the human character, and stifling or inspiring the human mind (pp.6–7). The human reaction to an intense outbreak, she points out, forces a culture to define itself: "In propitiating gods, administering herbs, vaccinating the uninfected, or bidding farewell to a hopeless case, survivors' responses reveal individual values and belief systems as well as the outlook of the times, whether sanguine, indifferent, or resigned" (p. 8). Because encyclopedias of this caliber furnish historical overviews and salient facts, they are essential to serious study.

A lineal precursor of my book is Charles-Edward Amory Winslow's *The Conquest of Epidemic Disease: A Chapter in the History of Ideas* (1943). In his survey of the human response to disease over two millennia, Winslow envisages the intellectual history of epidemiology from its earliest times as a "gradual evolution" in thinking (v), a phrase I take to mean the increasing complexity of human thought on the subject from age to age. As the subtitle suggests, the emphasis is not the lives of great scientists, nor the history of specific epidemics, but biomedical concepts— e.g., contagion, germs, putrefaction, the carrier, and quarantine — accretively defined through experimentation and in discourse.

One unavoidable difficulty with a survey such as Winslow's is that the linkages between ideas, from period to period, can at times be unclear. Because Winslow did not organize the text consistently under conceptual headings, some ideas are discontinuously presented, and some are even truncated. Of the eighteen chapters, covering nearly three millennia of epidemiological history, approximately a third are focused conceptually, for example, Chapter V: Primitive Concepts of Contagion, Chapter VIII: The Conception of a Contagium Animatum, and Chapter XVI: The Concept of the Carrier. But the remaining chapters are focused on social movements (Chapter XII: The Great Sanitary Awakening); on diseases (Chapter XI: The Enigma of Yellow Fever); and on great scientists (Chapter XIV: Pasteur). In certain instances, though the continuity of an idea can be followed (e.g., the idea of atmospheric causation, from tenth and eleventh-century

Arabic writers to Edwin Chadwick [1800–1890] and the great sanitary awakening in England), Winslow does not analyze its movement and transformations through time. Another example of this missed opportunity concerns the history of the human carrier: a truncated concept, it springs up in the text as if devoid either of antecedents or of an intuitive and inferential past. Winslow more than compensates for this unevenness by using primary texts as the bases of his discussions.

The third subgenre of epidemiological writing to which this study relates is the biographical survey. Paul de Kruif, in his representative work *Microbe Hunters* (1926), focuses on the lives and works of the germ theorists, the great biomedical scientists of the later nineteenth- and early twentieth century. Presenting the intellectual lives of thirteen eminent scientists, along with their collaborators, he devotes each chapter to their impact on a specific disease. Louis Pasteur's conquest of rabies, for example, is titled "Pasteur: And the Mad Dog," while Walter Reed's campaign against yellow fever is recounted in "Walter Reed: In the Interest of Science — and for Humanity!" Since insight and discovery are, in de Kruif's mind, of the greatest value, the ostensibly biographical apparatus of the book is deceiving. The portraits are actually studies in cognition, and the biographer stresses the importance to research of guesswork and of informed suppositions.

Although de Kruif's biographical survey has much in common with the intellectual history, *Microbe Hunters* (like *The Conquest of Epidemic Disease*) lacks an explicit statements pertaining to the intellectual progress of the discipline, to the unity of the corpus, and to the complex interrelationships of its phases, contradictions, and transitions. The problem stems from the way in which de Kruif presents each episode. Since discoveries are *narrated* rather than *analyzed*, it is up to the reader to outline etiological processes. An index to this shortcoming is the history of diphtheria research at the turn of the century, the overlapping phases of which (summarized here) are implicit in the text (pp. 178–200). The research history of this disease is quite complex, involving four major phases (and at least seven transitional ones) and the efforts of three major scientists and a host of associates: (1a) Löffler finds an anomaly: germs in the throat of diphtheria decedents are nowhere else in the body; (1b) he infers that the throat colony produced a lethal toxin; (2a) Pierre Roux (1853–1933) and Yersin try to filter the unknown factor from the blood; (2b) tests are positive: diphtheria is induced in lab animals through inoculation; the toxin is successfully isolated; (3a) Emil von Behring (1854–1917) counteracts the disease in some animals by injecting an iodine solution; (3b) he suspects that the blood sera of surviving animals have protective qualities; (3c) he stimulates immunity in healthy animals, injecting blood sera from surviving animals into those artificially infected with laboratory-grown diphtheria; (3d) some inoculated animals resist the disease; (3e) he deduces that an immunizing property exists in the blood of chemically-treated animals (discovered by Jules-Jean Vincent Bordet [1870–1961] in 1898 and known today as *antibodies*); (3f) von Behring manufactures inoculum in the bodies of large animals; and (4a) Roux, moving from animal testing to human therapy, attains promising results.

Since de Kruif does not break down the discovery-process for each disease into cognitive phases and investigative steps, the reader may not perceive the coherence of each campaign and the importance to each of intuition, of precedent, and of experimental innovation. Nor are parallels between one campaign and another clearly shown. By focusing on primary texts (as did Winslow), I hope to provide some insight into the process of discovery and into the relationship between scientific investigations.

The present work incorporates aspects of the encyclopedia, of the intellectual history, and of the biographical compendium. Its scope is chronologically broad (spanning three millennia), and it covers one-dozen illnesses, more than thirty select authors, and nearly fifty primary works. As an intellectual history, it has both a unifying principle and conceptual foci, and, like the biographical compendium, presents the complex processes that have led to great discoveries. The book is primarily concerned with the human experience of epidemic disease, from antiquity to the present day, and the various means through which this experience has been conceptualized and communicated.

1. THE HANDS OF DAGON
Epidemic Anomalies in I Samuel, 5–6

To illustrate how the pre-conceptual viewpoint operates in an ancient text, I will consider the epidemiological description in *I Samuel*, chapters 5 and 6. Its author(s) and redactors preserved the pre-conceptual explanation for the plague that God punished the Philistines for stealing the Ark of the Covenant (Davies, 1:222–26).

The writings of the Old Testament clerical historian, Abiathar, who lived during King David's reign (c. 900 B.C.), show that anomalies can tell us much about biomedical phenomena, such as the origin, cause, and effect of epidemic disease (Herbert 3; Corney 1:6–7). The Philistines and the Jewish priest-historian, Abiathar, believed that epidemics had a supernatural rather than natural cause. For the biblical pre-conceptualist, pestilence was an instrument of chastisement, exercised either against elected transgressors for their wrongdoings or against adversaries of the elect. In *I Samuel*, chapters 5 and 6, the Philistines interpreted the epidemic to be punishment for having transgressed against Jewish religion. As a result, unusual natural and physical occurrences, specifically a rodent infestation and enlarged lymph nodes in the sick, were ascribed to divine wrath. Thus, the Philistines assimilated the disease into a theology of divine providence and of justice.

The account of the battle of Eben-ezer is one of the earliest epidemic texts in Western literature (Stinespring 1:248–49). *I Samuel*, chapters 5 and 6, the text discussed here, along with *II Samuel*, was drawn from an early document, likely written in 1000 B.C., and from a later one, possibly composed around 900 B.C.; some claim that it was written as late as 700 B.C. (Szikszai 4:201–02; Tsevat, Supp.:777–81). The author of the first source was Abiathar, a priest and contemporary of David, and an eyewitness of many of the events recorded in the text; the authorship of the second source is unknown. During the seventh century B.C., redactors may have conflated the two sources, and in 550 B.C., following in the tradition of *Deuteronomy*, the entire narrative was consequently re-edited (4:201–02). The historical content of these texts is more certain. *I* and *II Samuel* tell of how the Jewish nation developed from a confederation of tribes under a semi-theocratic government of judges into a unified monarchy, c. 1030–c. 973 B.C. (Trawick 95–110). I will refer to the author of the plague narrative in *I Samuel* as *Abiathar*, although it is probable that this work was of corporate authorship, as the text evolved over a 500-year period.

After the Philistines defeated the Israelites in 1141 B.C., they moved the Ark of the Covenant from one Philistine city to another, initially from Ebenezer, a site possibly northeast of Jaffa, to Ashdod, inland three miles from the coast and equidistant between Gaza and Joppa (Greenfield 791–95; McNeill 112–13; Marks and Beatty 8). Placing the Ark in the temple of Dagon, the Philistine god of corn (not of fish), they angered Yahweh who is said to have knocked the pagan statue down twice, severing the hands (I *Samuel* 5: 3–4) (Gray 1:756; Carlyon 311). Consequently, the frightened priests of Dagon abandoned the temple (verses 4–5). In retreat, but still possessing the Ark, the Philistines were then afflicted with a plague of some kind which, they thought, evidenced God's wrath for having stolen the Ark (verse 7). To assuage God's anger, they transported the Ark from Ashdod to Gath, a third Philistine city, near Judah; but, wherever they went, the plague remained intense. In Gath, people developed *emerods* or tumors in their "secret parts" (verse 9), suggesting enlarged lymph nodes in the groin, a symptom typical of bubonic plague (Zinsser 110; Harrison 3:821–2).

When the Philistines transported the Ark northward from Gath to Ekron, a fourth Philistine locale, the people there rejected it, presumably because they feared the consequences (Stinespring 2:69); however, even though they refused to accept the Ark, they, too, were stricken by the very same malady and believed that it had come directly from God (verses 10–12). While the populace of Ekron suffered, the leaders of the Eben-ezer caravan decided, after seven months had passed, that returning the Ark to the Israelites might be the only way of appeasing the God of Israel. With this thought in mind, Philistine diviners decided to convey it from Ekron to Beth-shemesh, along with an atonement offering.

Before undertaking their journey with the Ark, the Philistines of Ebenezer forged five golden emerods and five golden mice, each object minted to represent a Philistine lord and each of the five principal, Philistine cities (I *Samuel* 6: 4). The objects had religious significance. As anti-plague offerings to Yahweh, the tokens signified the subjection of Philistine authority and religion to a power surpassing that of Dagon. The golden offerings, in the shape of lymph nodes (emerods) and rodents, dramatize the impact of the disease on the minds of the Philistines: they interpreted this natural occurrence in supernatural terms, were deeply affected by the physiological manifestations of the outbreak, and associated the disease with the swellings, as well as with a rodent infestation. The Philistines could not have known that, during an outbreak of bubonic plague, certain rodent species, to which the disease was endemic, died off *en masse* when the disease became active. Once the rodents died, infected fleas abandoned the carcasses to feed on other mammals, including man, thereby spreading the disease ("Plague," CDC; "Plague," *Communicable Diseases*, 382–83).

Along with the golden lymph nodes and rodents, the Philistines created other unidentified images with which to glorify and to appease the God of Israel (I *Samuel* 6:4–5). The golden tokens of the Philistines were actually propitiatory gestures to Yahweh who, they sincerely believed, had sent the disease as punishment (I *Samuel* 6: 17). Acutely aware of Israelite history and of the idea that epidemics were divine instruments, the Philistines (according to Abiathar) even recalled Pharaoh's obdurate refusal to release the Israelites and the price in plague and vermin infestations that he and his people incurred for refusing to do so (6:6). Abiathar's reference is to *Exodus* 9:8–15 (Mihelic and Wright, 3:822–24). The Lord directed Moses and Aaron to gather handfuls of ashes from the furnace and to sprinkle the ashes towards heaven in the presence of Pharaoh (verse 8). The ashes, translated as "small dust" in the *KJV*, spread all over Egypt, afflicting both man and beast with blain and boils (verse 9–10). So widespread had the dissemination become that even Pharaoh's magicians, to whom he had turned for assistance, could not stand before Moses, since they too were covered with lesions (verse 11). Even with this dreadful event, Pharaoh remained the obstinate skeptic and refused to liberate the captive Jews (verse 12). The Philistines, on the other hand, were wary of the power of Yahweh and sought desperately to appease his wrath.

At this point in Abiathar's narrative, neither the followers of Dagon nor the Israelites causally linked the disease to the rodents, but the coincidence of the infestation and the disease troubled them. At least up until the time of their arrival in Ekron, the Philistines were convinced that they were paying the price for having desecrated the Ark by housing it in a Dagonic temple.

Despite the fear and trembling, the contrite Philistines gradually began to question their pre-conceptual conclusions, since auspicious gestures of gold and supplications were having no perceivable effect on the plague. They even entertained the possibility that Yahweh was not the author of the disease (I *Samuel* 6: 9). Consequently, they devised a logical course of action: if they brought the Ark to a Jewish settlement, the plague would surely end, since the object would be with its rightful owners (unless Yahweh chose to be vindictive). Carrying the Ark and golden offerings, the caravan wended its way northward along the coastline to the settlement of Beth-shemesh, a city on the northern border of Judah (6: 1–18). The plan, consistent with the logic of pre-conceptuality, seemed reasonable.

Beth-shemesh, at the time of the Philistine's arrival with the Ark, had long been a Jewish town (II *Chronicles* 28:18) and would remain so up until the end of King Ahaz's reign (c. 735–774 B.C.), at least three centuries *after* the Battle of Eben-ezer (Gold 101; Gray 1:401–03). After Ahaz's reign, it fell under Philistine economic and cultural control although Jews continued to live there. The Philistines' decision on Beth-shemesh as the terminus to their sojourn was a last-ditch measure: bringing it to a Jewish city, they thought, would not only confirm the belief that Yahweh had sent the plague, but it would also atone for their transgression (verses 8–9). The Jews of Beth-shemesh were certainly overjoyed to see the Ark. The Levites set up an altar and sacrificed cows (verses 14–18). But, despite these expressions of piety, the unexpected happened: plague ravaged the Israelites, just as it had the Philistines (I *Samuel* 6:19). This represents the first inconsistency in the pre-conceptual fabric of the narrative, one upon which Abiathar did not comment. The question for the modern reader is as follows: if the pestilence is an instrument of chastisement, why would it strike a Jewish city?

Using historical, etymological, and theological arguments, modern scholars have tried to explain the paradox of Beth-shemesh in terms supporting the pre-conceptual interpretation. One orthodox argument is that Beth-shemesh was a Philistine rather than Jewish city and, as such, was subject to the divine imprecation of plague (Gold 1:401; Gray 101). This is doubtful, historically, since the Jews had controlled the city from at least 1000 B.C. to early 700 B.C., a period inclusive of the events narrated in I *Samuel*, chapter 6. And, as stated above, they held that city up until the time of King Ahaz, at which time it fell into Philistine hands. According to this timeline, Beth-shemesh was in Jewish hands when the caravan arrived.

A complicated etymological argument has been used to incriminate the Beth-shemesh Jews and, thus, to explain why they were so afflicted. It claims that they violated the Law when they *gazed* on the tablets. Biblical scholars have differing opinions on this thesis, and I will mention them in passing without becoming too deeply involved in the debate. One line of thinking does not see the act of *gazing* on the Ark as being intrinsically transgressive. Reading the verb *to gaze* as the literal translation of the original Hebrew word, George B. Caird concludes that nowhere in the Bible is gazing on the Ark or on another sacred object considered so offensive as to warrant the deaths of thousands of Jews (I *Samuel* 6:19) (2: 912).

Other scholars find connotative associations in the infinitive *to gaze* that do indeed violate the Law. John Gray's opinion is representative of this view. Since, in Hebrew, the verb *to gaze* is related to the biblical word *vanity*, the activity is therefore impious. As Gray sees it, the Hebrew word for *vanity*, the state of mind causing one *to gaze*, is synonymous with delusion, emptiness, or idolatry (4:746). Hence, if gazing means vanity, and if the latter connotes idolatry, then the plague outbreak among the Beth-shemesh Jews was justified punishment for proscribed activities. Worship of the Ark as a material representation of God would have rendered the gazers culpable since Yahweh forbade such practices and had destroyed the statue of Dagon for that very reason. Representing God symbolically, an abomination believed to have been assimilated from Canaanite cults, was a reversion to natural religion (Gold 2:675–78). We are reminded of the statutes and judgments in *Deuteronomy* 12:1–4 against pagan idols and places of worship, all of which had to be destroyed. In *Deuteronomy*, chapter 13, verse 10, the Jews are enjoined to levy severe punishment on the idolater who tempts them to embrace forbidden beliefs: "Thou shalt stone him with stones, that he die; because he hath sought to thrust thee away from the Lord thy God, which brought thee out of the land of Egypt from the house of bondage" (*KJV*).

The idolatry interpretation, if applied to the Levites of Beth-shemesh, means that they venerated the Ark itself instead of venerating *the Author* of its commandments. A different verb but the same idea is present in the *KJV's* translation of the passage. Instead of gazing, the Beth-shemesh Jews in the *KJV looked into* the Ark: "God … smote the men of Beth-shemesh, because they *had looked into* the ark of the LORD, even he smote of the people fifty thousand and threescore and ten men; and the people lamented, because the LORD had smitten many of the people with a great slaughter" [italics added]. Like gazing, *to look into* the Ark implies more than inspecting or scrutinizing it reverentially. As F. F. Bruce explains, it refers to the proscribed experience of *seeing* God: "In earlier O[ld] T[estament] narratives seeing God is believed to be fatal"—though there are exceptions, such as in *Exodus* 24:10 (4: 261–2). David's own brother, Uzzah, was killed, presumably for taking hold of the Ark because an ox shook it (II *Samuel* 6:6–7): "And the anger of the Lord was kindled against Uzzah; and God smote him there for his error; and there he died by the ark of God" (verse 7).

Twentieth-century biomedical historians suspected I *Samuel*, chapter 6, of being an early account of bubonic plague, as seen through the eyes of contemporary victims (Philistine and Israelite alike) and of an eyewitness historian (Abiathar or a corporate author), and as mediated by redactors down through the centuries. The biomedical implications of the narrative and what it tells us about pre-conceptual thinking are evocative. Rodent hyperinfestation, the high fatality rate, the rapid dissemination of disease, and lymph-node involvement make an outbreak of bubonic plague plausible. The forging of golden mice and of lymph nodes, though not an unusual act for a culture that made idols, demonstrates how powerfully the disease affected the Philistines.

The forging of the golden tokens was a way of normalizing these anomalies, that is, of subsuming them under a natural religion that imposed coherency on the world. For this reason, the failure of ritual atonement to revoke the disease confounded the Philistines: Yahweh, it seemed, was not responding to their penitential acts. The communication of the disease to Beth-shemesh, an anomaly that has puzzled exegetes to this very day, perplexed both the Israelites and their adversaries. If I *Samuel* 6:19 were read in the light of these anomalies, the theological supposition that God wields disease as punishment either against the wayward elect or against the elect's adversaries is compromised. According to pre-conceptual reasoning, the receivers of the Ark should have incurred blessings or, at the very least, immunity from what plagued the caravan. But neither contrite Philistines nor devout Jews were spared.

The people of Beth-shemesh eventually arranged for the Ark's transfer to Kirjath-jearim, to the house of Adinabad, where, under the ministrations of Eleazar's son, it would remain for twenty years (I *Samuel*, 7:1–2; and Gold 3:37–8). Why the disease was not communicated, in turn, to the Jews at Kirjath-jearim is a matter for conjecture. A theological historian could say that since the Philistines relinquished the Ark and since the Kirjath-jearim community, unlike that of Beth-shemesh, received it with reverent orthodoxy, God's anger had been appeased. Others who are inclined to a strictly biological explanation could conjecture that the focus of the infection, the Philistines and their flea-infested caravan, had communicated the disease to the Beth-shemesh Jews but that the Philistines had not come into direct contact with the community at Kirjath-jearim, so therefore the latter did not contract the plague (although this explanation does not account for possible exposure to infected people at Beth-shemesh).

The consensus among biomedical historians is that the immediate cause of the epidemic was not desecration but an outbreak of bubonic plague or of a similar disease, probably originating in the Philistine camp and carried about in their caravans. This may be the reason why the plague followed the Ark caravan, making it seem that God was pursuing the Philistines vindictively: the followers of Dagon, in all likelihood, had witnessed a mass dying-off of plague rodents, the infected fleas of which spread to Philistine persons, camels, and belongings. The idea that the Philistine travelers themselves carried the plague from city to city is entirely plausible. A later instance of this phenomenon comes to mind. According to William H. McNeill, the Mongols' invasion of Yunnan-Burma after A.D. 1252 might have "inadvertently transferred the plague bacillus to the rodent population of their own steppe homeland," thereby inaugurating a chronic pattern of infection currently active in Manchuria (142). The idea that a migratory human population could transfer diseases to animals is indeed an ironic thought.

The story of I *Samuel*, chapters 5 and 6, represents only one aspect of Old Testament epidemiology, for the Jews had an intuitive understanding of infectious disease and a systematic way of managing outbreaks. I am referring to the instructions found in *Leviticus*, chapters 13–15, concerning a specific disease, perhaps a form of leprosy (Winslow 78–9; Harrison, 3:111–13; Hays 20–22). The context of its management, to be sure, was the Temple; and the clinician, a lawgiver. The approach to its management was pre-conceptual, for the disease was viewed as punishment for sin and considered incurable except through divine intervention, as in II *Kings* 5:7 (G. R. Driver 576). But the lawgivers still proceeded along rudimentary, scientific lines, mainly because they intuited that the disease was contagious, that the body could heal itself, and that isolation of the patient was essential to disease management (Winslow 78–9).

At the outset of the *Leviticus* text, a cleric diagnosed the disease and declared the person unclean (chapters 13–14). If in doubt, he isolated the person for seven days, after which time the individual was reexamined. If the lesion(s) had not worsened, the person was once again isolated as a precaution. At a certain stage in the process, in the absence of "raw flesh," the patient was recognized as being free of the disease. During the contagious period, however, the sick person had to publicize his or her condition with bare head, a covered upper lip, rent clothing, and proclamations. Not only did the Israelites sense the importance of quarantine, as those stricken had to dwell alone outside of the camp or city, but they also understood that whatever brought on the disease could somehow cling to clothing which had to be burned. In chapter 14, the writer described the ceremonial procedure used to release a person from quarantine, the management of infectious disease, in this context, being part of religious law. To see if the lesions were resolved, the priest reexamined the leper. He then sacrificed a bird as a sign of atonement. Fundamental understandings of infection, of contagion, and of isolation, as this example shows, can exist even in pre-conceptual texts.

Abiathar, Fleming, and the Penicillin Anomaly

Comparing works separated by three millennia requires a considerable degree of caution. If the comparison I am proposing works, however, Abiathar's ancient record will not seem so distant from our experience. Here is the question: what does the interpretation of plague symptoms in the first millennium B.C. have in common with the discovery of penicillin in 1929?

Abiathar's history of the Philistine plague and Alexander Fleming's discovery of penicillin both involved the interpretation of biological anomalies. Although Fleming (1881–1955) did not describe the effects of an epidemic, his work nevertheless correlates with Abiathar's text in terms of how a bacteriological anomaly is perceived and treated. Fleming, a Scottish bacteriologist, was corecipient of the Nobel Prize in Physiology or Medicine (with Ernest B. Chain [1906–1979] and Howard W. Florey [1898–1968]). His great contribution was published in 1929 in a paper titled, "On the antibacterial action of cultures of a Penicillium, with special reference to their use in the isolation of *B. influenzae.*"

While working with variants of staphylococcus, Fleming set aside a number of culture plates on a bench and examined them from time to time (185). The plates which had been exposed to air became contaminated with various micro-organisms. He noticed, on one plate, the presence of a large colony of mold and what seemed to be the dissolution or lysis of the staphylococcus colonies. Suspecting that the mold colonies had something to do with the dissolution of the bacteria, he decided to isolate the unusual organism for closer study. That done, he could then try to ascertain the properties of the bacteriolytic substance now present in the dish. Unlike the Philistines who assimilated natural anomalies into a supernatural design, Fleming detached the anomaly from its natural setting so as to break it down into its constituents; in that way, he could determine the processes of natural causation at work in the culture dish. The helpless Philistines, on the other hand, assumed that they understood the processes of supernatural causation and sought to relinquish the Ark in order to make amends for their transgression.

Although engaged in informal work, Fleming realized that he had spied a potentially important anomaly: the coextension of the mold and of the dissolving bacteria was a reason to follow through with further investigation, although Florey, the Australian pathologist, and Chain, the German-born, British biochemist, would be credited with isolating and identifying the antibiotic substance in the mold (*Random House Webster's Dictionary* 94, 171). The Philistines who had no awareness of the relationship between the disease and the rodents were conditioned by their culture and religious tradition: they identified the invisible cause as an angry deity whose wrath could be appeased through adulation and sacrifice. Fleming, on the other hand, had only time and effort to sacrifice. Unlike the Philistines or Abiathar, he suspected, as did others before him, that the coextension of these anomalies (the mold and the dying bacteria, respectively) strongly indicated that a cause-and-effect relationship obtained, and he inferred as much from the evidence. Furthermore, this inference, supported by the intelligent speculations of predecessors, led Fleming to isolate the more tangible anomaly (the mold) and to employ it under controlled conditions against other bacterial strains in the hope of finding out if, and how, it killed disease-causing germs (Beveridge 161). Fleming's endeavor, governed by the hypothesis that the mold could destroy pathogenic bacteria, owed its elegant logic to Robert Koch, whose postulates we shall discuss in chapter nine. The Philistines, on the other hand, were doing only what they knew how to do, that is, what their culture and traditions mandated: if the stolen Ark were the reason for the plague outbreak, then they had to get rid of it. And when they could not transfer it to other Philistines, they thought that all would be forgiven if they returned it to its rightful owners. In the course of their sojourn, ironically, they likely spread the disease to others.

Whereas the modern bacteriologist controlled the microbes he was studying, the Philistines and the Jews were at the mercy of a proliferating strain of plague. Fleming grew the subcultured mold for one to two weeks. After this period, the mold acquired "marked inhibitory and bacteriolytic properties to many of the more common pathogenic bacteria." The mold itself, which he observed very closely, underwent striking physical changes. It began as a white, fluffy mass, increased in size over a few days, and began to form spores. As the culture matured, it turned dark green and then black (185–86). In four to five days, its color was bright yellow, with reddish areas, as it diffused through the medium (186). Fleming tested the pH of the broth, finding it to be alkaline (8.5 to 9); in glucose or saccharine broth, the reaction was acidic. The mold grew rather slowly at 37 degrees C. (body temperature), grew more rapidly at about 20 degrees, and did not grow without oxygen (186). Fleming was convinced that the mold was a living organism having unique characteristics.

A crucial stage of the experiment had arrived. Fleming now needed to find out if molds other than *Penicillin rubrum* had antibacterial effects. Testing eight other strains of penicillin, he learned that only one produced inhibitory effects similar to those of the original mold (186). He worked methodically to reach this conclusion. The first step in the process was to cut a furrow in an agar plate and then to fill it in with a mixture of equal parts of agar and of mold broth. After solidifying the surface material, Fleming streaked various kinds of microbes onto the surface, at right angles to the furrow and towards the edge of the plate. This done, the mold secretions then could diffuse rapidly in the agar. In a few hours, before the microbes could show visible growth, the mold broth had spread out more than one centimeter and in sufficient concentration to inhibit growth of a sensitive microbe. After further incubation, transparencies appeared. Examination of this portion of the culture showed that nearly all the microbes dissolved. The mold affected a number of organisms, including *pneumococcus, B. influenza,* and *B. diphtheria,* and the inhibitory rates could be measured. These results must have been startling. The next step was a tricky biochemical procedure: to determine how much antibiotic was present in a standard unit of nutrient broth. Using a standardized unit of measurement, he added uniform concentrations of the agent to different bacterial suspensions and measured the effects on the bacteria in each instance; he found, for example, that staphylococcus was very susceptible to the activity of *P. rubrum.*

Another factor for which Fleming had to account was temperature: could differing levels of heat affect the potency of penicillin? The results were very specific. Heating the penicillin in a temperature range of 56 to 80 degrees C. for one hour had no effect on its antibacterial power. Boiling it for a few minutes, however, reduced it to less than one-quarter strength if it was immersed in alkaline fluid; the reduction was much less if the penicillin was suspended in neutral or in slightly acid solution; autoclaving it for twenty minutes at 115 degrees C. destroyed it.

Passing a penicillin solution through a filter did not diminish its potency. Even when the broth evaporated at low temperature, potent penicillin could still be extracted as a sticky mass; in fact, its active element could be extracted with alcohol. Once extracted, penicillin's rate of inhibitory activity could be carefully studied. Planting mold spores in a 500 cc. flask containing 200 cc. of nutritive broth, he incubated the solution at different temperature levels, from 1 to 20 degrees C. (room temperature), which enabled him to measure its inhibitive power on staphylococcus. During his experiments, he learned that time depleted penicillin's effectiveness: at room temperature and after fourteen days, its antibacterial power diminished considerably; however, in a pH range from 9 to 6.8, its reaction was more stable. It turned out that the bright yellow fluid had the highest concentration of antibacterial substance. Penicillin was able to work against staphylococcus in a proportion of 1 to 800 units. Grown on solid medium, the felted mass could be harvested: even after having been immersed in salt solution for twenty-four hours, the extract continued to have bacteriolytic properties. If the extract was mixed with thick staphylococcus suspension and incubated for two hours at 45 degrees C., the opacity of the suspension diminished, and after 24 hours an opaque suspension became almost clear. The bacteria were dead.

It remained to be seen precisely how, and to what degree, penicillin affected the growth of bacteria. Four experiments yielded valuable results. On agar plates, it inhibited *staphylococcus pyogenes* and *streptococcus pyogenes* the best. The more concentrated the penicillin, the better the inhibitory effect, except in the cases of *streptococcus faecelis*, *E. coli*, *Salmo-nella*, *pseudomonas*, *proteus*, and cholera (188). The coli-typhoid group resisted penicillin, but it had a negligible effect on *Shigella* and *B. pseudo-tuberculosis rodentium*. Its action was most manifest on the diphtheria group and on *pyogenic cocci*.

As to how the mold killed, he determined that it belonged to a group of slow-acting antiseptics, and its power was amply demonstrated against staphylococcus, which it destroyed in a little over 4.5 hours in a concentra-tion that was 30 to 40 times stronger than what was necessary to inhibit such a culture in broth. As far as toxicity went, Fleming injected 20 cc. of pure penicillin intravenously into a rabbit to discover that this dosage was no more toxic than the same quantity of the mold in broth. Twenty grams of peni-cillin had no adverse effects on a mouse. Moreover, if large infected areas in man were constantly irrigated, no toxic symptoms occurred. When *P. rubrum* was tested *in vitro*, it inhibited the growth of staphylococcus in diluted strength of 1 to 600. In the final analysis, Fleming found that penicillin had advantages over antiseptics and was more powerful than carbolic acid.

In Fleming's work, the cultivation and systematic analysis of a bacte-riological anomaly proved that *P. rubrum* had antibiotic properties. For the Philistines, on the other hand, two striking epidemiological anomalies—rodent hyperinfestation and enlarged lymph nodes—were interpreted not as clues to understanding the physiological effects of the plague but as dis-connected manifestations of an angry God.

An anomaly in biomedical research, as I noted in the Introduction, is an irregularity or deviation from what is traditionally expected, and the ability to determine the potential value of such a deviation in the labora-tory is contingent on training in the discipline and on one's thorough famil-iarity with established scientific methods and precedents: thus, if one anticipates the outcome of a scientific procedure, this knowledge prepares the investigator to recognize, and to evaluate the worth of, something out-side the norm. This situation accurately describes Fleming's experience with penicillin, as it does that of ancient and of classical historians who viewed epidemics pre-conceptually, and who therefore tried to account for wide-spread disease in terms of their view of the world. As pointed out, Flem-ing's tradition allowed him to determine penicillin's effect on bacteria, whereas that of Abiathar and of similar writers precluded an understand-ing of what was behind an outbreak since its origin and cause were thought of in supernatural terms. With the intention of searching for anomalies and of discovering how the ancients perceived them, we will now turn our attention to epidemic portrayals in Greco-Roman and in early Christian literature.

2. THE FIERCE ONSLAUGHT OF FATE
Greco-Roman Pre-Conceptuality

The earliest Greek accounts of epidemic disease are embedded in mythological history. In works such as *The Iliad*, outbreaks were not portrayed as random events. On the contrary, they evidenced the power of mythological beings who wielded disease punitively. Let us begin by looking at a famous passage in *The Iliad*.

Homer's *Iliad* (c. 700 B.C.) contains a famous example of the gods inflicting disease on man as punishment for transgression. Chryses, a priest of Apollo, pleads for the return of his daughter, whom the Greeks kidnapped during a raid. Founder of an Apollonian temple, the priest had regularly administered ritual offerings and remained a devout follower (I: 36–42). Agamemnon, leader of the Greek forces, claimed the priest's daughter as a war prize, rejecting her father's petition to free her. The forlorn priest, upon returning to his homeland, invokes the intercession of Apollo against the Greeks and against his daughter's abusers. His invocation is heard. A pestilence arrives and is attributed to Apollo. The disease itself is metaphorically depicted as a torrent of arrows, the "shafts ranging everywhere along the wide coast of the Achaians [Greeks]" (I: 383–84). Apollo's epidemic strikes down mules, hounds, and human beings, and funeral fires burn unceasingly (I: 47–52). The irate deity drives this "foul pestilence along the host, and the people perished, / since Atreus's son had dishonored Chryses" (I: 9–11).

In the Homeric world, the plague evokes a reaction from soldiers and priests rather than from an established medical profession. Hence, after assembling his warriors, Achilles orders the prophet Kalchas to ascertain the reason for the god's anger. The seer then interprets "the design of the archer" (I: 385), that is, the provocation behind the epidemic. The prophet is also directed to sacrifice animals to Apollo so that the "bane" may be driven from them (I: 62–7). The Greek warrior becomes convinced that the disease is of divine origin and explicitly intended as retribution. Before Kalchas reveals the truth, however, he asks for a solemn oath that he will be protected from reprisals. This secured, he identifies Agamemnon's behavior as the cause of the outbreak. The warrior resents the accusation, refuses to relinquish his captive, accuses Achilles of desiring the priest's daughter for himself, and makes the insulting proposition of exchanging her for Achilles' mistress Briseis.

The supernatural balance of power is maintained when Athena promises Achilles a threefold compensation for the transgression and for the insult he has had to endure. Swearing not to fight for the Greeks again, Achilles eventually relinquishes Briseis to Agamemnon, invokes the goddess Thetis, and requests Zeus's direct intervention in the conflict. Zeus then favors the Trojans over the Greeks, the former profiting from Achilles' conspicuous absence from the battlefield. Consequently, Achilles' honor is restored. After Agamemnon releases the priest's daughter, she is placed onboard a black ship, along with sufficient hecatombs to appease the plague-wielding god (I: 142–43). Once Odysseus returns Chryseis to her father, the plague ends, although the heavenly squabbles continue. Unlike the story of the stolen Ark, the return of Chryseis revokes the god's anger and removes the plague. Like the story Abiathar tells, the Homeric depiction of epidemic disease is defined entirely in terms of a preconceived cosmic design and of warring deities.

Historical and archaeological discoveries support the idea that Homer was a pre-conceptualist, but his portrayal of the god Apollo is somewhat unusual. To a degree, the idea of Apollo as a *bringer* of disease is anomalous. Robin Lane Fox points out, in *Pagans and Christians,* that Apollo, the god of medicine, is actually considered a protector against plague, a role diametrically opposed to that which he plays in *The Iliad* (231–34). At Didyma, an Apollonian cult existed to protect against plague and, in the 250s B.C., was considered instrumental in staving one off. Apollonian oracles on plague, found in Pergamum, Callipolis, and Caesarea Trochetta (in Lydia), implored the god's protection. A cultist, according to Lane, had to draw water from seven fumigated fountains, to sprinkle it on their houses, and to erect an image of Apollo in the middle of the plain. With bow in hand, the archer would then shoot at and drive away invading plagues. In Callipolis, Lane continues, a similar statue was set up to ward off the plague; instead of watery libations, animals were also sacrificed to subterranean gods, their spiced flesh being immolated on wine-sprinkled pyres. Indisputably, ceremonies such as these were intended to stem rather than to invoke outbreaks.

Lane points out that, even though hymns to Zeus and invocations of Apollo's son Asclepius had no effect on the disease, the Greeks remained faithful to the gods. To them, the inefficacy of their supplications meant the gods were dissatisfied, not powerless. Once the plague ended, relieved adherents credited Apollo for intervening. The ineffectuality of the gods was not interpreted in heterodox terms; rather, in the minds of adherents, the gods' presumed motives were accommodated to the ebb and flow of the outbreak. As a result, pre-conceptual rationalizations made it impossible for the Greeks to understand disease biologically: epidemics were signs of divine anger, the survival of an Apollonian cultist was a reward, and disease that struck an enemy was a sign of favor.

The kind of detailed documentaries of Thucydides and of Hippocrates, which we shall discuss in chapter four, had a negligible effect on the imaginative literature of Rome. As late as the first century B.C., pre-conceptuality still prevailed as a way of situating, and of accounting for, the epidemic event in the natural order. The pre-conceptual design itself, as we shall discover, was not always theological or mythological in orientation.

Titus Lucretius Carus (c. 99–c. 55 B.C., Roman poet and philosopher, best known for his didactic poem, *On the Nature of Things*, situated the epidemic event in a godless cosmology. According to the theory governing his poem, all of creation, including the human soul, is made up of atoms, indestructible particles operating in accordance with natural laws. In Book I, both the soul and the body are said to be materialistic aspects of the selfhood. The world itself came into being not through divine fiat but, rather, through the random combination of atoms. The fundamental principles of Lucretian physics, derived from the atomistic thought of Democritus, are expressed in the lines: "nothing ever by divine power comes from nothing" (I: 148–9); and "nature / Resolves all things back into their elements / And never reduces anything to nothing" (I: 215–17). Although "Nature forbids anything should perish" (materially, that is), the atoms or "seeds" of which all things are composed can be shattered, penetrated, or broken up with the application of sufficient force (I: 221–25).

The Lucretian cosmology claims to liberate man from superstition and from systematic religion. To contend that heavenly bodies are divine and indestructible is illusory (V: 114–16). Neither can one describe the gods physically: "far removed / From our senses," they are imperceptible (V: 146–9). Nor have divine agencies fashioned the world for the use of mankind, for that would presume, unfoundedly, an intimacy between man and the supernatural (V: 156–64). Creation, moreover, has no inherent plan or *telos* (V: 197–99), while mankind occupies an indifferent world, naturally resistant to his inroads, and human history records man's incessant struggle against inhospitable geography, bad weather, and wild animals. To cultivate the earth, mankind has had to labor, often fruitlessly, against the environment.

These hardships have inspired man to create wondrous beings in order to explain the order of the heavens. Thus, in locating "the gods' abode" in the sky (V: 1194–1202), man imagines himself in control of sidereal powers, the worship of which is folly (V: 1194–1202). "True piety," from the Lucretian perspective, "is for man to have the power / To contemplate the world with quiet mind" (V: 1203–04), the only trustworthy avenue to truth being the observation of natural phenomena. Lucretius would likely have rejected the Apollonian practice of correlating the gods' moods to the phases of widespread disease, so his vision had a revolutionary undercurrent.

The epicurean interpretation of nature could be thought of as preferable to theological pre-conceptuality which locates the ground of disease causation in the heavens rather than in nature, and which defines the epidemic experience in moral and in theological terms. It is superior, additionally, because it emphasizes the need to observe and contemplate nature (a practice concurrently at work in the Thucydidean tradition). The epicurean, Diogenes Laertius, in his *Letter to Herodotus*, seems to have been criticizing the Homeric idea of disease, as exemplified in *The Iliad*, that an epidemic can be a vehicle of divine chastisement rather than an amoral, natural occurrence. Thus, Laertius has much in common with Thucydides, when he states that it is necessary "to observe all things in accordance with one's sense-perceptions" and according to "our actual feelings." Only from this standpoint can one genuinely hope to arrive "at a general view about the things which are non-evident" (text 2.38, p. 6).

Although Lucretius criticized mythical understandings of natural events, and although Laertius extolled the value of recording firsthand experience, they both accommodated observations of nature to a preconceived, philosophical system. I therefore consider them to be secular preconceptualists. This viewpoint, as I understand it, encompasses the biology of epidemic disease, the processes of which are apprehended in terms consistent with speculative cosmology. In regard to epidemics, the epicureans merely substituted a philosophical and atheistic explanation for a mythological or religious one.

Assigning a hypothetical cause to "the nature of diseases" (VI: 1090–1091), Lucretius formulated a philosophical etiology in which disease agents are mobile particles or atoms. The imagery should not suggest that he was thinking of aggregated protons, neutrons, and electrons; rather, in his formulation, disease is caused by irreducible, living contaminants (VI: 1093–96). In deadly mists or clouds, these particulates would arise from putrid material, drift from region to region, and eventually descend upon unsuspecting victims (VI: 1096–1102). From this description, it appears that Lucretius was an early proponent of the *miasmatic* theory of disease. The theory has had a long life, extending well into the nineteenth century when fevers were blamed on poisoned air exuding from rotting animal and vegetable matter, and on soil and standing water (Porter 10–11). The word *malaria*, an artifact of miasmatic theory, derives from the Italian phrase *mala (=mal') aria*, meaning bad air. As late as the eighteenth century, malaria referred to "the unwholesome condition of the atmosphere which results from the exhalations of marshy districts," as well as to fevers allegedly arising from this source (*OED* X: 78; "malaria"). The first English usage of the word is attributed to Horace Walpole who wrote, in a letter of 1740, about "A horrid thing called the mal'aria that comes to Rome every summer." Walpole would have been surprised to learn that the disease was, in fact, endemic to Roman swamps and flared up seasonally, as mosquitoes transferred the infectious organism to man directly or from host to host.

Echoes of Thucydides' description of the 430 B.C. plague of Athens are audible in Lucretius' text. Even though Latin literature belongs to the pre-conceptual heritage and to the Homeric tradition, generally Roman writers could not resist interpolating a raw, Thucydidean passage into a pre-conceptual text. Lucretius was no exception. Within an atomistic cosmos, the Roman poet imagines a plague drifting over the Mediterranean, that is, over six hundred miles from Egypt to Athens. Derivative and graphic, lines 1145 to 1214 describe the eyes of victims glowing red (line 446), their throats turning black, sweating ulcers choking them (VI: 1146–1150), lungs filling with fluid (VI: 1115–54), and the breath becoming fetid. Ulcers appear to have been burnt into the flesh (line 1167), and "fire" seems to have spread across the limbs. Febrile inflammation occurs, and ulcerations penetrate vital organs (line 1169). To relieve these symptoms, sufferers immerse themselves in wells. Those who are about to expire exhibit familiar symptoms: panting, labored breathing, yellow spittle, hoarse coughing, twitching, trembling, cold extremities, pinched nostrils, sunken eyes, hollow temples, grinning mouths, tensed foreheads. Death ensues on the eighth or ninth day (VI: 1180–1198). Anyone surviving the respiratory attack succumbs to gastrointestinal symptoms. A "copious stream of putrid blood," aptly named the "black flux," quickly debilitates the hardiest person (VI: 1200–04). The pestilence disfigures survivors, destroying extremities and even the eyes (VI: 1205–12). The balance of the text (VI: 1230–85) follows the Athenian closely and without improvisation. Lucretius does not try to reconcile the atomistic theory of contagion with Thucydides' vivid description of symptoms and of devastating effects (to be discussed in chapter four). But the Roman poet's imaginative descent into the midst of a raging epidemic is a significant departure from his earlier, cosmological speculations.

Virgil's (70–19 B.C.) terrible plague of animals in *The Georgics* (III:

478–566), the third text in our survey, might have paralleled an outbreak of anthrax in the Alpine region north of the Adriatic, but precise historical identification of the disease is problematic (Wilkinson, 3:97n). Virgil's treatment of the origin and cause of the disease, however, belongs unmistakably to the Homeric tradition. Once again, gods use the epidemic to punish man. One member of a triumvirate of nasty sisters, whom the Greeks called Erinyes or Furies (Allecto, Megaera, and Tisiphone), is Tisiphone who, unleashed from Stygian darkness, begins to destroy ruminant animals. The Furies, along with other monsters, are the offspring of mother Earth who had been inseminated by the blood of Jupiter, whom his son Cronus had castrated (Grant 87). Vindictive instruments, they carry out Juno's dictates. A vengeful Tisiphone is also behind the plague outbreak of Aegina in Ovid's *The Metamorphoses*. There, as a monstrous creation, she is associated with venomous snakes, poison, and madness (III: 483–565).

In *The Georgics*, the infection emerging from the netherworld ravages both man and beast, which suggests that the infectious agent comes from the soil. Apparently, Virgil understood that contagion could take place through physical contact with the agent. Thus, if anyone donned a garment made from the fleece of an infected sheep, it would not take long for "feverish blisters / And filthy sweat" to run down his "stinking limbs" (III: 563–65). Blistering would be followed rapidly by fever, "the accursed fire" (III: 566). At this point, however, the poem ends. There is an interesting shift in emphasis here, largely due to the influence of Thucydides: Virgil is concerned with an agent that causes disease, and the supernatural machinations are in the background. The disease, whatever it is, does not descend from the heavens in the form of metaphoric arrows. Instead, it is an organic toxin, something coming from the soil that produces necrotic blisters, that strikes man and beast, and that contaminates animal furs. All of these allusions, obviously based on experience, point to anthrax: it comes from the soil, causes black lesions, and spreads from contaminated animal products ("Anthrax," CDC). Even today, anthrax remains a genuine threat in its natural state because, in Bernard Roueché's words, "not all susceptible animals are vaccinated, not all infected carcasses are properly destroyed, not all processors of hides and hair and bristle and bone take the trouble to sterilize their products" (188). In light of this commentary, it appears that Virgil had a rudimentary idea that a soil-borne pathogen attacked man and that animals carried the infectious agent.

Ovid's (43 B.C.–c. A.D. 17) plague in *The Metamorphoses* (7: 523–671) was likely indebted to Thucydides, to Virgil, and to Lucretius (Kennedy, 418n.). A fusion of pre-conceptuality and of observed effects, the passage in question refers to a "fearsome plague" (VII: 529) that had annihilated the people (and every mammal) on the island of Aegina. It was the hand-iwork of a vindictive goddess. Juno (Hera), the sister-wife of Jove, was enraged at her consort's adulterous relationships with mortal women, one of whom, Aegina, is the mother of King Aeacus. According to Aeacus' account, the plague was the direct result of "Juno's unfair rage" (VII: 529–30): the goddess hated the people of Aegina because they not only adopted the name of Jove's mistress, but also because they were the bastard race of this adulterous union.

Traversing familiar ground, Ovid alludes to an insidious pestilence and to the failure of every remedy against it (VII: 533–34). The "vile infection" is associated with stifling atmosphere (as black clouds weigh down upon the earth), and with an acrid south wind (VII: 535–40). In what may be a reference to Virgil's image of the snake-charmer Tisiphone, the poet attributes the toxicity of the disease to thousands of swarming serpents, polluting rivers and fields with their venom (VII: 541–44). The miasmatic and herpetological imagery aside, the poet stresses the idea that the disease's "power" is amply manifested in its invisibility, virulence, and spontaneity (VII: 544–45). Echoing Virgil, he describes how it initially kills dogs, birds, sheep, cattle, horses, and boars. Because scavengers avoid rotting carcasses, Ovid associates the disease with putrefaction, the "effluence" of which "spread[s] the infection far and wide" (VII: 562), a notion in keeping with miasmatic theory, probably borrowed from Lucretius via the Hippocratic tradition.

The disease works its way, inexorably, upward through the animal kingdom, eventually striking man (VII: 563). Moving from the farmlands into the heart of the city (a route reminiscent of the Athenian pestilence), it is known by its effects, once again suggesting the influence of Thucydides: high fevers, inflamed intestines, shortness of breath, flushed skin, furred and swollen tongue, gaping mouth, and epidermal sensitivity (VII: 565–573). The fate of health-care workers is a familiar concern. Physicians die as rapidly as their patients: "the more closely and faithfully men served the sick," the quicker they move down "their road to doom" (VII: 574–78). Abandoning hope, some indulge their lusts; multitudes die near water as they try to reduce their fevers; and unbearable discomfort forces people to the ground where they writhe about (as per Thucydides). Since "the cause" of the disease is hidden, frantic patients run wildly or simply wander "half-alive / Along the streets," while the prostrate vainly beseech the heavens (VII: 578–97).

Thucydides' plague description had a lasting influence on the Roman psyche: poets, philosophers, and dramatists replicated the description as a set-piece, an authoritative account lending authenticity and power to their creative works. The influence of Thucydides on Roman epidemiological literature indicates that documented observations of pestilence were more riveting than any pre-conceptual narrative could possibly be.

Lamenting the deaths of his people and his inexplicable survival, Ovid's king Aeacus communicates his frustration and suicidal thoughts to Cephalus in a rhetorical question: "What heart had I? Was it not natural / To loathe my life and long to join my own [people]?" (VII: 598–99). It seems that the people vainly seek Jove's intervention against Juno whose behavior vexes Aeacus, especially since Juno is his progenitor. Since nothing appeases the gods, and since sacrificial animals die before ritual blood-letting, the Greeks, like the Philistines, are perplexed. Divination through the reading of animal viscera and entrails, believed to be a means of disclosing divine warnings (VII: 650), provides no insight into the gods' motivations since the plague destroys internal organs. The failure of the ceremonial antidote leads to desperation. Without the medical arts or religion to save them, some scornfully deposit cadavers near shrines and altars while others, dreading the plague, commit suicide (VII: 652–56).

Another motif likely to have been inherited from Thucydides is the effect of the epidemic on interment practices, an important aspect of Greek religion. Under these conditions, expediency overrides tradition; ceremony is discontinued. It had even become difficult to find burial ground and pyre-wood. These eventualities would have important consequences. If the deceased were not interred on family soil, and if religious rituals were not performed, the Greeks believed that the spirits of the dead would wander aimlessly (VII: 612). Ironically, in this instance, pestilential devastation directly altered a pre-conceptual ceremony.

When the population of Aegina is destroyed (all with the exception of the royal family), Aeacus implores his divine father Jove to repopulate the realm. One can infer that, by this time, Juno's rage had been spent, for her plague had destroyed virtually every living thing on the island. The deeper implication is that Jove would not arrest Juno's natural wrath until it was satisfied. Juno recedes from the foreground after transforming ants into a tribe of men called Myrmidons.

An anomaly appears in the midst of Ovid's pre-conceptual epidemic. The uselessness of ritual as a means of appeasing angry deities is plainly in sight, but the reason for its ineffectuality is not. Ovid does not question the potency of the gods or consider the possibility that the epidemic reflects divine caprice. Nonetheless, the failure of prescribed rites to assuage the gods' anger suggests one of two orthodox possibilities: either Juno's wrath had to run its course, or the divine motivation was inscrutable. Either conclusion reflects the belief of Greek and Roman worshipers that epidemics issued invariably from the gods, who had absolute power to inflict punishment or to relieve suffering.

Annaeus Seneca (c. 3 B.C.–A.D. 65) interpolates into his version of *Oedi-*

pus several epidemiological passages traditionally ascribing disease causation to retributive gods. Sophocles (c. 495–c. 406 B.C.), nearly five hundred years earlier, depicted the plague-afflicted populace of Thebes as languishing before the Apollonian altars, their supplications seemingly ignored. Unlike Homer's Apollo, that of Sophocles drove the plague *away* with arrows (lines 203–04; italics added). The chief priest describes the dire events to the newly-arrived King Oedipus: "The fever god has fallen on the city, / And drives it, a most hated pestilence / Through whom the home of Cadmus is made empty. / Black Hades is enriched with wails and groans" (lines 27–30). According to the Delphic oracle, the epidemic is the effect of Oedipus's unwitting commission of parricide and of maternal incest, and Thebes is suffering the consequences. Creon declares that the murder of a prominent individual brought the plague to the city. Oedipus agrees with him but thinks that highwaymen slew King Laius and that the gods' rage will be calmed and the epidemic revoked if the murderer(s) are punished: "release would come / From this disease only if we make sure / Of Laius' slayers and slay them in return / Or drive them out as exiles from the land" (lines 306–9). Of course, he does not yet know that it is the inescapable fulfillment of his own fate that has brought on the epidemic, unquestionably a pre-conceptual state of affairs, and that only his own death or exile will relieve his people of this burden. Ironically, believing that the epidemic derived from mortal corruption and exudations, he prays to Apollo for deliverance from "everything polluted by the dead" (line 313).

Seneca's Oedipus follows much the same path of self-discovery as did his Greek namesake. After departing Corinth so as to prevent the fulfillment of the prophecy concerning his parents (that he would kill his father and marry his mother), he realizes that he can not circumvent his fate. The Theban pestilence, in each drama, functions as a natural symbol for the fulfillment of the oracle. Unaware of the fact that his life is morally and socially fated, Oedipus tries to uncover the cause of the pestilence since its presence usually means the gods are displeased. Given the gods' attitude towards him, Oedipus has reason to be nervous. Ironically, he is anxious because the plague has thus far spared him. The original oracle in mind, he wonders if "the fates" are preparing something far worse for him (lines 28–32).

Seneca's outbreak, like the brooding atmosphere of the Sophoclean original, is miasmatic: thus, "a heavy, black fog" overshadows the citadels with "hellish aspect" (lines 46–9). Describing the effects of the outbreak, a passage from Thucydides extends from line 50 to 71. Thucydides, we shall see in chapter four, did not characterize infectious disease as a black cloud. But Seneca does recapitulate interesting aspects of the Greek original, including virulence and high mortality, the psychological impact, the futility of the medical arts, and the overturning of custom and religious ceremony. Blighting the corn harvest, the cloud indiscriminately destroys citizens of "every age and sex" (lines 50–2). The "persistent bane" and high mortality rate dulls Theban emotions (53–9). The rites attending cremation are desacralized: the bereaved undertake burials rapidly, some even casting their loved ones on the pyres of strangers (64–5). The wretched, under these extreme conditions, exhibit neither grief nor shame. Religious supplications and the medical arts seem useless: "Neither prayer nor any skill avails the stricken" (lines 69–70); and "the healers themselves fall victim to the plague" (line 70–1).

Though Oedipus destroys the Sphinx that reveals the riddle of his fate, he cannot annihilate it. Its decomposed matter, transformed into disease particles, alights into the atmosphere, the disintegrated "pest" and "fierce onslaught of fate" becoming the epidemic of Thebes (lines 106–09, 124–26). To decontaminate the air, priests sacrifice bulls, but nothing works (lines 133–45). The ecologically-pervasive destruction creates congenital malformations (lines 146–59). For instance, when Tiresias's daughter Manto reads the entrails of cattle in order to find the root of the present crisis, she is shocked at the sight of monstrous fetuses and of mangled cattle bolting from altars to attack the priests (lines 385–92). The ecological catastrophe in Thebes, then, is not a natural phenomenon; rather, it is an outward manifestation of Oedipus' terrible fate of which he had been unaware. The oracles, however, will eventually enlighten Creon as to the terrible truth: "the plague-fraught south-wind with its destructive blast" (lines 632–33) is not in itself the source of the plague. The problem, rather, is inherent in the human condition. The source of the dilemma, known today in Freudian terms as the Oedipal Complex (lines 633–39), engenders the epidemic, and the person of Oedipus is the focus of the outbreak. If Oedipus leaves Thebes, Creon observes, then "Ruin, and Pestilence, Death, Suffering, Corruption and Distress, fit company for him, shall depart together" (lines 649–55). Enmeshed in historical necessity and without free will, Oedipus is the immoral source of a natural pestilence.

In his depiction of epidemic disease, Seneca regresses on the pre-conceptual continuum from the miasma of Lucretius to the anthropocentricity of Homeric myth. The Senecan interpretation of infectious disease has in common with the Old Testament the idea that supernatural powers use disease as a weapon against mankind, except that in the case of the Senecan Oedipus the gods neither chastise the faithful nor defend them against their enemies. The deities of Seneca's universe are malevolent; and, in the cosmos over which they preside, man is a helpless, irredeemable creature.

The cultural memory of great plague events in the Mediterranean region have in common the experience of their sudden onset, of many fatalities, and of helplessness before an invisible terror, known only in its effects. From 790 B.C. to A.D. 5 (the year of Seneca's death), more than a dozen occurrences are mentioned in the contemporary literature by writers such as Herodotus, Plutarch, Livy, Marcus Terentius Varro, and Strabo of Pontus (Snodgrass 13–18). It is therefore not difficult to understand why the Greeks and the Romans extrapolated intellectual constructs from these circumstances. Mythic beings and philosophical concepts corresponding to, or accounting for, the natural experience of plague would expectedly be motiveless, malign, and inscrutable.

Roman writings on infectious disease in whatever form (philosophical poetry, drama, history, and treatises) contributed little to the Greek corpus beyond recapitulating passages from Thucydides' work. The Greek historian's writings either are subsumed under mythological narratives or are used to heighten dramatic effect. Consequently, one finds in Roman texts familiar opinions about the causes of disease: the retribution or capriciousness of the gods, the inalterable determinism of malevolent fate, or the randomness of an atomistic cosmos.

3. The Sins of the Nation
Early Christian Pre-Conceptuality

The convention that supernatural powers employ diseases either to punish human disobedience or to protect the elect is conspicuously present in the plague accounts of chroniclers such as Eusebius of Caesarea (c. 263–339), of St. Bede (673?–735), and of St. Gregory of Tours (539–94). Although their writings place the human experience of pestilence within a providential context, and although they tend to interpret epidemics as instruments of good and evil in redemptive history, important variations on the Old Testament formula of a vengeful God, as exemplified in I *Samuel*, chapter 6, occur in these texts, usually where the historian presents epidemiological material *without* affirming supernatural causation.

For the Christian historians surveyed below, epidemic disease is evidence of *eschatology*, a doctrine pertaining to the end of each individual life and of human history, according to God's revelatory texts (H. P. Owen 3:48–9). In several of these texts, however, one finds clinical or epidemiological observations incongruent with the all-encompassing design of theological history. These are anomalies. Indiscriminate disease contradicts the idea of divine chastisement, which implies selectivity on God's part and immunity for the faithful. On the one hand, apologists have accounted for Christian suffering as a divine mystery, intended either to purify the sufferer spiritually or to inspire fearful pagans to convert to Christianity. In other instances, Christian historians present anomalies without trying to account for them at all. The inclusion of anomalies in early Christian texts suggests either that pestilential events were too perplexing to ignore or too difficult to explain in conventional ways.

Bishop Eusebius of Caesarea's (c. 260–340) theology of history portrays Christianity and the inception of Constantine's monarchy as convergent, watershed events in God's plan for man (Sinnigen and Boak 494). The genre of theological history, to which *The History of the Church* belongs, assesses "the uniqueness and the universality of God's providential action in history, and the various phases of the divine plan" (Hug 7:26). For Eusebius, epidemic disease is literally an act of God. The Bishop includes an interesting plague commentary that takes place during Galerius Valerius Maximinus' (Maximin) (d. 313) persecution of the Christians. During his reign, Maximin (308–313) persecuted the Christians, tried to revive paganism, but met his downfall when he allied himself with Maxentius against Licinius and Constantine.

Eusebius describes Maximin as a bitter enemy of the Eastern Church (9.1:357). A participant in the pagan revival, he erects an image of Zeus and invents "devilish rites, unholy initiations, and loathsome purifications" (9.3:360). Moreover, to vilify the Christian community, he manufactures false affidavits, charges them with immorality, and organizes accusers to bear false witness against them. The rescript expresses the hope that Rome would be purged of Christian impiety, and that reverence will be accorded exclusively to "the immortal gods" (9.7: 364).

According to the narrative, God reveals himself to be an ally of the Christian minority (9.5:361–63). Famine and plague strike abruptly. Eusebius describes how this outbreak produces malignant pustules or "carbuncles" (9.8:365). Resembling smallpox, the disease spreads over the entire body, attacking the eyes and causing blindness in hundreds. Of the greatest importance to the theologian of history is the idea that the coincidence of famine and plague invalidates Maximin's faith in paganism: his unfounded belief that devotion to idols and the persecution of Christians will confer immunity to natural disaster (9.8:365). Hundreds die in the city, and the pestilence consumes every household indiscriminately (9.8:367). The wealthy rulers, governors, and officials come to a swift end. Mourners fill the streets, and entire families are wiped out. Eusebius, however, does not comprehend the outbreak to be a mysterious natural phenomenon, one without apparent origin or cause. Its origin and cause, in his mind, derive from Maximin's anti–Christian policy. The ordeal highlights the "limitless dedication" of the Christian minority as they serve the famished and the sick.

In ascribing the cause of the plague to pagan abuses, and in identifying it as God's punishment, Eusebius is certainly using the Old Testament formula. The false dichotomy he erects between the Christians and the pagans, however, significantly undermines the historicity of the narrative. Several historians argue that, while the persecution was in effect, some Roman officials and civilians actually *protected* their Christian neighbors from the persecutors (Sinnigen and Boak 494; italics added). Eusebius believes unshakably, however, that the debacle under Maximin was a spiritual trial for the Christian community (9.8:368), rather than a political outgrowth of a Caesarian struggle. From a secular viewpoint, one can say that the disease beset the Christian community in the fourth century A.D. in much the same way as pestilence had beset the people of Beth-shemesh.

Using Livy's *History of Rome* as a source, St. Augustine of Hippo (A.D. 354–430) in *The City of God against the Pagans* disparaged the Roman gods for their impotence in the face of "fearful" plagues, the worship of these deities having been of no avail against the plague of 399 B.C. Augustine uses the *ubi-sunt* convention derisively to criticize pagan religions. This rhetorical convention, usually found in verse, asks: where are the transitory things of life so mistakenly overvalued? (Thrall and Hibbard 497). The plague of 365 B.C., a periodic wasting disease described by the Christian historian Paulus Orosius of Braga, Spain (Snodgrass 16), evokes a similar Augustinian refrain: "Where were [the deities], when the great plague claimed such a host of victims, amongst them that same Furius Camillus [then defender of the republic]?" (III. 17:112–13). A third outbreak, possibly venereal in nature and attributed to "poisons" spread by Roman matrons, received no supernatural relief while another disease, in 293 B.C., forced the Romans to their own altars to invoke the aid of Aesculapius, the legendary Roman physician (to the Greeks, *Asclepius*), to whom temples would be built in Epidaurus, Cos, Pergamum, and Rome (III. 17:113); but supplications to the god of medicine were futile. Thus, St. Augustine indicted pagan gods for being unable, or disinclined, to mollify Roman suffering from 399 to 293 B.C.

A prominent Christian exegete, hagiographer, and historian of the sixth century, St. Gregory of Tours (539–94), attempted with varying success to demonstrate that epidemic disease reflected divine dissatisfaction with a sacred people. Even though St. Gregory read human history providentially, that is, in accordance with God's omniscience and eternal will, and even though he linked Frankish to sacred history, one can infer from his writings (V.33–4: 295–98; and IX.21–2) that outbreaks ran their courses, irrespective of piety or of apostasy.

In St. Gregory's view, because count Nantinus transgressed against the Church, he incurred God's wrath in the form of disease (V.36, pp. 299–301). But was Nantinus an incorrigible adversary of God and deserving of this kind of punishment? One can only answer that question if events leading up to his demise are viewed closely. According to St. Gregory, Marachar, bishop of Valennes and Nantinus' uncle, built and furnished churches, as well as Church houses. In the seventh year of his episcopate, his enemies poisoned him, but "God in His justice did not allow him to go long unavenged" (p. 299). Eventually, the chief conspirator Frontonius died of an undisclosed cause and "by divine judgment." To replace Marachar, the bishops consecrated Heraclius of Bordeaux.

Meanwhile, with the ulterior motive of avenging his uncle's death, Nantinus had been pursuing the courtship of Angoulême (p. 299). Once appointed to the court, and under the pretext of revenge, he harassed Heraclius for harboring his uncle's murderers. In addition, he occupied the estates that Marachar had bequeathed to the Church, believing that no one had the right to possess the property of a benefactor whom the clergy had murdered. Nantinus then killed a number of laymen and executed a priest who, he thought, was implicated in the plot against his uncle (pp. 299–300). Run through with a javelin, and hung alive from a post, the priest, to his last breath, denied any involvement. An irate Heraclius promptly excommunicated Nantinus. But, at a council of bishops, convened in the city of Saintes, the vengeful Count reconciled himself with Heraclius, promising to do penance and to return Church property that he had wrongfully seized (i.e., according to St. Gregory). But, upon his arrival at Angoulême, Nantinus looted and destroyed the Church buildings that he had allegedly occupied illegally. Consequently, Heraclius excommunicated him once again. After Heraclius' death, however, Nantinus bribed and flattered his way back into communion. A few months after his reinstatement, he contracted dysentery and confessed his guilt. Gregory of Tours interprets the Count's deathbed confession as "incontrovertible proof that [Nantinus] was being punished to avenge the holy Bishop" (p.300).

On moral and theological grounds, the story of Nantinus exemplifies the weakness of pre-conceptuality. He is made to believe that dysentery was God's punishment for having attacked the corrupt bishop Heraclius, the man who harbored Marachar's killers and who enjoyed ill-gotten gains. From this dubious perspective, God is portrayed as a kind of partisan advocate who resembles a Greco-Roman demigod. It is clear that St. Gregory had little sympathy for Nantinus' vengeful campaign against the bishopric of Heraclius, even though the latter harbored those who murdered bishop Marachar. In this political struggle, dysentery is more than a natural phenomenon: it is a manifestation of moral corruption.

The A.D. 580 plague outbreak in Auvergne, as St. Gregory sees it, had a supernatural origin (V.33–34, pp. 295–96). It was augured by unusual events: a flood drowning cattle and destroying crops; a bright light in the sky disappearing in the East; the thunderous sound of a crashing tree heard over a fifty-mile radius; an earthquake undermining the city walls; avalanches cascading down the peaks of the Pyrenees and crushing cattle and inhabitants; a sidereal fire burning villages; and, near Chartres, blood issuing from bread, while a hailstorm "scourged" the city of Bourges. This succession of unusual phenomena convinced many that a supernatural event was imminent. To the early medieval mind, the etiology of disease transcended nature and was unquestionable proof of a teleological design.

St. Gregory did not explicitly link the events of 580 together in an effective pattern, so the reader is able to differentiate biomedical information from legend. On the one hand, we have extraordinary prodigies while, on the other, we have an outbreak throughout Gaul of what may have been dysentery (V.34, p. 296). People suffer from head, neck, and back pain, vomit green or yellow material, and blame it all on poison. Countryfolk believe they have internal boils, and some exhibit suppurating tumors in their shoulders and legs. The epidemic, beginning in August, fatally afflicts children, and King Childerbert II himself loses his wife and two sons; the belated contrition of the royal family over having exploited the poor does not ward off the disease.

In A.D. 588, a severe epidemic characterized by inguinal swellings broke out in Marseilles and quickly spread to Saint-Syporean d'Ozon, a village near Lyons (IX.21, pp. 509–10). This description is characteristically pre-conceptual, but it is especially noteworthy for containing an anomaly that contradicts the theological explanation of disease. In Saint-Syporean d'Ozon, King Guntram sought a pre-conceptual remedy to a pestilence by ordering the people to fast on barley bread and pure water and to keep vigils. The King is even endowed with curative powers. One story is of a woman whose son is afflicted with paroxysmal malaria (symptoms likely reflecting the growth cycle of plasmodia). She is reported as having pulled threads from the King's cloak while in public, with steeping the threads in hot water, and with giving the infusion to her son. The thread tea is claimed to have cured the disease. St. Gregory also states that the mere mention of King Guntram's name expelled demons.

At this point, the pre-conceptual structure unhinges. According to St. Gregory, the epidemic began on the Marseilles docks, specifically on a Spanish ship that had put into port "with the usual kind of cargo, unfortunately bringing with it the source of infection" (IX.22, pp. 510–11). This is a startlingly modern assertion to find in a pre-conceptual context. To the idea of the transportation of the epidemic via maritime commerce, the anti-plague measures of King Guntram stand in stark contrast. As it turns out, quite a number of the town's people purchased objects from the cargo; as a result, in a short time eight people in one house became ill, and their house was abandoned, implying that they carried the disease. The idea of contagion, in the Marseilles passages, has neither moral nor supernatural significance and is extrinsic to theological history. Some time passed before the residential quarter and the entire town "like a cornfield set alight" (IX.22, 510–11) was swept with pestilence.

Throughout the ordeal, Bishop Theodore of Marseilles, who resided in Saint Victor's Church, along with seven poor folk, remained to pray and keep vigils, all the while "imploring God in His mercy to put an end to the slaughter and to allow the people some peace and quiet" (p. 511). In two months, "the plague [supposedly] burned itself out." Thinking the worst over, the people who had fled the city returned to Marseilles, only to discover the plague recrudescing with great lethality. This anomalous event dramatically contradicts the pre-conceptual idea that devotion was the surest measure against plague.

Pre-conceptuality informs *The History of the Franks*, but the epidemic events described in the text do not support this outlook convincingly. Although King Guntram is believed to have had curative powers, and although the Church rightfully supplicated God for assistance in the midst of the epidemic, St. Gregory explicitly states the possibility that commerce, not divine wrath, was the direct source of the outbreak. Moreover, he neither ignores nor discounts the fact that the plague unpredictably reappeared in Marseilles, despite the piety of its residents who obviously were not being punished for transgressions.

Since these anomalies do not support the theological prescription, it is reasonable to conclude that St. Gregory had a rudimentary understanding of contagious disease as a purely natural phenomenon. This is an interesting point. If we are interested in knowing where the idea of contagiosity originated, Girolamo Fracastoro's *Contagion, contagious diseases and their treatment* (1546) is regularly cited as a seminal text. Fracastoro (1478–1553), a physician in Verona, distinguished between three fundamentally different types of contagion, the second of which is most relevant to our discussion of St. Gregory's narration. The second form occurred by direct contact with contaminated objects or "fomes," that is, with "clothes, wooden objects, and things of that sort, which though not themselves corrupted can, nevertheless, preserve the original germs of the contagion and infect by means of these" (70). According to Fracastoro, the germs remained on the surface of, or within, inanimate objects, persisting there for "a very long time without any alteration" (71). He used tuberculosis as an example of an infectious agent surviving on the surface of manufactured objects. But he also acknowledged that the long-term survival of the agent in droplets or in secretions was unlikely and that, in cadavers, the agent retains its virulence, but only for a short time.

A degree of caution is called for when initially reading Fracastoro. One is inclined to think that he was ahead of his time. He should not be considered a lineal precursor of Pasteur, for Fracastoro's word for germ, *seminaria*, did not refer to micro-organisms at all but to chemical processes involved in contagion (Winslow 133; Litsios 63–9). What is noteworthy about his work, as it relates to St. Gregory's thinking on the subject, is the idea that contagion can occur through direct contact with a sick person, through fomites, and at a distance (the notion of atmospheric bodies of infection) (70–1). St. Gregory's narratives demonstrate that, as early as the sixth century A.D., pre-conceptuality could not adequately account for the origin and cause of epidemic disease

Although it is difficult to state with absolute certainty that Gregory of Tours' observations contain original epidemiological insights, there is no doubt that he linked the tainted cargo in Marseilles to the pestilence. Unknown to the historian, the vector carrying the disease to the eight index cases in Marseilles was not the shipboard rat but the fleas infesting clothing, bales of fiber, or furniture. By recording the facts, however, St. Gregory adumbrates Fracastoro. That the eight infected persons in Marseilles ignited a major outbreak suggests that primary bubonic plague, acquired through flea bites, had gradually become pneumonic; thus, of the original eight carriers, several survived long enough to communicate the disease to others, not through fleas on their bodies or in their belongings, but through aerosolized exhalations. People rather than fomites, therefore, had become the carriers.

The other interesting idea in St. Gregory's plague historiography is that disease diminishes naturally rather than through the intervention of divine agencies. The unanticipated resurgence of the Marseilles plague suggests as much, since the disease had no discernible theological purpose. On this ground, I believe that St. Gregory's description of the Marseilles epidemic anticipates a kind of discourse emphasizing the apriority of natural process over dogma. The histories of Bede and of St. Gregory suggest, on the one hand, that the early medieval mind subscribed to the idea of divine punishment through natural calamities while, on the other hand, recognized the epidemic to be an inexplicable natural event having nothing to do with transgressions against moral or religious codes. An apologist, it is possible, might account for the disjunction between the course of an epidemic and its ostensibly divine purpose by saying that a refractory disease either is God's chastisement or is a means of spiritual purification. But this dual rationale loses cogency in the face of a devastating plague that destroys randomly and unpredictably. St. Gregory of Tours' commentary is significant for providing clinical details, for emphasizing that symptoms are important to the classification of disease, and for exploring, however briefly, epidemiological possibilities outside the scope of pre-conceptuality.

The English historian and Benedictine monk, St. Bede or Baeda (673?–735), wrote extensively on theological, historical, and scientific subjects. His theological works are patristic commentaries on the Scriptures, and his biographical writings include hagiographies, notably one on St. Cuthbert.

The *Ecclesiastical History of the English Nation*, a primary source for English history, A.D. 597 to 731 and his major work, records the establishment of Christianity and of Anglo-Saxon culture in England.

Bede portrays epidemics in three distinct ways. One is simply to record the occurrence and to refrain from speculative commentary on it, which is the strategy of the observational writer. He alludes, for example, to a disaster in Constantinople in 446. At that time, famine preceded plague; consequently, the city fell into disrepair. So widespread were these conditions that the "stench of rotting corpses" contaminated the city and (in his view) contributed to a disease outbreak spreading "among men and beast alike" (54). In this context, Bede does not explore the interrelationship between famine and plague or the effects of the disease on the city. He subscribes to miasmatic theory when he writes that the putrefied corpses worsened the epidemic.

The portrayal of disease as an act of divine retribution against either apostasy or pagan hegemony identifies Bede as a pre-conceptualist. He went so far as to compare the English Church of the fifth century A.D. to the Israelites of the first millennium B.C. In 446, he thought that plague was an instrument of supernatural justice. Because the Britons trusted in "God's help where no human hand could save them," they resisted Irish and Pict barbarians (p. 54). Irish and Scottish pirates were forced to depart British soil while the Picts remained pacified in the north. A period of great abundance ensued for the Christian Britons because they had become a favored people; however, they did not appreciate that God was the source of their great blessings. For the people and the clergy were cruel and contemptuous of the Gospels, as well as slothful, quarrelsome, and self-indulgent.

Bede believed that, when the Britons' moral behavior declined, devastating disease broke out. So many Britons died that "the living could not bury the dead." A terrible retribution, apparently, had overtaken the wicked nation, threatening them with physical and spiritual death. The historical coincidence and the intensity of the disease, according to Bede, were divinely decreed "as punishment on their wickedness" (p. 55). The pillaging of the Britons at the hands of Germanic tribes further evidenced God's displeasure with a perfidious community.

The British king, Vortigern, recruited Germanic mercenaries, notably the Angles and Saxons, to protect his realm from local enemies. According to the *Anglo-Saxon Chronicle*, the king invited the Angles to settle in the southeast on condition that they defeat the Picts; the Angles were successful in this regard (pp. 12–13). But they also reported to their homeland that the Britons themselves could be easily defeated. Eventually, the Angles and the Saxons turned on their British clients, conquering their lands, and pillaging the countryside. The rapacious Saxons destroyed public and private buildings, slew priests at the altar, murdered and enslaved the people, and tried to uproot Christianity. Once again, Bede thought that the disaster represented "God's just punishment on the sins of the nation, just as the fires once kindled by the Chaldeans destroyed ... Jerusalem" (p. 57). Bede's juxtaposing of Israelite (612 to 582 B.C.) and of British history (A.D. 446) demonstrates the theological orientation of his historiography. Just as the Babylonians carried the Jews off into captivity, the Germanic tribes enslaved the British Christians. After many years of inconclusive warfare, however, the British became victorious, around the year 500. As a resident of the powerful Germanic kingdom of Northumbria, Bede, whose narrative extends as far as 731, revised the role of the Anglo-Saxons, who become the just instruments of punishment against the sinful Britons for having failed to convert the Germans (Breisach 90).

The conventional formula of a retributive deity as the wielder of disease is ironically inverted in the record of 665. In that year, a plague among the East Saxons precipitated a relapse from Christianity to paganism. The ironic inversion of the pre-conceptual formula (i.e., in its Judeo-Christian form) is that the people believed that pagan gods, angered over their conversion to Christianity, were punishing them! To appease the old gods, and hoping for supernatural protection against the disease, the Saxon king Sighere rebuilt the ruined temples, restoring idolatry. Upon learning that part of the province relapsed to paganism, the Christian king Wulfhere dispatched bishop Jaruman to reconvert Sighere. Jaruman was eminently successful; however, it is unclear from Bede's narrative whether the East Saxons abandoned Christianity because they perceived it to be an ineffectual antidote to the disease, or because they thought their abandoned gods vindictively wielded an epidemic against apostates (pp. 201–02).

If one were to accept the veracity of the East Saxons' story (that an epidemic actually drove them from Christianity to paganism), then this exemplum raises questions about the supernatural premise informing the Britons' experience in 446. The irony in the story is that God's perceived failure to intervene during an outbreak of endemic disease caused the East Saxon Church to backslide into paganism. A Christian apologist could just as well have turned the story on its head: God's failure to rescue Sighere's people was punishment for failing the test of faith, yet they were given sufficient grace to embrace Christianity again.

4. SET DOWN ITS NATURE

Eyewitness Reporting in the Age of Pericles

In this chapter, we look back to the fifth century B.C., to the beginnings of an intellectual approach to epidemic disease that focused, not on the preconceived belief-system, but on the clinical symptoms of pestilence, and, consequently, on how it impacted all levels of society. The observational writings of Thucydides and of Hippocrates exemplifying this focus contain few speculations on the origin or cause of epidemic disease. Instead of speculating on what they experienced, these writers and their emulators were intent upon capturing the epidemic experience in all of its frenetic reality, and, through the selection of essential scenes and details, each attained a unity of effect in their writings.

Thucydides

In 430 B.C., Thucydides (460–400 B.C.), historian of Athens, wrote in his *History of the Peloponnesian War* of an unprecedented epidemic, emphatically not the weapon of vindictive gods (110). Instead of employing pre-conceptual reasoning to make sense of the event, the Greek historian wrote of his first-hand experience, emphasized observed effects, and did not conjecture on matters of causation. For this reason, Thucydides' description of the plague of Athens is a benchmark in the development of epidemic discourse: the emphasis is on the observed effects of a biomedical disaster and not on how these events verify doctrinal tenets.

At the beginning of the narrative, Thucydides personifies the epidemic into a faceless, unpredictable power moving relentlessly along the western coast of the Red Sea and eventually across the Mediterranean Sea. The historian abruptly shifts his focus to clinical effects. Manifested without warning, the illness leaves people helpless. Physicians succumb to it as rapidly as do their patients, and no "human art" affects it. Religious supplications,

47

especially the practice of "divination," prove useless during the crisis. According to the historian's sources, the disease is believed to have come from Ethiopia; from there, spreading into Egypt and Libya, it fell upon Athens like a predator. It attacked the populace of Piraeus who thought the Peloponnesians had somehow poisoned their water supply. When the disease reached the "upper city," the death toll increased significantly. By this time, it was obvious that this was no man-made disaster.

An eyewitness to the epidemic, Thucydides "set[s] down its nature" with a practical end in mind: clinical information of this kind could be used in the future (110). I paraphrase his observations here to show that he included impressive symptoms and unusual behaviors, though there is no guiding idea as to diagnosis or treatment. The historian, however, had an acute sense of the disease as a historical phenomenon and of his unique position as documentarian.

The symptoms of this disease are "violent," that is to say, acute and severe (110). Inflammations of the tongue, eyes, and throat occur at its onset. Sneezing and hoarseness rapidly give way to acute respiratory distress, nausea, and bilious discharges. Dry retching and intestinal spasms are common (111). Blistering skin prostrates sufferers who can no longer endure being clothed. Fever drives some mad and into the streets. Some hurl themselves into rain-tanks for relief. The course of the infection is unpredictable. At times, those who weather its onset have significant setbacks and die. Generally, when the disease affects the bowels, patients decline rapidly, due to severe diarrhea, ulcerations, and dehydration. Thucydides suspects that the disease spreads through the body from the respiratory to the gastrointestinal system. Survivors usually bear signs of the disease: lost fingers, toes, eyes, and limbs, as well as neurological damage. The historian perceives that the disease is contagious. When scavenging animals shun the dead, Thucydides is startled at the instinctive aversion; from this observation, he infers that the disease is communicable and that the infectious agent inheres in corpses.

The futility of public health efforts to which Thucydides alludes at the beginning of the narrative is brought on by the ineffectiveness and vulnerability of the health-care providers. The epidemic disorientates logical thinkers who try to predict its course. Not only do all remedies fail, but the disease is unpredictable: healthy people die quickly while the weak survive. In the historian's judgment, the emotional weight of the illness contributes significantly to an unfavorable outcome: people who lose hope are at the greatest risk. Because public health authorities are themselves at considerable risk when caring for the afflicted, the public well-being is seriously shaken. An ethical quandary arises: to shun the patient precludes recovery;

to help the patient is futile; to intervene puts one at grave risk (112). The rate of mortality increases until "men die like sheep" (112).

At this point in the narrative, the historian describes how the body reacts to the infection. This sudden shift in focus may suggest that the narrative is disunified, but it is important to realize that recapitulations and abrupt turns are characteristic of the eyewitness report which captures striking events as they happen. In the process, Thucydides recognizes a curious anomaly: survivors appear to be immune to reinfection, a suspicion encouraging health workers and civilians in this category to help the sick. Another interesting distinction is that some of these survivors believe (erroneously) that they have become immune to *all* diseases. Of course, neither Thucydides nor the Athenian health-care establishment understood the mechanism of immunity or the idea of antibody protection, but many Athenians, including the historian, intuited the idea of naturally-acquired immunity, what is know today as the primary immune response (that is, when a person, exposed to a live, attenuated, or dead pathogen, acquires resistance to a disease).

Even though Thucydides does not analyze the demographic dimension of the crisis, his observations in this regard are acute. One deduction he draws is that the rate of mortality increased significantly when war refugees from the countryside migrated to the city to live in crowded, poorly-ventilated shelters (112). In makeshift towns, with their appalling conditions, the plague has its severest effect. The dead are stacked in the streets, and the sick wander about the outskirts of the city. Delirious refugees gather at large fountains for relief while, others set up camps at sacred locations.

The urban populace grew careless of sacred and of profane interests (113). There was little time for pre-conceptuality in Athens. Carelessness over religious obligations is evident with respect to burial rites, an important part of Greek religion and culture. The disease forces the people to expedite interments: some deposit relatives on any available pyre. According to J.B. Bury, since the right of property had a religious meaning for the Greeks, interments took place on private property. The Greeks believed that the dead possessed the soil within which they lay, and that the land around the sepulcher belonged to the living family whose duty it was to protect the ancestral tombs (46). Greek burial customs and family plots were therefore intertwined with family life and tradition (Murray 250). More than an instance of dejected expediency, then, the behavior of the Athenians in Thucydides'narrative dramatizes how seriously the calamity influenced culture and tradition.

The historian does not ignore the behavioral impact of the plague. The rich and propertied Athenians are shocked to see the lower classes acquiring the material possessions of well-to-do decedents. Having no safeguard against this eventuality, the well-to-do often squander their wealth rather than to allow it to be looted. Seeing nothing to be gained in honorable living, citizens become self-indulgent, believing that neither divine nor civil law has any jurisdiction over them. Many cease to rely on the supernatural for help against the plague, whereas some insist the pestilence is a divine instrument, the fulfillment of an oracle foretelling a Dorian war and widespread mortality or famine. Those recalling the oracular verse believe it demonstrates that the gods favor the Peloponnesians over the Athenians since the former seem to resist the disease. Thucydides, on the other hand, finds no merit in these assumptions, the Dorian oracle, for instance, having been contingent on the obscure meanings of oracular words. He understands that the trauma of these events makes esoteric sources inviting but maintains critical distance from the experience, even when ill himself.

The possibility that an epidemic can alter the course of history or divert the schemes of great armies has intrigued historians. The plague of 430 B.C. definitely affected the course of Peloponnesian War, but Thucydides does not explicitly say so, nor does he read the plague into a prescribed historical design. Hans Zinsser comments that the outcome of the war owed as much to the plague as it did to "force of arms" (122). For William H. McNeill, the mysterious plague of 430–429 B.C. was instrumental in Athens' failure to defeat Sparta and the Peloponnesian League (94). Although Thucydides had no opinion on the subject, it remains to be seen whether the disease was a turning point in the fifth century.

The outbreak certainly compromised the Athenians' war-making efforts; for example, their fleet was prevented from attacking the Peloponnesians because of it. According to the historian, the Peloponnesians were thought to have withdrawn from Athens to escape it (115). The plague affected politics. After it crippled an Athenian army under general Hagnon (son of the Periclean loyalist, Clinias), the people blamed Pericles (495–429 B.C.) for these misfortunes (115). When Sparta rejected Athenian peace overtures, the populace, once again, chastised Pericles who had recently returned from an unsuccessful campaign in Epidaurus (his indictment and acquittal for the misappropriation of funds did not enhance his public image). In his famous address to the people, the emperor (who had already lost two sons to the plague, and who would succumb to it himself in 429 B.C.) acknowledges that the epidemic is an unanticipated cataclysm. An inscrutable and virulent enemy, it strikes a primal chord in the Athenian mind (119). Using the formulaic phrase, the "hand of Heaven," to convey the inscrutability of the pestilence, he urges his people to endure it resignedly. The Spartans, on the other hand, have to be faced with determination and fortitude. Bearing their sufferings, he asserts, will publicize their honorable characters before their enemies (119). Even though Pericles uses the language of pre-conceptuality, his attitude towards the epidemic is a modern one: he rhetorically extrudes the disease from the war crisis because it is beyond their control and, like any other natural calamity, has to run its course.

Thucydides' description of the epidemic is noteworthy for its emphases on salient phenomena. With astonishing acuity, he writes about symptomology, public health, demography, behavioral psychology, culture, religion, and history. Unconcerned with fitting the disaster into a pre-conceptual framework as a way of normalizing it, Thucydides acts the role of a news reporter who catalogues experiences discernfully, while omitting distractions and irrelevancies. The Greek historian sketches scenes boldly but neither conjectures about, nor elaborates on, what he records.

Hippocrates

Hippocrates' writings complement Thucydides' history: the former, also an eyewitness documentarian, emphasizes the effects of a medical catastrophe. While Thucydides documents prominent features of the outbreak from the perspective of one who is both victim and recorder, Hippocrates of Cos (c. 460–c. 370 B.C.) experiences infectious diseases at the bedsides of patients, whose medical histories he documents. Socrates Litsios has recently observed that, "A key characteristic of the Hippocratic approach to medicine is the careful observation made of the history of individual sickness" (8). Like the historian, however, the Greek physician does not employ clinical data as the raw material of inference, at least as far as his famous work *Epidemics* is concerned. Yet he was aware that this needed to be done and that a theoretical method for the understanding of epidemic diseases was wanting. I would, therefore, like to consider Hippocrates' attempts to describe a method for the comprehension of epidemic disease.

In *Epidemics*, Books I and III, Hippocrates compiles information on forty-two cases of acutely ill patients (twenty-five of whom died). Book III may have been written in 430 B.C., the plague year of Thucydides' text (Jones 143); external and internal indicators suggest that the date of composition is early fifth century B.C. (Jones xxxi–xxxii). Modern scholars have tried to discover the nature of the disease or diseases afflicting the people of Thasos. Convinced that the forty-two records contain ample information for diagnosis, Zinsser identifies an array of diseases, including streptococcal infections, typhoid, poliomyelitis, encephalitis, tuberculosis, diphtheria, and sundry skin infections (114–17). While W. H. S. Jones, on the other hand, posits that the writings in the Hippocratic corpus are concerned almost entirely "with endemic disease and do not describe plagues, not even the great plague at Athens" (lvi), Marks and Beatty contend the book deals specifically with an Athenian plague, although its exact nature (either typhus or bubonic plague) is uncertain (31–32). Since the Greeks classified diseases in terms of symptoms, McNeill doubts whether these infections can be definitely identified (89). In view of the inexactness of the texts and of the absence of diagnosis, the nature of the affliction(s) has remained a matter of ongoing debate. The present chapter is concerned not with diagnostics but with *the manner* in which the effects of the disorders were evaluated and understood.

Hippocrates believed that observation, diagnosis, and treatment were closely intertwined activities. In his treatise, *Ancient Medicine*, he criticizes an approach to health science not based on observation; clearly, he was no pre-conceptualist. To the contrary, the "main task" of pre-Hippocratic and of Hippocratic writers, as W.H.S. Jones states, was explicitly "to free science from superstition and from philosophic hypotheses" (xxiii). Thus, an inquiry with an absolute viewpoint, one to which observed phenomena were made to conform, risked obscuring information about an infectious disease. According to Hippocrates, one should avoid the *postulate* (i.e., an absolute criterion) as a starting point, since it narrowed "the causal principle of diseases" down to one or two choices. A postulate, he rightly believed, is rigidly deductive and can not accommodate valid observations not fitting the prescribed system. The definition of postulation used here adumbrates the modern usage of the term in logic: a postulate is "claimed, taken for granted as, or assumed to be, true on the basis of reasoning, discussion, or belief; above all, it is an unproved assumption ... thought to be self-evident" (*OED* XIX: 1178; "postulate").

Whereas pre-conceptualists such as Abiathar and Homer postulate about epidemics, Hippocrates subscribes to the use of both "a principle and a method" in the understanding of infectious disease (*Ancient Medicine*, 6). Since principled methodology is built upon and conformable to precedent, "a competent inquirer" is encouraged to use "knowledge of the discoveries already made" as "starting-point[s]" for further exploration (*Ancient Medicine*, 17). Hippocrates' philosophy of knowledge sounds very modern, foreshadowing as it does the opinions of Beveridge, of Kuhn, and of Medawar. The Greek physician was rightly convinced that one had to be familiar with earlier theories of medicine in order to recognize and to explore new phenomena.

To *theorize* is Hippocrates' word for investigating a biomedical problem in the context of earlier work. A *theory*, he states in his *Precepts*, is "a composite memory of things apprehended with sense-perception" (313). This idea has interesting implications if applied to Thucydides' description: the latter's proclivity for discussing impressive aspects of the epidemic experience raises the likelihood of his having had prior experience with, or knowledge of, such an event. In other words, how did he know which aspects of the outbreak were significant and worthy of recording and which ones were not?

Unlike the postulate, the theory depends upon empirical support for validity. Even though Hippocrates was no rationalist and did not believe that "reason, rather than sense" constituted the "foundation of certainty in knowledge" (*OED* XIII: 169; "rationalism"), he had more in common with Thucydides, who refrained from conjecture, than with Pythagoras and Plato, whose philosophies of knowledge substitute insight for sense perception (Reichenbach 32). The Hippocratic idea of *theory*, then, is equivalent to the modern meaning of *hypothesis*, each term signifying a premise, "confirmed or established by observation or experiment, and ... propounded or accepted as accounting for the known facts" (*OED* VII: 513; "hypothesis").

Hippocrates' case studies consist of detailed observations over time. Although, for the most part, the records in *Epidemics* I and III are devoid of diagnosis, they are nonetheless very interesting. The course of Meton's illness is particularly revealing:

Case VII

Meton was seized with fever, and painful heaviness in the loins.

Second day. After a fairly copious draught of water had his bowels well moved.

Third day. Heaviness in the head; stools thin, bilious, rather red.

Fourth day. General exacerbation; slight epistaxis twice from the right nostril. An uncomfortable night; stools as on the third day; urine rather black; had a rather black cloud floating in it, spread out, which did not settle.

Fifth day. Violent epistaxis of unmixed blood from the left nostril; sweat; crisis. After the crisis sleeplessness; wandering; urine thin and rather black. His head was bathed; sleep; reason restored. The patient suffered no relapse, but after the crisis bled several times from the nose.

[*Epidemics* I. 200–01]

One shortcoming of this representative casestudy is that Hippocrates did not articulate or explore inferences. Many questions could have been asked about Meton's disease: why did he fight off the infection in five days? What infection did he have (it caused bleeding)? Could Meton's case be grouped with similar infections? What about Meton's survival and care that could be applied to others? What about his symptoms? How did they relate to those experienced by the remaining forty-one patients?

Though the exant medical records are inconclusive, G. E. R. Lloyd nevertheless asserts that Hippocrates' "theoretical assumptions and interests," especially with respect to the cause of disease, inform his clinical observations (58). Reading *Epidemics* in conjunction with *The Book of Prognostics* (400 B.C.), I think, puts Lloyd's opinion to the test and reveals the way in which Hippocrates arrived at judgments from compiled symptoms (Part 22:1). In *Prognostics*, for example, he states that naming a disease is not as important as recognizing its distinctive, physiological effects (Part 25:1). Compiling common symptoms facilitates disease taxonomy; and taxonomy, in turn, enables the physician "to treat those aright who can be saved." With accumulated knowledge, the physician can anticipate the disease's course since he or she has become familiar with its symptoms (Part 1:1). A clinician who records the manifestations of disease in great detail obviously perceives its documentary value as a comparative and future resource.

So what do we make of the *Epidemics* as a discrete document? Ostensibly, it was intended neither for diagnosis nor for prognosis. Instead, the physician-speaker was more of a spectator or medical reporter whose primary objective, as one scholar put it, was "to discover the sequences of symptoms [and] to set down the successes and failures" of the individual in his or her struggle against disease (Jones 144). On these grounds, *Epidemics* can best be described as a history of immunological responses rather than of medical interventions. Hippocrates focuses primarily on the clinical effects of disease on patients. The importance of his method lay in its "consistent doctrine of medical theory and practice" which was "free from both superstition and philosophy" (Jones xxi).

Both Thucydides and Hippocrates wrote vividly about the diseases they experienced. While the soldier-historian recorded the effects of the catastrophe as a detached participant who intimately experienced the plague, the physician did much the same thing but at the bedside of his patients. Each created a document indispensable to our understanding of the plague events of fifth century Greece. And neither of them contorted the facts to fit a preconceived formula. The observational modality, exemplified in the writings of Thucydides and Hippocrates, emerged in the fifth century B.C. and developed concurrently with the older, pre-conceptual tradition.

5. THE PROVINCE OF HUMAN REASONING

Eyewitness Reporting and the Plague of Justinian

The eyewitness descriptions in this chapter achieve a unified effect through the authors' selection of meaningful scenes. Not to be confused with *descriptive epidemiology* (the study of "the amount and distribution of disease within a population by person, place, and time" [Mausner et al., 119]), the type of discourse under scrutiny here permits the reader to apprehend the disruptive effects of epidemic disease vicariously. Writings in the lineage of Thucydides treat the physiological, psychological, social, cultural, and political consequences of epidemics but do so superficially since descriptive passages are embedded in the history of a broader period (as with Procopius) or are subordinate to a larger work (as with Boccaccio). The most distinguishing feature of this kind of writing is that, unlike pre-conceptual historiography which assimilates epidemics into a system of belief or of knowledge, the eyewitness account has immediate, dramatic appeal in and of itself.

Procopius and the Plague of Justinian: A Hybrid Form

An early medieval example of the observational modality is Procopius' account of the plague of Justinian, which struck Asia Minor, Africa, and Europe in the late spring of A.D. 542, and which arrived in Constantinople, the capitol of the Byzantine Empire (Kohn 188–89; Snodgrass 20–1). The historian Procopius (d. A.D. 565?) recorded his experience in his great work the *History of the Wars*. The outbreak, the first pandemic of plague on record, was named after emperor Justinian I (483–565; Byzantine Emperor, 527–65) (McNeill 109–10).

The account in question is a turning point in the history of epidemiological thought: in it, graphic description supplants pre-conceptual thought, and the cumulative effect of the disease is riveting. At the outset of the narrative, the historian writes of a scourge of great magnitude and ferocity, nearly annihilating "the whole human race." Its overwhelming effects, he believes, suggest its supernatural origin. From this orthodox standpoint, he decries natural philosophers whose explanations for the epidemic were deceptive and outlandish. He criticizes the sophists, itinerant Greek teachers (5th century B.C.) known for their venality, and the astrologists who explained natural events in terms of the movements of celestial bodies. In the spring of A.D. 543, with the plague established in Byzantium, Procopius subscribed to a supernatural etiology. Thus, he uncritically cites the testimonies of those claiming to have been physically assaulted by apparitions, and to have developed disease precisely where they were struck (p. 455). Yet, at this juncture, he encountered a conundrum similar to that which faced Bede, Gregory of Tours, and others: piety did not ensure immunity; hence, exorcisms failed (p. 455), and those hiding in Christian sanctuaries were not spared (p. 455–56). In some cases, pre-conceptual thinking made matters worse; for example, the sick were shunned because they were thought to be possessed by demons. When in need of aid, they desperately banged on neighbors' doors, but the neighbors were too terrified to answer. Procopius states that people who dreamed of demonic attacks, or who claimed to have heard disembodied voices foretelling their suffering, inevitably became sick. To most of the people, however, the disease did not announce its coming.

The philosophical turn from pre-conceptuality to empiricism (i.e., to knowledge derived from sense experience) occurs at this point. Procopius rather suddenly abandons popular beliefs for medical matters. Victims, he begins, develop fever at any time of the day. During the incubation period, the disease is especially insidious in that disarming symptoms (fever, discoloration, languor) create a false sense of security. However, between one and three days, enlarged lymph nodes appear in places like the groin (p. 457). A "diversity of symptoms" then besets the sufferer. Some fall into deep comas while others become violently delirious. Characteristic symptoms include insomnia, hallucination, paranoia, and delirium.

The historian observes that, although the caretakers are under great duress, they do not contract the malady from the sick or the dead, which implies that the atmosphere is not the source of the disease, as was commonly supposed (p. 459). Even though Procopius neither elaborates on specific observations nor speculates on the general idea of contagion, his comments illustrate the fundamental difference between the observational and the pre-conceptual modalities, as well as between the former and etiological discourse which involves the systematic analysis of disease causation. Perhaps intuiting the importance of etiological thinking, Procopius refers to autopsies of plague victims.

In spite of the desperate conditions described above, medical workers serve diligently. Some lives are saved; but, for many, nothing can be done (461). Agitated patients, at times, fall from their beds, thrash on the floor, and have to be restrained. Fever drives many to immerse themselves in water, even into the sea. Some starve to death; others hurl themselves from buildings. Some patients not suffering from high fevers or delirium die from mortified lymph nodes, an excruciating condition.

Though sudden and frightful events perplex physicians, they still are inclined to discover how the disease damages the human body. Procopius alludes to their findings, namely that dissected lymph nodes contain "a strange sort of carbuncle" or encapsulated mass (461). Certain clinical features do not bode well for a patient; for instance, those having lentil-size carbuncles (approximately one-half centimeter) die almost immediately (perhaps because the infection had spread into the bloodstream) (463); others vomit blood and quickly perish. Medical prognosis in such cases, however, is unreliable. Some hopeless cases survive; some hopeful ones do not. Some benefit from baths; some uncared for patients recover. The plague is both elusive and unpredictable: "in this disease there was no cause which came within the province of human reasoning" (463). Yet persistence pays off as medical workers gradually meet the challenge through trial and error.

Although the narrative begins with a pre-conceptual orientation, its emphasis on descriptive effects identifies it as belonging to the lineage of Thucydides. Like Hippocrates, Procopius does not ask questions (e.g., in cases in which bathing helps, is cold water used to lower a fever? Or: who survives without intervention, and what are the conditions?). The great number of patients and the confusion overwhelming the Byzantine medical establishment make it difficult to distance oneself from the crisis and to analyze events objectively. But, despite the chaos, Procopius still draws noteworthy inferences: for example, pregnant women are especially vulnerable to the infection (a fact that Hippocrates had observed); and recovery is assisted if engorged lymph nodes are surgically drained.

Procopius comments on the intensity of the disease at various points in time. The infection peaked after three or four months, but, by that time, the morbidity rate (the total of infected cases) had increased, until "the tale of the dead" reached 5,000 per day and eventually exceeded 10,000 per day (likely an inflated statistic). Like Thucydides, Procopius tells of how the plague overturns burial customs. Since both historians lived in religious societies, it is quite conceivable that each witnessed the impracticality of elaborate obsequies. Or perhaps Procopius turned to the Greek narrative for dramatic effect? Whatever the case may be, in the Byzantine narrative, each family reverently buries the deceased; but, as the disease intensifies, burial rites and customs are abandoned; and bodies are thrown expeditiously into the nearest tomb (II. xxiii: p. 465).

The abandonment of interment ritual is an index of the overall collapse of social and domestic life. If servants and slaves die, the rich are left unattended; consequently, when the well-to-do die, no one is around to bury them. So dire has the situation become that the Emperor Justinian allocates funds for the burial of rich and poor alike, but trench-burial, for some, is the only alternative. The situation becomes quite deplorable.When public grave-diggers run out of usable land for this purpose, they mount towers in the fortifications of Sycae (modern Galata), tear the tower roofs off, and throw the bodies into the building (p. 467). As a result, the rotting corpses are piled, one on top of the other, to the very top of the building, at which point the grave-diggers mindlessly re-attach the roofs; the stench inevitably pervades the city (p. 467). Another method of disposal is to dump bodies on skiffs bound for unknown destinations.

The plague alters Byzantine social behavior dramatically. Factionalism and feuding abate considerably, as foes join together to remove the dead. The profligate experience moral conversions and embrace religion (pp. 469–71). Fear obviously motivates them, for, as soon as "the curse" (i.e., the plague) wanes, so too does their piety. They revert to "their baseness of heart," displaying villainy and lawlessness. The ubiquity of the disease invites personification: once again, Procopius calls it a malevolent entity arising from the mysterious East (p. 471).

The plague is also an important dimension of the ongoing war between Rome and Persia, the history of which is Procopius' primary concern. The degree to which it is a major factor is revealed if one reads the passage carefully. Significantly, the historian does not contend that the disease is a divine instrument against non-Christian forces. For Procopius, the plague, like famine, storm, or earthquake, is an environmental factor over which man has no control. If exploited, it can conceivably work to the Romans' advantage; however, it is not exploited as a tactical element (II. xxv: pp. 479–89). The Persians initially are forced to retreat from their strongholds because of the disease; however, instead of using the retreat to their advantage, the Romans attack in an undisciplined and precipitous fashion, allowing the plague-stricken Persians to regroup and to counterattack successfully. The details of the conflict follow.

Before the outbreak, the Persian emperor Chosroes migrated northward, from Assyria to Adarbiganon, to plan an invasion of the Eastern Roman Empire through Persarmenia, but, having second thoughts, he decided to seek peace. When the Roman peace emissary Valerianus learns that the retreating Chosroes desires peace, he informs Justinian (who had recovered from the plague himself). Justinian decides to invade enemy territory and to press the advantage. The Romans plan a convergence of armies to attack Persarmenia in force. As the commanders gather their forces in Armenia, Chosroes is still in the process of retreating from plague-ridden Assyria to Adarbiganon which at that time is plague free. Perceiving that a retreating army is vulnerable, the Romans prepare the three-prong assault. However, before the synchronized attack is launched, a commander named Peter commits his forces unilaterally. As a result, the element of surprise is lost. On the next day, Roman allies, the Eruli, learn of Peter's decision and follow him into battle. With little choice, Martinus and Valerianus follow suit. Since the assault is staggered rather than concerted, the Romans' numerical advantage is also neutralized. Eventually, the Roman armies meet in enemy territory, but, by that time, the Persians at Doubios have had time enough to prepare (p. 479). Nabedes, the Persian commander, establishes a strategic stronghold near the village of Anglon in an inaccessible mountainside fortress. Nearly four thousand Persians hide in trenches, assume flanking positions, and await the inevitable Roman advance (p. 481).

After plundering the countryside, the Roman general Narses assaults this precarious site but does so without conferring with the other generals, and without knowing the Persians' deployment. Advancing in confusion and disorder, with baggage trains ready for plunder, they attack successfully at first, but flanking Persians of whom the Romans are unaware drive them into headlong retreat. The lack of Roman discipline startles the Persians who wonder if this unexpected maneuver is actually a ruse to draw them out of their redoubts for a Roman counterattack. The fleeing Narses, however, has no such plan, and the retreat turns into a rout.

An ecological determinant, the plague forces the Persians to retreat, which provides an opportunity for them to regroup. But the more immediate cause of the Persian victory at Doubios, in my opinion, is military incompetence and a breakdown of discipline. Thus, the Roman generals Peter and Narses, *not* the pestilence, are directly responsible for the disaster. What Procopius does not say about this debacle is most important. For the historian, the epidemic is neither an expression of God's wrath against Byzantine civilization or against Justinian, nor is it a phenomenon warranting serious speculation on his part. All he does is to record what he perceives.

Although Procopius begins his narrative from an ostensibly pre-conceptual standpoint, he does not skew historical events to support doctrinal assumptions (e.g., the plague of Justinian and the military defeat of Roman forces as the consequences of apostasy). Procopius' treatment of epidemic disease stands midway between pre-conceptuality and the observational modality.

6. The Vast Estates
The Decameron of Giovanni Boccaccio

Giovanni Boccaccio (1313–1375) wrote *The Decameron*, his master-piece of one hundred novellas, under the shadow of the Black Death, a pandemic devastating Europe from 1345 to 1351, and killing an estimated 25,000,000 people or one-third of the entire population of the Continent (Kohn 27–8; Snodgrass 32–46; Ziegler 13–29). His description of one of worst pandemics in history, second in mortality rate only to the influenza pandemic of 1918, juxtaposes the ubiquity of morbid disease to the imaginative celebration of life.

My purpose here is to discuss Boccaccio's contribution to the heritage of Thucydides and its place in that tradition. As a preamble to this discussion, I will speak briefly about the medical theories on plague current at the time. Medieval biomedical scientists, forced to theorize about the disease, came to some interesting conclusions about its causes. Contrary to popular belief, medical and civil authorities, notably in Italy, went to great lengths to control the plague. In the provincial Italian city of Pistoia, located in the region of Tuscany, administrators formulated ordinances and provisions, in the spring of 1348, to control its spread ("Pistoia"; Ziegler 54–6). They believed that decomposing cadavers, of which there were many, were infectious and remained so until putrefaction and exposure to the elements destroyed whatever it was in the body that caused the malady. The plague particles in decaying bodies, they conjectured, when released from corpses, contaminated ground, water, and air. Although the causative leap from putrefaction to contagion via the natural environment was certainly rational, it did little to stem the plague. But the Pistoians should be credited for having acted on the basis of a biological supposition, namely that, if the source of the Black Death were the foul atmosphere, aerial pollution had to be minimized. One obvious way to do this, which harkens back seven hundred years to Byzantium, was to remove corpses from premises and to bury bodies in trenches that were six- to eight-feet deep. Despite its theoretical limitations, the Pistoian ordinances were intelligently formulated.

The civil authorities of Pistoia could not have known that the plague is caused by a microbe, known today as *Yersinia pestis* ("Plague," CDC; "Plague," *Communicable Diseases*, 381–87); that this organism is endemic to regions populated by certain species of rodents, especially the so-called black rat (or *Rattus rattus*); that, at times, rodent populations are decimated by epizootics; that during these outbreaks, rats die by the hundreds; that the pathogen can not spread farther than the rodent population without a natural vehicle or vector to communicate infected rodent blood to man; that certain species of flea contract the plague germ from infected blood and regurgitate it into bite-wounds inflicted on human beings; that infected human beings (and other susceptible mammals) replace the rat in the cycle as carriers of disease; that the plague spreads through the body from the localized site of infection, entering the bloodstream and the lungs; and, finally, that the airborne bacteria are communicated via this route and develop into pneumonic infection, the most lethal form of the plague.

Of these hidden realities, which Western science would not elucidate for another five and one-half centuries, the Pistoians knew nothing. Instead, they proceeded empirically: since the plague destroyed bodies (they reasoned), it came from and resided in decomposing tissue. There was some precedent for the interconnection between putrefying corpses and disease. In 1155, at the battle of Tortona, for example, the Emperor Frederick I Barbarossa was able to pollute the Guelph's water supply by hurling corpses and carcasses into it (Snodgrass 29). The medieval mind, it seems, made the connection between putrefaction and contagious disease on the basis of what they sensed: they did not have the slightest idea that through decomposition bacteria, fungi, plants, and lower animals utilize the remains of dead tissue as a source of nutrition (Burdon and Williams, 336); that, on a biochemical level, enzymes break down polysaccharides, lipids, nucleic acids and proteins into smaller elements (336); that micro-organisms absorb these by-products, to use as sources of chemical energy (336); and that the very same polysaccharides, lipids, nucleic acids, and proteins assimilated from the dead tissue allow complex organisms to metabolize compounds in their own systems (336). The foul gases to which medieval science ascribed such virulence are actually the by-products of putrefaction and not the source of plague: trace elements and nitrogen are absorbed by higher plants, becoming the basis of fertilizer; ammonia, hydrogen sulfide, volatile amines, putrescine, and cadaverine, the by-products of protein decomposition, harmlessly fill the air (336). The Pistoians would have been amazed to learn that putrefaction is essential to life. And they could not have suspected that the flea, *Xenopsylla cheopsis*, acquired the plague bacillus from rats and, as the primary vector, carried it in its system.

The plague tractates of the period contain interesting variations on the idea of contagion. Jacme d'Agramont, Gentile da Foligno, the Faculty of Medicine of Paris, along with the Islamic physician Ibn Khatimah, were some of the chief contributors to the corpus. While most contended that the plague spread through corrupted air or during extremes of temperature, concepts inherited from Hippocrates and Galen, physicians such as da Foligno explicitly state that the plague is spread from person to person and from community to community (Winslow 96–114). Khatimah warns, specifically, of the danger posed by fumes issuing from the sick (101). And Guillaume de Machaut counsels that, if one can not escape a pestilential area quickly, then every effort should be made to avoid the sick whose breath is a source of contagion (102). Even though medieval writers did not understand the role of the flea in the cycle of plague transmission, they had a rudimentary notion of how pneumonic plague occurs.

Evidently a student of Thucydides, and possibly an eyewitness to the plague in 1348 Florence, Boccaccio (like Procopius) did not interpolate theories into the *First Day (Introduction)* of *The Decameron* but chose, instead, to describe the effects of the disease and how it rapidly destroys the city. Judging from style, rhetoric, and content, some scholars believe that Boccaccio's *Introduction* is actually a work of fiction rather than an eyewitness report, one that amalgamates the writings of other plague authors and historians, notably those of Thucydides and of Lucretius. So, before I discuss the content of the *Introduction*, I would like to outline these opposing views and then, in the light of probable sources and of rhetorical evidence, consider the text's historical authenticity.

Some believe that *First Day (Introduction)* is an eyewitness report. Carlo Muscetta subscribes to this interpretation (159), as does Philip Ziegler who calls it "the most celebrated eye-witness account of any pestilence in any epoch" (46). There is biographical support for this thesis: Boccaccio was in Florence during the plague outbreak, in March or April of 1348, and his father, an official involved in public health, kept him well informed of the crisis (Branca 76). Today, biomedical writers tend to accept the thesis at face value. Among its advocates are Christopher Wills who identifies Boccaccio's "experience of the plague in Florence" to be the source of his description of pigs rooting through discarded clothing (66) and J. N. Hays who states that Boccaccio *reported* the decline of morality in Florence (51; italics added).

Two aspects of *First Day (Introduction)* challenge the assumption that it is an eyewitness report: first, since it resembles historical works in the lineage of Thucydides, it might be derivative; and, second, rhetorical conventions identify it as an artificial rather than eyewitness document. On the basis of these suppositions, a counterthesis has gradually emerged.

Thomas G. Bergin, though accepting the idea that Boccaccio was an eyewitness of the plague, questions the intermingling in the text of reportage and of formulaic elements (290–91).G. H. McWilliam, translator of *The Decameron* and author of the excellent Introduction for the *Penguin* second edition, is not convinced that Boccaccio was present in Florence during the plague crisis of 1348. Boccaccio's plague description, he believes, is too "heavily dependent on literary antecedents, especially that of the eighth-century historian of the Lombards, Paul the Deacon," to be an eyewitness document; in addition, McWilliam finds "no external evidence to support Boccaccio's contention that he was an eyewitness to the terrible suffering to which the Florentines were subjected" (nearly 75,000 out of 100,000 citizens died [xliii–iv]). As far as contemporary sources (oral or written) are concerned, Boccaccio could easily have received firsthand communications about the disaster from his father who, as Florentine Minister of Supply, was "actively engaged in implementing the emergency measures decreed by the Florentine government to combat such pressing problems as shortage of food and inattention to customary standards of hygiene" (McWilliam, intro., xliv).

Although no compelling evidence exists that Boccaccio was on the scene, he was not insulated from the horrors and grief associated with the plague. Indeed, he lost close friends, literary acquaintances, his second stepmother, and his father (presumably from plague as well) (McWilliam xliv). McWilliam does not question the factual authenticity (albeit secondhand) and the philosophical evocativeness of the text (cxii–cxiii). Unquestionably, the plague shook Florentine civilization and culture, and Boccaccio imaginatively conveys this reality (cxii–iii). In the final analysis, McWilliam maintains that *First Day (Introduction)* "is not to be read as the eyewitness account [Boccaccio] claims it to be," largely because (in his opinion) it is based upon earlier plague descriptions (Paul the Deacon's, for one), and because it exhibits rhetorical devices (e.g., anaphora and the *ubi-sunt* motif), identifying it as a literary artifact (Notes [*First Day*], p. 804). In the paragraphs to follow, I will look closely at the bases of McWilliam's thesis.

First, I doubt that *First Day (Introduction)* is heavily indebted to earlier histories, such as the eighth-century *History of the Langobards*. A comparison between the sources and the *Introduction* suggests that Boccaccio was acquainted with classical plague texts but *not* explicitly reliant on them. If one compares the *Introduction* to these precursors in terms of geography, of epidemiology, and of social effects, this position gains support.

Although both the plagues of Thucydides and of Boccaccio originated in the East, on the question of geography, Boccaccio's scope is narrow and vague, whereas Thucydides' is wide and specific. The latter, for example, writes that the Athenian plague originated in Ethiopia, arrived in Egypt and Libya, and eventually broke out in Greece (110). The 1628 Hobbesian translation of the text reflects the same geographical pattern, as the plague is said to have originated in that part of Ethiopia, "that [lies] upon Egypt and then fell down into Egypt and Africa" (II. 47:115). In view of modern geographical borders, one can only speculate as to why Thucydides situated Ethiopia in close proximity to Egypt and Libya (nearly 1100 miles separates Cairo from Eritrea). The important point is that Thucydides, unlike Boccaccio, was concerned with the plague's capacity to spread over vast regions and even over mountains and large bodies of water. Although he did not know *how* the plague spread, he intuited the epidemiological importance of recording its place of origin and the regions where it appeared. Boccaccio's description of the Florentine plague, on the other hand, is not concerned with geography, a fact attenuating the argument for direct indebtedness

More cogent dissimilarities between the two texts exist. Thucydides and Boccaccio appear to have been writing about different diseases altogether, a premise to which some modern historians subscribe. One historian, in particular, believes that Thucydides' plague can not be definitively diagnosed since the inflammation, upper-respiratory symptoms, alarming discharges, disfiguration, and virulent contagiousness characterize an array of infectious diseases, including typhus, smallpox, typhoid, measles, and perhaps even bubonic plague (McNeill 287). The Florentine outbreak, on the other hand, exhibits distinctive symptoms, associated with the bubonic plague (enlarged lymph nodes, subcutaneous bleeding, but not the acute inflammatory response observed in Athens). From a diagnostic perspective, then, Thucydides is vague; Boccaccio is more precise.

The Athenians and Florentines react to the respective epidemics in a similar fashion, but this does not strengthen the argument for Boccaccio's direct indebtedness to Thucydides, for panic, abandonment of family and neighbors, moral decline, and the decimation of health-care workers can be expected in a city beset by an uncontrollable epidemic. In addition, both writers deal with the ideas of contagiousness and immunity but only tentatively so. In Athens, unlike in Florence, survivors are reputedly immune to reinfection and, as a result, are better able to help the sick. In Boccaccio's text, on the other hand, no such immunity is observed. Like the Athenians, the Florentines theorize about contagion, as did the Pistoians. They think, for instance, that human breath, clothing, and objects carry the infective agent, recalling Boccaccio's image of pigs dying instantly upon exposure to infected clothing.

Both writers treat the profound effect of the disaster on funeral rites. But this, too, is equivocal evidence of indebtedness, for interment rites are important in both Periclean and medieval culture. The alarming accumulation of dead bodies in the midst of a virulent epidemic would overtax mortuary resources anywhere, past or present. On this subject, though, Boccaccio provides more detail than does Thucydides. Both writers mention that circumstances preclude ritual. A difference in detail between the texts supports the argument that Boccaccio is not following Thucydides closely. Human migration patterns are reversed as peasants rush to Athens, not recognizing it as the disease focus, while panicked Florentines self-deceptively flee to the countryside.

The plague narrative of Paul the Deacon (c. 720/30–799), which McWilliam considers a principal source of the *Introduction*, has more in common with Procopius' rather than with Boccaccio's work. An eighth-century historian and member of a noble Lombard family, Paul describes a 566–67 outbreak in Liguria (a region in Genoa) (Marks and Beatty 48–50). Although *The History of the Langobards* is not wholly original, its plague descriptions are quite realistic, despite traces of pre-conceptuality. Like Procopius, Paul mentions premonitory and ineradicable signs mysteriously appearing on dwellings, doors, utensils, and clothes; inexplicably, these "marks" become more prominent with each attempt to remove them (conversely, Boccaccio mutes the supernatural influence).

In terms of symptoms (with the exception of high fever), Boccaccio's work resembles that of Paul, possibly because both writers are describing the effects of bubonic plague. In 566, the Ligurians develop lymphatic swellings in the groin resembling "a nut or date." This manifestation is followed by "unbearable fever," with death ensuing on the third day. If one survives the third day, the prognosis improves greatly. It is widely observed that many abandon their homes in fear. Shepherds desert their flocks, while crowded villas and fortified places are depopulated. Parents leave their children; young adults, their aged parents. And some die in the midst of funerals. Paul speaks explicitly of human extinction and of the epidemic returning the world to "its ancient silence." Agriculture suffers, rural areas are used as cemeteries exclusively, and homes become "places of refuge for wild beasts." These dire conditions affect the Romans in Italy and extend as far as north as Bavaria.

In a second outbreak, Paul cites "mystical portents," such as a deluge in Venetian and Ligurian territories. Other events are equally foreboding: men and animals die, estates fall to ruin, and floods demolish roads and highways, along with the walls of Verona. Adding to the misery, the River Tiber overflows its banks. At this point, Paul seems to have borrowed a page from Roman myth when he speaks of how the streams are alive with serpents (snakes do swim when flushed from their nests) and of how a giant dragon (perhaps an allusion to *The Revelation of St. John the Divine*) passes by the city to descend into the sea. These preliminaries usher in the epidemic. In 590, Pope Pelagius II died from a disease that causes inguinal swellings. Deacon Gregory who was elected pope then ordained a sevenfold litany, imploring God's mercy against the disease, but the new pope also succumbs to the plague in 604. Paul tells of a third epidemic devastating Ravenna in 589 and, in 617–18, of a fourth striking Rome. He also describes a plague which breaks out in Rome and in much of Italy (Kohn 280).

Since Paul the Deacon does not differentiate sufficiently between portents and symptoms, his writing more properly belongs to the Judeo-Christian tradition than to the kind of secular, observant record associated with Thucydides. Observations in the early Christian texts are often subordinated to supernatural causation and motive, although anomalies appear (e.g., Gregory of Tour's description of the Marseilles plague) that are not subsumed under the theological scheme.

McWilliam believes that the presence of rhetorical conventions in *First Day (Introduction)* (i.e., the *ubi-sunt* convention and anaphora) proves that Boccaccio wrote a literary artifact or a reconstruction rather than an eyewitness report of rapidly-unfolding events. These conventions, in my view, do not necessarily invalidate the argument that Boccaccio experienced the plague firsthand; they might simply have been worked into a substratum of first- and of secondhand observations. Let us look at each trope.

The *ubi-sunt* convention, used primarily in verse to reiterate the formula "Where are" (or "Whither has gone...") certain overvalued aspects of life, emphasizes the idea that material comforts and high station are transitory. A homeless exile, in the Old English poem *The Wanderer*, conveys this elegiac sentiment after he loses everything of value to him (Greenfield 215):

> Whither has gone the horse? Whither has gone the man?
> Whither has gone the giver of treasure? Whither has gone the
> Place of feasting? Where are the joys of the hall? Alas, the
> Bright cup! Alas, the warrior in his corselet! Alas, the
> Glory of the prince! How that time has passed away, has
> Grown dark under the shadow of night, as if it had never been!
>
> [74; trans. Gordon]

Boccaccio's use of this formula follows:

> Ah, how great a number of splendid palaces, fine houses, and noble dwellings, once filled with retainers, with lords and with ladies, were bereft of all who had lived there, down to the tiniest child! How numerous were the famous families, the vast estates, the notable fortunes, that

were seen to be left without a rightful successor! How many gallant gen-
tlemen, fair ladies, and sprightly youths, who would have been judged
hale and hearty by Galen, Hippocrates and Aesculapius ... having break-
fasted in the morning with their kinsfolk, acquaintances and friends,
supped that same evening with their ancestors in the next world.

[*First Day (Introduction)*, 13]

The *ubi-sunt* interrogation, along with the anaphora or "How"-formu-
lation, reflects a terrible truth: the plague destroys households, does not dis-
criminate between rich and poor, and kills rapidly. The references to
Hippocrates and Galen, though formulaic, suggest that Boccaccio had in
mind the emphasis these classical physicians placed on direct observation.
The allusion to Aesculapius, ancient Roman god of healing, admittedly
harkens back to Homeric myth (specifically, to the Greek god of medicine,
Asclepius) and to pre-conceptuality, but the reference does not undermine
the historicity of the fourteenth-century narrative. The allusions and conventions certainly reveal self-conscious craft, but they may simply have been
interpolated into the eyewitness report. Since the *Introduction* is the first of
nine days on which the characters tell their stories, its language had to be
congruent with that of the main text. Congruity between the *First* and the
Second to *Tenth Days* was, therefore, a thematic necessity for Boccaccio, since
the imaginative reconstitution of life expressed in the one hundred novellas was a means of creative transcendence over the insufferable reality gripping Florence in 1348. A world of imminent, widespread death is transformed
into what Francesco De Sanctis aptly calls "the carnival-like freedom" of
imaginative creation (223). Bergin is most certainly correct to say that, "The
exuberant vitality of the work may well be seen as a reaction against the horrors of the dreadful scourge" (158).

Boccaccio's plague narrative is not consonant with the idea that the epidemic is instrumental in the fulfillment of biblical prophecy. Before Christ's
Second Coming, according to such an exegesis, demonic forces are expected
to wreak havoc on mankind. Adverse natural events, such as earthquakes,
storms, and meteor showers, are considered portents of the plague; and the
plague is given eschatological meaning (the interpretation refers to the seven
plagues of *The Revelation of St. John the Divine*, chapters 15 and 16, especially 16, verse 2). As the plague worsened, the biblical interpretation gained
relevance. The dire predictions associated with biblical pre-conceptuality
also had terrible social repercussions, one of which was the scapegoating of
vulnerable segments of the population. Lepers, the poor, the clergy, and especially the Jews, were blamed and persecuted for having brought the calamity
(Cohn 87). In view of the estimated 25,000,000 deaths, it is not difficult to
imagine the panic and fear gripping the fourteenth-century mind.

The plague experience of 1348 demanded an accurate record, and Boccaccio assumed the dual role of witness and of historian. His account of the public reaction to the plague's relentless devastation resonates throughout the *Introduction*. Initial counter-measures, though rigorous, are misdirected, all wisdom and ingenuity failing to halt its spread. Even though refuse is cleared away, the sick isolated, and the public informed about prevention, nothing works. Quarantine (from the Italian, *quaranta: forty* days in isolation) makes sense in principle, but how it is to be implemented is unclear. Generally, public service information based on arcane theories has little effect.

By early spring, the plague takes a terrifying turn. We are familiar with the symptoms from our reading of Procopius, the most obvious being apple- or egg-shaped lymph nodes (called *buboes*; hence, *bubonic* plague) in the groin and armpit that can grow to the size of apples or eggs and that are called *gavoccioli*. These widely disseminated abnormalities give way to black blotches under the skin and to bruises on the arms and thighs. Florentine physicians, just like their Athenian and Byzantine predecessors, are unable to treat these alarming symptoms. Like their ancient colleagues, they quickly learn that, after the appearance of symptoms, patients survive about three days. At this point, Boccaccio reflects on the idea of contagiousness. Some think that casual contact, even conversation, communicates the infection. Those in close contact with the sick, such as family members and health-care workers, are especially susceptible; infection is possible, some believe, through clothing and objects.

The plague also affects the emotional health of the people. Fears and fantasies consume the terrified Florentines. Individuals behave in extreme ways. Some people shun the sick altogether. Others avoid them and live abstemiously. Florentine families disintegrate: brother abandons brother; the husband, his wife; and, unbelievably, parents leave their children (9). Indigent parents are left to depend on the charity of friends and neighbors. Some evacuate the city altogether, leaving their homes, relatives, and estates. In their headlong flight to the countryside, they mistakenly believe they can outrun the disease (8). Although Boccaccio enunciates the conventional opinion that the plague is the result of God's wrath towards the Florentines, it is unlikely that this is an expression of pre-conceptuality on his part. The weight of the social description suggests that the reference is formulaic, the author's genuine interest being the effects of disease on corporate and on domestic society.

Along with the fear and panic, there is a need to alter funeral rites, and in this we are reminded of Greek and of Byzantine predecessors. No longer do Florentine mourners and clergy gather at the home of the deceased to take part in elaborate processions to church. To expedite matters, a grave-digging fraternity organizes itself. The diggers who come from the lower ranks of society bring the deceased to the nearest church, often for per-functory rites, and bury the dead in the nearest available plot. These quick burials are usually reserved for those with money. Deceased commoners and the middle-class who can not afford expedient interment are left to decom-pose in their homes. Fear of contamination forces some neighbors to remove bodies from these domiciles and to leave them outside front doors for the disposal crews.

At the height of the plague, thousands of cadavers are regularly stacked in the street. Funeral biers are set up for some, but most are taken away on plain boards, two or three at a time, in a most undignified manner. Some-times family members are removed and buried together in this way. Boc-caccio remarks that the deceased are handled like dead goats (Thucydides compares corpses to so many dead sheep). It even becomes impractical to bury the dead in consecrated ground according to long-established tradi-tion because there is not enough land. As a result, mass-burial trenches are excavated and filled with hundreds of bodies. Even the trenches cannot accommodate the vast numbers of dead, so hundreds of cadavers are stacked like ship's cargo. In the city, "the cruelty of heaven" is having its most unpleasant effect. From March to July 1348, the pestilence claims more than 100,000 lives. Boccaccio acknowledges the exaggeration, but the numbers are undoubtedly high.

The rural poor have no way of escaping the plague as an ill-wind sup-posedly carrying the disease blows through Florence into the scattered ham-lets and countryside. Having neither physicians nor servants, the peasants collapse by the wayside, in the fields, and in the cottages. Like the city pop-ulation, the rural poor grow apathetic, disregard their affairs, and neglect their possessions. Some squander their assets, seeing no need for them with the future foreclosed.

Writings in the descriptive modality share certain common traits. Pro-copius and Boccaccio, like Thucydides, avoid teleological commentary. Instead, they are most concerned with concrete details such as disease symp-toms, the ideas of contagion and of immunity, the effect of the disaster on the health-care establishment, the problem of public and of private inter-ment, and the impact of pestilence on human behavior. Thucydides and Boccaccio refer to demographic shifts occurring because of plague, while the former, along with Procopius, considers the influence of the outbreaks on current wars. It is difficult to gauge the degree to which the Christian writers are indebted to the Greek historian. Conceivably, the startling effects of plague on society and on culture, described in each narrative, are to be expected under such conditions. Thucydides' enumeration of symptoms, of health-care efforts, of human misbehavior, and of factors such as war and famine no doubt form a paradigm for the epidemic narrative as it developed over two and one-half millennia from the descriptive to the etiological modality.

7. PERSONS OF THOUGHT
Nathaniel Hodges and the London Plague of 1664–1665

As we begin to discuss the genesis of investigative work and its discursive modalities, we must be mindful of three points: (1) systematic biomedical thought emerged from the observational tradition; (2) it gradually displaced (but did not eliminate) pre-conceptuality; and, (3) at its inception, it greatly depended on common sense, on intuition, and on popular wisdom.

A great variety of epidemiological writings appeared in the early seventeenth century. These works (chronicles, compendia, and treatises) are generically and methodologically diverse. Works containing statistics, clinical observations, anecdotal discoveries, and genuine methods for the management and prevention of diseases such as plague began to appear with regularity. In her chronological outline of the period, Mary Ellen Snodgrass mentions a number of overlooked contributors. John Graunt, for one, surveyed epidemics in the first half of the seventeenth century in his *Natural and Political Observations Made upon the Bills of Mortality* (1662) (73). In 1629, the Dutch naturalist Jacobus Bontius of Leiden published his professional experiences with cholera and beriberi while in the Dutch East Indies (1629) (78). The court physician Theodore Turquet de Mayerne wrote a twenty-volume set of case histories on plague and famine, unpublished at his death in 1655 (79). Father Antonio de Calancha of Peru observed, in 1633, that the cinchona bark (from which quinine would be made) relieved the symptoms of malaria (81). Paul Barbette, a surgeon and anatomist, published a *Treatise on Pestilence* (1678), which was a clinical account of the 1655 plague outbreak in Amsterdam (89). Important work on the efficacy of quarantine was done in Naples and in Rome during the 1656 plague. Cardinal Hieronymi Gastaldi wrote an influential compilation, *Treatise on Averting and Avoiding Plague* (1684), which contains mortality statistics and the positive results of quarantine and of sanitation

(89); during this period, these practices first emerged as essential means of comprehending the epidemic experience. Thomas Sydenham (1624–1689), a physician called "the English Hippocrates," practiced *nosology* (the systematic classification of diseases). He described diseases in an effort to define them "as distinct entities," and his work contributed greatly to the genesis of modern bacteriology and epidemiology (Stolley and Lasky 24). And William Petty (1623–1687), an anatomist, understood that hypotheses required supportive data (i.e., statistics such as records of mortality) describing the effects of disease on a community (25–7).

An unappreciated figure in the early development of epidemiological thought was the physician, Nathaniel Hodges, clinical practitioner during the London plague of 1664–1665. Hodges whose opinions exemplify the seventeenth-century perspective on infectious disease wrote an extraordinary pamphlet on his experiences, which belongs to the heritage of Thucydides. Just as Procopius valued observation over dogma, Hodges offered valuable insights into public health, and his thinking will be the focus of this chapter.

An eyewitness to the disaster, Hodges describes an epidemic that turned out to be the worst on record for that city since the fifteenth century (nearly a dozen outbreaks preceded it), and that was responsible for 75,000 to 100,000 deaths (20 percent of the population). Historians trace its origin to Holland, which had experienced intermittent occurrences of the disease up to 1664–1665 (Kohn 196–97). Believed to have been transmitted in bales of cotton and to have gained a foothold in the slums of St. Giles-in-the-Fields (a London outer parish), the pestilence spread from the west, to the south, and then to the east. After the Great Fire (September 2–5, 1666), it disappeared from London, although it subsequently emerged in France, where it eventually subsided. Hodges' pamphlet, *Loimologia: or, An Historical Account of the Plague in London in 1665: with precautionary Directions against the like Contagion*, a work to which Daniel DeFoe was greatly indebted in *The Journal of the Plague Year* (1722), is a pivotal text in the corpus of epidemiological writing and the focus of discussion here.

Living in a pre-conceptual world where medical science was rudimentary, Dr. Hodges intended to report impartially on his firsthand experiences (101). Adopting an ostensibly neutral vantage point, he is reminiscent of Thucydides and of Procopius who wrote about epidemics without explaining causes. In the course of his report, however, Hodges unexpectedly exchanged the self-appointed role of distanced observer for that of critical historian, who could not ignore the hysteria, misinformation, and crime that exacerbated the medical crisis. As a critic of society, he enunciated three very sound measures in support of public health: the revamping of quarantine procedures, the stamping out of dangerous remedies, and the controlling of criminal activity. Hodges implied that the medical establishment of London, along with the civil authorities, needed to formulate a coherent strategy against the plague, one having the twofold aim of managing the disease and of avoiding social chaos. *Loimologia* is important for combining descriptions of the calamity and ways of mitigating its effects.

The plague's geographical origin had long been suspected. Dutch merchants picked up contaminated cargo in Smyrna, a seaport in western Turkey on the Gulf of Izmir, brought it to Holland, and then to England. The idea of contaminated cargo (the nature of the contaminant being unknown to contemporaries) was not an original idea and is as old as St. Gregory's history. Hodges' thinking on the subject adumbrates certain aspects of Dr. Richard Mead's (1673–1754) *Discourse on the Plague* (1720). According to Mead, the disease is communicated not only through the air and infected persons, but also by "Goods transported from infected Places" (quoted by Winslow 183). In the early winter of 1664, after three people had died of the illness, and as rumor and hysteria swept the city (Nicholson 72), Hodges conjectures that the disease is spread specifically by inhaled droplets of something that, for want a better word, he calls "venom." On the basis of this assumption, he questions current quarantine practices. If the disease is indeed communicated this way, then it makes no sense to shut up entire families in poorly-ventilated quarters, virtually guaranteeing that everybody will get sick. Hodges' idea is to quarantine the town but to do so by sending infected people into the suburbs: in this way, the sick would be isolated in the country while those in contact with them would be sequestered under hospitable conditions. This simple solution would safeguard family members from infection, would identify carriers, and would give the sick the best chance of recovery. Unfortunately, this practice was not put into action. The reason for inaction is not clear. Because the medical establishment had not yet proven the mode of contagion conclusively, it was difficult to plan an effective public-health strategy. Every other strategy failed, and Hodges voices his frustration over the fact that even the aggressive efforts of the College of Physicians came to naught. The failure of conventional medicine opened the door to untested remedies and to quackerie, one especially nasty regimen having been imported from France. For this reason, Hodges is disdainful of illicit practitioners. Because the public was not informed about the disease, rumors and misinformation had a breeding ground. The doctors themselves had no concrete understanding of the plague cycle, Hodges' insights notwithstanding.

To the public's credit is the fact that they were cognizant of the long history of plague in London (eight outbreaks: 1499–1500, 1563, 1578, 1593,

1603, 1625, 1636, and 1664–65) and, on the basis of this record, tried to predict the plague's recrudescence. According to Hodges, the popular belief is that it appears at twenty-year intervals, as if through some intrinsic necessity. Without rejecting this idea outright, he cautions that "persons of more judgment" are skeptical of its predictability. The persons of judgment are right to be skeptical. Although the plague is brought to London via maritime traffic from infected European ports, from 1563 on it sprung up in London at irregular yearly intervals (15, 16, 10, 22, and 11 years, respectively), on average every thirteen years, which meant the latest visitation was overdue by about sixteen years.

Hodges is fully aware that the reappearance of plague is profoundly affecting the minds of the London populace (102). It is not clear as to whether he means that fear breeds confusion, although he is certain that misinformation and false claims stir up the public. One dubious source of information is astrology, the practitioners of which base their predictions on the conjunction of stars and on the appearance of comets. Though "persons of thought" pay no attention to astrological signs as predictors of disease, the uneducated masses believe these claims and can not be persuaded that during the conjunction of certain planets both good and bad things occur. Hodges sensibly concludes that, "The mischief was much more in the predictions of the star-gazers than in the stars themselves" (102–03).

The magistracy to whom public care is entrusted decides to act after watching the morbidity rate increase on a daily basis and the infection spread to nearby parishes. They belatedly close infected houses so that no one would accidentally come in contact with sick people at their homes or in the street (just as Hodges suggests). The strategy of containment had become policy. Encouraged by this, Dr. Hodges continues to criticize whatever makes the situation worse. The quarantine sign posted on homes, for example, is quite alarming and recalls the plagues of Exodus: a red cross is painted on the door of an infected house, and the ominous statement LORD HAVE MERCY UPON US is inscribed on the door. Actually, the biblical analogue is ironic. In *Exodus*, Moses warns that all the firstborn of Egypt, whether man or animal, would be slain unless the Jews are freed (verse 11:5). An essential part of the Passover instruction is that blood markings (from the sacrificial lamb) are to be placed on Jewish residences to distinguish their homes from those of the Egyptians and to deflect God's wrath away from the former: "For the Lord will pass through to smite the Egyptians; and when he seeth the blood upon the lintel, and on the two side posts, the Lord will pass over the door, and will not suffer the destroyer to come in unto your houses to smite you" (12:23). Significantly, God's destroyer is a *"plague"* of some kind (12:13; italics added). In Egypt, ironically, warnings protected Jewish residents in their homes from an intrusive disease; but, in London, biblical signage is employed to protect visitors from plague-stricken residents *inside* of homes.

To make matters worse for Londoners, guards are posted to prevent ingress or egress, to provide food and necessities for the sequestered families, and to open the house up forty days after recovery. Yet the plan has no effect on the plague. The disease continues to spread, and healthy people are forced to remain in close quarters while the sick suffer greatly (104). If someone enters the house on the 39th day after recovery, the waiting period recommences for a 40-day cycle before the person is released. Once again, the author refers to the susceptibility of those caught in this useless bind: "the dismal apprehension [i.e., the quarantine] laid them under, [and] made them but an easier prey to the devouring enemy."

Hodges detests those who exploit these stressful conditions. So-called nurses who are supposed to care for the sick sometimes strangle them, making it look as if the illness was responsible (104). Other nurses actually infect the healthy with purulent material taken from plague lesions and then burglarize the homes. This is an ironic perversion of variolation, at the time an unregulated procedure rooted in folk medicine. Because homicidal nurses infer that plague exudates can be injected into healthy people to induce disease, they are aware that secretions, rather than the atmosphere, can communicate the malady. Hodges does not see the medical acumen in their crimes. He trusts in divine justice to right the scales and sees evidence of this when nurses, engaged in "wicked barbarities," are stricken with plague themselves (104). This observation is the extent of Hodges' pre-conceptuality.

Quarantined houses and their pre-conceptual adornments frighten neighbors away or dissuade them from helping those who are stricken. Because of the foreboding signs and the writing on the doors, even domestic helpers flee, hastening the deaths of those within. Ironically, plague contagion seems to diminish once the doors are opened and the houses aired out (just as Hodges suspected) (105). Although civic and public cooperation has not been realized, and although Hodges criticizes the city's response to the pestilence, he remains cognizant, and supportive, of the government's desire for order.

In future, better procedures need to be formulated. Proper accommodations outside of the city, Hodges points out, should be set up for forced seclusion of those not yet infected. If they continue to live healthily at that locale, everyone would benefit: the uninfected would be spared forced exposure, and the community would have an effective way of distinguishing between sick people and asymptomatic carriers (106). Rather than to be abandoned, the plague-stricken should be sequestered in "convenient apartments." This plan would relieve the fears of neighbors who would otherwise have fled to the countryside. Hodges' humane plan contrasts with contemporary instances of quarantine. One example of the kind of warehousing common in the seventeenth century was going on in the city of Genoa where, in 1650, a pesthouse and quarantine system had been established that was policed by German mercenaries. According to Mary Ellen Snodgrass, the building housed fifty-five diagnosed patients and two hundred thirty-eight who may have been exposed to the disease (88).

Even though the majority of the populace flees London, the plague does not abate. Hodges personifies it, at this juncture, as a "cruel enemy" returning with redoubled fury to kill its victims (106–07). In one week, eighty people die, forcing the magistracy to take emergency action. The first activity, a pre-conceptual one, is to require a monthly fast for public prayers, "to deprecate the anger of heaven" (*deprecate* meaning to implore, not to depreciate, God's power) (107). Hodges suggests that the supplications may have been effective, for moderate breezes in the summer of 1665 arise presumably to "carry off the pestilential steams" (apparently, he subscribes to the atmospheric theory of disease) (107).

The King orders the College of Physicians to write a general directory, and a number of the faculty is required to tend to the sick. But even their expertise proves fruitless as the disease overwhelms them, killing eight or nine. In August and September, the plague worsens considerably, killing between three and five thousand each week. In a scene reminiscent of Thucydides' Athens, Hodges relates that the dead decompose in their beds, and that the ravings of delirium and pain can be heard in the street (108–09). Some of the infected, driven mad by the disease, expire in the street, while others die suddenly in the marketplace.

In September, the disease kills twelve thousand, an incredible number. Desperately believing the very air infected with plague, residents create large bonfires. Though Hodges has his doubts about the effectiveness of this remedy (citing Hippocrates as an authority), the fires are kindled nonetheless. Either the suffocating fumes or the heavy humidity (he believes) contribute to an unprecedented number of deaths that night (four thousand are said to have died). Unscrupulous chemists and quacks, once again, fill the void that the physicians leave. Their medicines are more lethal than the plague itself, but many of the opportunists contract the disease as well (111). The French claim they possess an effective medicine, which they share with the British. Hodges relates how he was cautioned in its use and for good reason. The French remedy proves toxic (112). The art of medicine and the public health certainly suffer from these concoctions and at the hands of charlatans who profit from them. Hodges criticizes colleagues who flee the city, for their absence leaves the people with little recourse than to solicit peddler medicine and to consult well-intended but ignorant folk healers. Obviously, it is better not to have physicians at all than to be under the care of the unlearned whose efforts interfere with one's natural ability to fight off disease (113).

Hodges' history demonstrates that the biomedical knowledge of his times was insufficient and that the readiness of authorities to respond to a disease emergency was wholly ineffective. Without understanding the etiology of the disease, the medical establishment enacted no effective countermeasures, even though dedicated medical people did what they could to arrest the epidemic. Hodges found it difficult to suppress his frustration as the disease spread relentlessly through the community. From that standpoint, he is very much like Thucydides. The best course of action, for Hodges, was to record information for posterity so that the insights and the aberrations of 1665 would not be forgotten. For this reason, whenever Hodges perceived gross errors of civic judgment, as in the quarantine regulations, as in the impotency of his colleagues (many of whom died trying to stave off the epidemic), as in the intrusion of charlatans, murderers, and thieves, and as in the detrimental effects of superstition, he spoke out sensibly. His critique underscores what could have been done to weather the epidemiological challenge: even if the agent of disease is unknown, theories have to be explored and information gathered from every source. *Loimologia* is precisely that kind of resource.

London in 1665 was not completely in the dark about the disease. Since plague was transported via shipping, maritime traffic from plague locales could be interdicted or at least inspected; if the plague made its way into the country (in the reputed form of pathogenic atmosphere), other things could have been done: like Pistoia three centuries before, London could have destroyed stray animals as a sanitary measure; consequently, general sanitation would also have eliminated a food source from plague-carrying rodents; and, where infection appeared, rural housing rather than urban quarantine would have lessened the risk of aerosolized dissemination. A centralized authority, even though limited in resources and in knowledge, could have quelled rumors, diminished hysteria, and counteracted quackery and the spread of illicit medicine. Strict licensing of medical practitioners would have helped to identify homicidal nurses; and the presence of an effective police force and coroner would have kept public order and would have expedited interments. These measures, expressed or implied in Dr. Hodges' tract, form a coherent public-health strategy that seventeenth-century London had within its grasp. *Loimologia* is an index of an emergent form of biomedical writing: Hodges virtually eliminated pre-conceptuality in favor of descriptive material and critical views on the management of extensive disease.

8. THE TOPOGRAPHY OF INFERENCE

In the history of human efforts to understand epidemic disease, *inference* has been a fundamental intellectual response and the linchpin of experimentation. To appreciate why this is true, we have to begin by understanding what the term means and how it differs from *hypothesis*. *To infer* is to derive "from assumed premises either the strict logical conclusion or one that is *to some degree probable*" (*Random House* 682; italics added). Understanding inference to mean an assumption about the origin and cause of an outbreak, I will demonstrate how it operates in the history of three epidemic diseases, bringing discoveries to light, and establishing medical praxis.

At the outset, we need to make a distinction between *inference* and *hypothesis*. A hypothesis, precisely defined (from the Greek, *hypotithenai*: "to put under, suppose"), is a *kind* of inference, that is, "an assumption made ... in order to test its logical or empirical consequences" (*Merriam-Webster* 363). As a way of describing intuitive thinking about epidemic disease, one can see that inference is a cognitive activity, whereas hypothesis is a statement of intent and of purpose, one designed to prove, to modify, or to disprove a guiding supposition experimentally. With this distinction in mind, one can see that biblical and Greco-Roman writers did not hypothesize about the origin and cause of pestilence; instead, they inferred ideas about epidemic disease from a fund of observation, of popular knowledge, and of personal experience.

In antiquity, inferences about the cause of epidemic disease sprang from a heritage of folk medicine and of custom that had conditioned the way in which the malady was perceived. Smallpox immunization is a case in point: scholars have traced its origin as far back as A.D. 1000 in China to acute observations about susceptibility from which crude immunization practices were devised (I. and J. Glynn 48). Yu T'ien-Chih, in *Miscellaneous Ideas in Medicine* (1643), referred to the Chinese practice, begun in 1567, of inhaling ground smallpox scabs or matter through an ivory or silver tube (Snodgrass 65). To this ancient tradition, Edward Jenner owed much. Childbed fever, the second disease I will focus on, has afflicted humankind since time immemorial, but my immediate interest here is how inferences about disease causation, informed by circumstantial evidence, led to experimental proof and then to therapy and prevention. The journey of discovery can be a contentious one, as the life of Ignaz Semmelweis illustrates. The absence of microbiological proof did not hinder John Snow in his efforts to stop a cholera outbreak. Mortality statistics, demographic information, residential interviews, the opinions of colleagues, an understanding of public-works infrastructure, and the ocular assessments of water samples provided Snow with enough information to urge a practical remedy: the incapacitation of the Broad Street water pump, the focal source of contaminated water. At each juncture in his investigation, he relied on inference.

Jenner et al.: Smallpox

Pre-conceptual cultures devised ingenious ways of dealing with smallpox. The Japanese, for example, invoked the twelfth-century hero, Tametomo, to aid in the recovery of a smallpox victim; because he was believed to have slain the smallpox demon, his image was thought to have curative properties (Tucker 13). The west African Yoruba tribes had a different strategy: instead of invoking an intercessor against the demon, they worshiped a smallpox deity called Sopona, presumably to protect themselves against epidemics (13). The practice of deifying the disease can be found in many cultures: the Brazilian god Omolou was endowed with power over the disease. All the major religions of China recognized and revered the smallpox goddess, T'ou-Shen Niang-Niang. In northern India, Hindus built shrines and temples in honor of the smallpox deity, Shitala Mata (13).

The efforts of primitive people to expel smallpox from villages greatly impressed Sir James George Frazer (1854–1941), Scottish classicist and anthropologist. Practices such as these were religious in nature and involved displacing the disease, imagined to be an invisible, evil entity. An African tribe called the Ewe, for example, tried to expel smallpox using clay effigies of the villagers that were placed on low mounds and accompanied by food and water. The hope was that the smallpox spirit would take the food and clay figures in lieu of infecting people; the rationale was to lure the spirit out of town and then to barricade the town against its return (571–72). The natives of Formosa ritualistically drove the smallpox demon into a sow, cut off the animal's ears, burning them or the carcass in the belief that, in so doing, they could destroy the disease (626). When pox appeared, the Kumis of southeastern India sealed off their village, killed a monkey, hung its carcass at the village gate, mixed its blood with river pebbles, sprinkled the mixture on houses, and swept the threshold of every house with the monkey's tail, all the while adjuring the fiend to leave (636–37). The Patagonians, unlike the besieged Kumis, abandoned their villages to the smallpox demon. In their retreat, they left the sick behind, slashed the air with weapons, and doused themselves with water in the frantic hope of distancing themselves from the disorder (637–38). Like the Formosans, the villagers in Munzerabad, a district of Mysore, in southern India, tried to conjure up the smallpox demon and drive it into a wooden image. They proceeded from village to village with the idol, believing that, along the way, they absorbed smallpox entities into it. When all were captured, the people threw the idol in the river (652).

In the primitive mind, two strategies against smallpox predominated. One was to embody the virus as an evil entity and a second was to invoke a counterentity or personage believed to have legendary powers to drive the spirit of disease away. In Frazer's examples, the religious authorities of each village separated the people from the disease-entity, either by abandoning the contaminated locale, or by trapping the spirit in an effigy, or by eliminating the disease through animal sacrifice.

The Puritans who settled in New England in the seventeenth century thought of themselves as an elected people, and they, too, entertained a pre-conceptual view of epidemic disease. Using *Psalm* 2:8 as a mandate ("Ask of me, and I shall give thee the heathen for thine inheritance, and the uttermost parts of the earth for thy possession" [*KJV*]), they conceived of themselves as being divinely-ordained to inherit the land they invaded and to dispossess the native people whom they encountered. The 1617 outbreak that ravaged the Algonquian natives in Massachusetts prompted John Winthrop (1588–1649), physician and governor of the Massachusetts Bay Colony, to write in his journal that smallpox was God's way of reducing the Native American population (ninety percent of whom died as a result) so that, in 1620, Puritans could resettle Indian land (Snodgrass 76). And Cotton Mather (1663–1728) sermonized that the deprivations Native Americans suffered because of smallpox proved they had been cursed by God (Snodgrass 82).

The inhumane aspect of pre-conceptuality did not characterize all the New England narratives on smallpox. William Bradford's (1590–1657) description of a smallpox event in *Of Plymouth Plantation*, to which we now turn our attention, does not fit the formula entirely; rather, it is a very humane and moving text, made so primarily by the author's strict adherence to the facts as smallpox decimated the Pequot Indians. There is no biblical justification here, only a revolting depiction of what a virulent strain of smallpox can do to non-immune people.

The smallpox epidemic striking the Pequot Indians of the Connecticut River in the spring of 1634 recurred over a seven-year period, afflicting Native American tribes along the St. Lawrence River and Great Lakes into Canada. At that time, the British had constructed a trading settlement just north of a rival Dutch outpost in what would later become Newtown (today's Fairfield County, southwestern Connecticut) (Kohn 66–7). There, infected Dutch traders, immune to smallpox from earlier exposures, communicated the disease to the Native Americans. The most famous firsthand account of the *Pequot incident* (as I choose to call it) is that of Governor Bradford, who had come to New England in *The Mayflower* in 1620, who remained governor of Plymouth Colony for most of his life, and who maintained amicable relations with indigenous people. The description belongs to the heritage of Thucydides. A firsthand narrative, it stresses the physiological and social effects of an epidemic on its victims.

In *Of Plymouth Plantation,* we read that the Pequots living in the vicinity of the English trading houses suddenly fell sick of smallpox, and that some 900 out of 1000 died most miserably. Bradford describes a nightmare vision: hundreds of Pequots are prostrated with what might have been flat, hemorrhagic pox, the most virulent form of the disease (176–77; see Preston 25–48). Since they lacked proper bedding and linen, the victims lay on hard mats which contributed greatly to their sufferings. The viral strain they had contracted from European traders caused diffuse pustules which clustered together in sheets, came to a head, and ruptured, to exude virulent sera all over the body. Destroyed in the immune system's response to the virus, the skin pealed off, and the resulting exudates adhered to the fiber mats. Thus, writes Bradford, "a whole side will [flee off] at once." With the skin pealed from their bodies in swathes and shreds, the victims were left covered with "gore blood." The spectacle of hundreds of human beings undergoing this dreadful process was, for Bradford, too "fearful to behold." The loss of skin and blood making them susceptible to other infections, they died "like rotten sheep."

The outbreak stripped the Indian settlement of the most basic necessities. Since so many were incapacitated, they could no longer care for themselves. Consequently, they neither started fires, nor procured drinking water, nor buried the dead. Since it was no longer possible to gather firewood, for fuel the ambulatory victims burned their trays, dishes, and bows and arrows. In short order, the Pequot settlement deteriorated to the point that the people ate uncooked food with their hands. In just a few days, a previously thriving hunting and gathering society, one that had been developing a trading economy, had been reduced to prehistoric inertia, having lost the ability to hunt for food and to prepare cooked meals, activities essential to their cultural life. Those with enough strength crawled to get water from a lake; some died on the way; and others, on the way back to the villages.

The rapidity with which the disease decimated the Pequots evoked the settlers' compassion. Every day, they brought firewood, water, and food to the Indians, along with whatever else was needed for their survival and dignity; they even buried the Pequot dead. No doubt the Puritans' assistance must have saved some lives, although only ten percent survived. The Pequot chief Sachem, along with his entire family, did not. According to Bradford's narrative, these particular Puritans did not quote Scripture; they lived it and tried to help their suffering neighbors.

The early settlers of the northeastern United States did not understand the mechanism of immunity that protected them from smallpox. This idea would prove to be one of the most significant inferences in the history of medicine. Drawing a conclusion from known or from *assumed* facts or statements is to infer (*OED* VIII: 257; "inference"), and this was precisely what had happened during the early history of mankind's experience with smallpox. Custom and popular knowledge became the groundwork of the therapeutic praxis of immunization.

The idea of stimulating one's internal defenses against smallpox by actually taking the material of the disease internally, in the forms of pus, exudate, or sloughed off scabs, would have struck the Ewe, Yoruba, or Kumis, along with any number of God-fearing Europeans and Americans, as insane. But an inferential tradition advocating this very practice antedated, by millennia, primitive tribal and Puritan thinking. Jonathan B. Tucker explains that, although quarantine was the primary means of controlling the disease up until the 1700s (14–15), deliberately inducing an attenuated infection gradually became another means to that end. The practice of stimulating immunity against smallpox through the inoculation of virulent excretions into a person dates as far back as the first millennium B.C. in China where smallpox scabs were ground into powder and snorted (Beveridge 38). According to Tucker, "It had been observed in India and China [i.e., from 1000 B.C. to A.D. 1000] that pockmarked survivors *never again contracted the disease*" (15; italics added). The transition from observation to inoculation, undoubtedly, was one the most momentous leaps of faith in medical history.

Before discussing this history in broad outline, I will define two key terms. The first is *variolation*. Entering the English lexicon in 1805, it refers to the practice of taking pus or scabs from patients with a mild form of smallpox, and of inoculating uninfected patients with small quantities of this material (*OED* XIX: 52; "varolation"; Tucker 15; I. and J. Glynn, 4–5). As I mentioned above, Tucker traces the practice back to 1000 B.C. or before but, contrary to Beveridge, says that it had originated in India, not in China, and that the praxis spread from the subcontinent to Tibet where, c. A.D. 1000, Chinese Buddhist monks in Sichuan province employed it (Tucker 15). Another historian points out that variolation gained a foothold in northern Turkey as early as 131–136 B.C., as an outgrowth of the practices of Mithridatus VI, King of Pontus (northern Turkey) who said he could immunize against a poison by absorbing small quantities of it (Messadié 209). The British Royal Society, in 1700, was the first organized body to report about the Chinese practice (I. and J. Glynn 52). By the eighteenth century, the Turks were extracting serum from skin lesions of mild cases and then injecting this material into healthy people, a practice reported to have conferred immunity (52). Ian and Jenifer Glynn succinctly trace the migration of the variolation procedure from Turkey, to Europe, and finally to America (52). The Greco-Italian physician, Timoni, communicated his experiences with variolation to the Royal Society in 1713, and the Greek physician Pylarini, in 1716, wrote a similar account. Timoni's paper came to the attention of Cotton Mather who had earlier discoursed on smallpox as a divine instrument against the heathens. Timoni's paper which Mather came across in Boston reminded the clergyman of something his slave Onesimus had said about being inoculated against smallpox while in Tripoli (52). Mather wrote down Onesimus' story and sent it to the Royal Society, with a call for the institution of variolation in times of epidemic (52).

Variolation had its dangers. In fact, the use of live smallpox virus was quite risky, for the dosage could be too strong and induce the disease, overpowering the immune system and defeating the purpose. It could spoil or harbor other virulent organisms. European physicians systematized the practice in Turkey, but these dangers lurked in the background and, as Edward Jenner observed more than a century later, manifested themselves occasionally. Yet the praxis endured because the effects of the disease outweighed the risks.

Whether the seemingly unnatural practice of variolation originated in China, India, or ancient Pontus is not as important as understanding the tentative conclusion, drawn from assumed fact, that the physical stuff of infection protected against, or stimulated resistance to, a subsequent bout with the disease. For our purposes, it is important to remember that casual observations about recurrent disease led to the inference that inoculated exudate had protective properties. Voltaire remarked, in 1733, that once one had the pox (even if the first instance was severe), one had a mild case the second time. It seemed logical to him that if a mild first case were induced, then perhaps a naturally-acquired infection would be mild. The logic was impeccable and had its roots in a past millennium.

The eighteenth-century praxis of smallpox immunization brings us to a second key term. Whereas in *variolation* live smallpox virus is used to stimulate the immune system against the naturally-occurring disease, in *vaccination* (a word entering the French lexicon in 1800; and the English, in 1803) immunity to smallpox is achieved through the inoculation of cowpox (a related disease) into healthy patients (*OED* XIX: 5; "vaccination") Cowpox is usually not fatal to humans, but it can be contracted and, at that time, was an occupational hazard for dairy farmers. Some suspected on the basis of anecdotal evidence that immunity against smallpox, the far greater hazard, could be attained in a safer way with the use of cowpox, hence, the term *vaccination* (from the Latin *vacca*, for cow).

A second representative text, which is quite interesting, was written by an eighteenth-century physician, the Englishman Thomas Dimsdale (1712–1800) (I. and J. Glynn 78–81). While treating Catherine II of Russia (1729–1796) in October 1768, Dimsdale wrote a detailed account of the procedure. He knew from common practice that the pox material (i.e., scabs, exudates) caused the disease, smallpox; that its inoculation into a healthy patient was likely to confer immunity to the disease; and that the patient became immune after enduring a period of discomfort. Though the entire procedure was undertaken in a controlled environment, Dimsdale, of course, had no inkling as to how the disease spread, as to how it affected the body, or as to its intrinsic properties. But observation, anecdotal evidence, and popular tradition suggested that, despite its risks, *engrafting* (as the procedure was known at that time) protected the patient from the disease. Thomas Nettleton is officially credited with the first use of the term in a medical context: in his 1722 paper, "Inoculation," he writes that, "This Distemper is raised by an *Ingraftment* from the Small Pox"); Lady Mary Wortley Montagu, in the letter discussed below, used the term informally in 1717 (*OED* IV: 818–82; "engrafting"; italics added).

The Empress' inoculation record tells us much about the history of epidemic discourse. It exemplifies the use of the Hippocratic modality featured in *Epidemics* I and III, with three important distinctions: that Dimsdale knew that the material at his disposal was smallpox exudate, that it caused a mild form of the disease, and that it could be used to immunize the patient. Unlike Hippocrates who, as far as can be ascertained from the extant texts, did not diagnose his patients' maladies during the epidemic in Thasos, the Empress' physician deftly used the pathogen itself as prophylaxis.

The record below illustrates how systematic and predictable the variolation treatment had become. Minor symptoms, intensifying from days one to eight, usually peaked on the ninth day, the patient becoming progressively more comfortable for the duration of the treatment period. From

October 21 to November 1, the variolation experience gradually resolved itself, as the (no doubt) anxious Dimsdale looked on:

> *Tuesday, Oct. 21:* numbness under one arm; pain in back and feet; evening: all complaints moderated. More pustules appeared around the incision, and the circumference of the wound itself looked [redder] than before. One pustule was also discovered in the face and arms, and the fever was entirely gone.
>
> *Wednesday, Oct. 22:* More pustules appeared, and advanced according to my wishes.
>
> *Thursday, Oct. 23:* sore throat.
>
> *Friday, Oct. 24:* The pustules continued to maturate in the most favorable manner.
>
> *Saturday, Oct. 25:* throat pain abated; towards evening some of the pustules, which at first appeared, began to change their color to a darker hue.
>
> *Sunday, Oct. 26:* In the evening most of the pustules in the face put on a brownish color.
>
> *Monday, Oct. 27:* all the pustules were now become brown.
>
> *Wednesday, November 1:* returned to St. Petersburg in perfect health.
>
> [Dimsdale, "An Account"]

The Empress's reactions mirror on a small scale the progress of a naturally-acquired smallpox infection: the incision sites became inflamed and reddened over a six-day period, paralleling the widespread rash that the natural infection caused. Whereas in the full-scale infection, virus-filled pimples united into sheets of infected skin, the inoculation brought on diffusive lesions at the injection site, with only a few on the face and arms; the natural contagion, in contrast, covered the body, even to emerge internally on the mucous membranes and in the mouth. Pimples containing an opaque serum filled with white blood cells, dried up, turned brown, and sloughed off. This process also occurred in naturally-acquired infection but spread all over the surface of the body.

Lady Mary Wortley Montagu (1689–1762), an international socialite, writer of travelogues, and smallpox survivor herself, recorded her experiences in Constantinople in 1717, at the court of the Ottoman Empire while with her husband, the British ambassador. Her letter to Sarah Chiswell is the third document in our survey. In Adrianople (northwest Turkey), she narrated the amazing variolation practices of that culture.

Lady Montagu who lost her brother to the disease and was disfigured by it herself (I. and J. Glyn 53) writes ingenuously in the letter that smallpox, so dreaded in Europe, is in the Ottoman Empire "entirely harmless," being made so by virtue of "engrafting" (their term for inoculation). A group of old women, every September, visit those inclined to undergo the treatment. When the women arrive, the people have an engrafting session. With fifteen or sixteen recipients gathered together, one woman displays "a nutshell full of the matter of the best sort of small-pox," the shell containing serum removed from ripe blisters. The old woman, likely immune to the disease herself, and clothed not in a HAZMAT (i.e., Hazardous Material) suit but in simple peasant attire, courteously asks the patient to pick a vein which she promptly opens with a large needle and inserts into it "as much matter as can lie upon the head of her needle"; afterwards, she binds the wound "with a hollow bit of shell" and repeats the process four or five times. Called the Circassian method of inoculation, the procedure was named after the region in southeastern Russia where it was commonly practiced.

Turkish children play together on the day of inoculation and are unaffected by it up until the eighth day when fever forces them into bed for two days. While in bed, they develop about twenty to thirty lesions on their faces, but the lesions never leave scars, and the entire treatment is over in eight days with no after-effects. Every year, thousands submit to the procedure, the writer's tone suggesting that variolation is a kind of therapeutic diversion. Montagu affirms that no one had ever died of it, though this may have been ingenuous on her part. Nevertheless, vouching for its safety, she proposes to introduce the practice to England.

True to her word, Montagu introduced the Circassian method to Britain in 1718, in the process acquiring the help of renowned physicians. Upon returning to England, she had her four-year-old daughter variolated (Snodgrass 104; see also, I. and J. Glynn 43–6). Many people were successfully engrafted, but for various reasons, some died (Kohn 203). Even though engrafting carried risks, proponents believed its benefits outweighed them in times of epidemic, and this opinion had special relevance for children who were more susceptible to the disease than adults.

The introduction of variolation into England, astonishingly, was based on inferences drawn from popular practice and folklore, and not on scientific experimentation. The Princess of Wales (1683–1737) (later Queen Caroline of Ansbach), upon learning of the procedure, cautiously underwent inoculation (I. and J. Glynn 53–4). Voltaire (1694–1778), who survived smallpox pox in 1723, mentions in Letter XI.: "On Inoculation" (*Letters concerning the English nation* [1733]), that she offered four condemned criminals a chance not only to save their lives but to acquire immunity to smallpox (527–28). Each was engrafted, got through without complications, and received amnesty. Assured of the usefulness and of the relative safety of the operation, she allowed her own children to be inocu-lated, and thousands followed her example. Voltaire mentions how far-reaching the practice became. An unnamed Jesuit missionary, after reading Letter XI, inoculated Indian children at baptism, helping them in this life and the next (529). The bishop of Worcester preached the virtues of engraft-ing in London. And the College of Physicians publicly endorsed the oper-ation in 1755 after the epidemic of 1751 (Kohn 203).

Voltaire's commentary on variolation in Letter XI (1733), the fourth document in the series, offers an interesting contrast to Montagu's letter. Unlike writers who were content to describe the effects of disease or a ther-apy, Voltaire tried to explain to his readers how the immunization process worked. Unfortunately, in this regard, he relied on analogy, simply because science had no explanation. For him, the effect of smallpox exudate on the system is analogous to what "leaven does in a piece of dough"; that is, it "ferments in it, and communicates to the mass of blood the qualities with which it is impregnated" (524–25). Generally, Voltaire is correct: the exu-date gradually modifies the body (if we can call the immune response a modification), but that is as far as the analogy goes. The poorest Turks embraced inoculation to prevent the disfigurement of their daughters (525). The inoculation sessions in Montagu's letter, read in Voltairean terms, might therefore have had an ulterior motive, especially with respect to female chil-dren. The concern might not have been to protect their health but to keep them physically attractive. It seems that their fathers sold them at a young age into the service of the seraglios of sultans and Persian sufis. A daugh-ter with smallpox scars was not marketable.

More important, from the standpoint of epidemiological thought, was what Voltaire had to say about how observation could be the grounds of inference and the origin of therapy. In Europe, according to Voltaire, it was the Circassians who figured out that whoever survived the disease did not contract it twice in a severe form and that a second bout left no scars; thus, a mild encounter, presumably, had protective effects. These "natural obser-vations" even suggest that, "by insinuating into the child's body a pustule taken from the body of one infected with smallpox ... the experiment could not fail" (526). And he notes that, among the Chinese, the practice of snort-ing dried pox powder had been customary since A.D. 1500 (529).

Montagu's epistolary description of engrafting is a variant of Dimsdale's account: both documents record the clinical practice of variolation. The obvious differences between the two are discursive and clinical. Dr. Dims-dale composed an official, archival document. Clearly, the inoculation of Empress Catharine represented the state-of-the art in the practice of immu-nization; dietary and physiological details are chronologically noted, as one would expect for the medical record of a dignitary. The Montagu letter, though informal and personal, highlights the facts of the procedure as the author observed them. Lady Montagu marvels at how mundane the engrafting practice had become among the peasantry, the perils of a smallpox outbreak far outweighing the discomfort and risks of inoculation. And, as Voltaire observes, simple observations engendered the concept of immunity.

A practicing country physician, Edward Jenner (1749–1823) was not as enthusiastic as the Empress' physician or as Lady Montagu about the relative safety of variolation (Tucker 23–7; I. and J. Glynn 95–129). It was accepted practice at the time of his birth. While serving his medical apprenticeship, he learned of "the local belief in Gloucestershire" that contracting cowpox brought immunity to smallpox (Beveridge 38). Once again, simple observation revealed a fantastic possibility. Jenner discovered that local physicians were indeed aware of this folk belief but had discounted it, even though they were unable to explain why cowpox patients did *not* react to variolation (38; italics added). Could it be that the initial illness had desensitized them to the smallpox inoculum? And if that were true, then not only was this further proof that immunization worked, but also that there was a natural kinship between the two forms of pox.

Jenner eventually took the perilous step of using cowpox rather than the more dangerous smallpox for human immunization. Vaccination, therefore, appeared to be a safer alternative, but it needed to be tested. Jenner recorded his findings in his famous essay, *An Inquiry into the Causes and Effects of the Variolae Vaccinae, a disease discovered in some of the western counties, particularly Gloucestershire, and known by the name of The Cow Pox* (1798). In this classic etiological piece, he discusses the origins, causes, and effects of cowpox. He begins with the erroneous (but inconsequential) assumption that an equine hoof infection causes cowpox: according to the theory, those tending to horses manually spread the infection to cows; the ulcerated udders of the cows, in turn, give the disease to dairy workers (13–14). Via this route, an entire farm could be infected with cowpox. It was later determined that the equine disease was coincidental to cowpox, and that the bovine pox was communicated to man, occupationally, through broken skin or mucous membranes. The exclusion of the horse from the cycle had no impact on Jenner's trials or on his acute observations of how cowpox affected both man and beast: the latter strain was rarely fatal, though it could disfigure with sores and spread into the bloodstream.

Jenner sought to confirm two popular beliefs: contracting cowpox forever protects one "from the infection of the Small Pox"; and exposure to naturally occurring smallpox or to traditional inoculation with variola did not produce cowpox. Three of Jenner's twenty-two recorded cases, in particular, suggest that, like Dr. Dimsdale, he approached the inoculation procedure with a measure of confidence. In a way, he proceeded with the acuity of Hippocrates.

Joseph Merret, the first patient treated, was a farm servant who, in 1770, was thought to have acquired the equine infection and to have then passed it on to the cows that he milked (15–16). As a result, the lymph nodes in his armpits swelled and stiffened; consequently, he became indisposed, but he soon recovered. In April 1795, when a variolation program was undertaken in the Gloucestershire area, Merret and his family received live smallpox inoculations. Repeated inoculations, however, did not elicit a reaction from him, beyond localized inflammation and scabbing. Apparently, his bout with the bovine disease had conferred immunity on him. Confirmation of this came when his entire family acquired smallpox some time later; he alone remained uninfected. Merret's resistance to the bovine and human infections, Jenner strongly contended, derived from his exposure to cowpox twenty-five years earlier.

Case 17 was the most controversial in the group as Jenner began to inoculate pediatric patients (24–26). To observe accurately "the progress of infection," he selected a healthy eight-year-old boy, James Phipps, whom he inoculated with cowpox (*1801*: 5–6). The unsanitary process by which the vaccine was culled startles the modern mind. Jenner extracted it from a *sore* on the hand of a dairymaid, who presumably had picked up the disease from cow udders. Phipps received the material, on May 14, 1796, through two superficial arm incisions. Seven days after the inoculation, he complained of discomfort in the armpit nodes and on the ninth day got the chills, lost his appetite, and had a headache. After an uncomfortable night, he awoke on the tenth day relieved.

The most disturbing phase of the experiment was when Jenner attempted to ascertain if the child was immune to smallpox. Jenner decided to inoculate him with *live* smallpox exudates on July 1, in effect, subjecting Phipps to variolation. The boy received several slight punctures and incisions on both arms (today's patient receives fifteen needle punctures), and the matter was inserted. No infection developed. Jenner then had to make sure that the patient had achieved immunity, so several months later he *repeated* the experiment, "but with no sensible effect ... on the constitution."

These successes inspired Jenner to attain further proof of vaccination's efficacy. Thus, he took serum from Phipp's lesions and inoculated it into *another* person with no appreciable results, a process undertaken successively five times. The process raised the distinct possibility that immunity could be passed on from one human being to another without attenuating the vaccine. J. Barge was the fifth to receive the infection successively from William Summers who had originally contracted cowpox (29).

Critics of vaccination made their opposition known. Dr. William Woodville (1752–1805), conductor of large-scale vaccinations, published his findings under the title, *Reports of a series of inoculations for the variolae vaccinae, or cow-pox; with remarks and observations on this disease, considered as a substitute for the small-pox* (1799) (I. and J. Glynn 107–09). Woodville, the Director of London Smallpox and Inoculation Hospital, was startled to find that many of those receiving cowpox inoculations developed smallpox-like lesions all over their bodies, rather than only at the injection sites (as was typical of vaccinia). It was later determined that the vaccine (from cowpox) was contaminated with smallpox and with other infectious organisms (107). In the paper, "The Origin of the Vaccine Inoculation" (1801), Jenner answered Woodville's charges directly. In the course of the trials, Jenner learned that some patients who claimed to have been exposed to cowpox contracted it again, despite having undergone variolation. His explanation was that they probably never had the disease in the first place. After some inquiry, he concludes that since the cow is subject to varieties of "spontaneous eruptions upon her teats" (3), the farmers may have actually contracted a disease other than cowpox; thus, the reputed second exposure had actually been the first. Jenner was therefore able to distinguish between true cowpox, which conferred immunity against the human strain of the disease, and other conditions mistaken for cowpox which he grouped under the heading of *spurious* cowpox. In the process, Jenner also learned that the cowpox vaccine itself could become contaminated with organisms, causing a secondary infection, and that the vaccine could weaken naturally (4–5).

Holmes, Semmelweis and Puerperal Fever

Oliver Wendell Holmes, M.D. (1809–1894), in "Border Lines in Medical Science" (the Address to the medical class of Harvard University, November 6, 1861), compared the medical professional to the topographer who sets out to map an intellectual *terra incognito* (211). Just as the topographer represents surface features of a region on maps and gathers information while surveying terrain from "elevated points," the biomedical scientist triangulates an area of inquiry that enclosed "infinite unknown details." Within these parameters, he drops a plumb-line (suspended lead measuring the depth of water or of subsurface space), which symbolizes the formulation of theory. The plumb-line, penetrating the surface of the ground, scoops up small quantities of sand, a procedure analogous to experimentation. Thus, to penetrate the abyss, according to Holmes' analogy, is to explore the unknown depths of medicine.

Holmes hoped to encourage the graduating class of 1861 to move ahead boldly. With their state-of-the art education, the new doctors stood on the threshold of a renascence in biomedical thought. The process through which this new face of reality was to be quarried, however, demanded a scrupulous attention to detail and, above all, indefatigable patience.

As a biomedical topographer, Holmes outlined the parameters of puerperal-fever research in the well-known essay, "The Contagiousness of Puerperal Fever" (1843 and 1855); in so doing, he placed himself squarely in the midst of the debate on the idea of contagion. In the mid-nineteenth century, a sizable portion of the medical community rejected the idea that diseases such as puerperal fever could be spread from person to person. Holmes subscribed specifically to contagionist theory, one variant of which was that disease could be communicated through exhaled particulates (that is, effluvia). Holmes' paper antedated by nearly two decades the advent of the germ theory of disease, the greatest breakthrough of all, which emerged from the work of Louis Pasteur, of Robert Koch, and of many others.

Puerperal infection, we now know, occurs in the birth canal and in other structures during the postpartum period. It was a very serious condition before the availability of antibiotics but today can be treated, usually with success. It is caused by a number of bacteria, such as streptococci, staphyloccci, *Clostridium perfringens*, *Bacteroides fragilis*, and *Escharchia coli*, most of which live in the vagina naturally (Ryan 915–16). Infections occur when there is a rupture of the membranes, traumatic labor, caesarean section, unsanitary vaginal examinations or delivery, retained products of conception, hemorrhage, maternal anemia, or other predisposing condition (915–16).

Holmes rightly believes that a contagious agent caused the disease (402–03). Dismissing authoritative resources of the day, such as William Potts Dewees' *Diseases of Females* or the standard text on the subject, the *Philadelphia Practice of Midwifery*, Holmes affirms: "*The disease known as puerperal fever is so far contagious as to be frequently carried from patient to patient by physicians and nurses*" (403; author's italics). *How* the disease spreads, whether from the "atmosphere the physician carries about him into the sick-chamber" or from the physician's hands, is not Holmes's primary concern (404); rather, he is more interested in summarizing anecdotal opinions supporting the idea that health-care workers unknowingly carried the infection to patients. The disease was first reported by the gynecologist Philippe Peu in 1664, during an epidemic in the maternity ward of a Paris hospital, and in the 1750s doctors believed that the disease was communicated through breast-milk (Snodgrass 91, 114).

The testimony of the Scottish obstetrician, Dr. Gordon of Aberdeen, in a *Treatise on the Epidemic Puerperal Fever of Aberdeen* (1795), was that women who came down with the illness had been cared for by a practitioner, previously in contact with patients who had the disease. Such a sequence of events, interpreted according to the argument *ex post propter hoc*, could not prove transmissibility. But, on the basis of seventy-five cases, Gordon thought otherwise: everyone who had come into contact with a sick patient "became charged with an atmosphere of infection," and this *charge* was, in turn, communicated to every pregnant woman who happened to be "within its sphere" (405; italics added). According to Gordon's imagery, the obstetrical ward was a chamber filled with infectious particles. But he was not entirely convinced that the source of infection was a cloud of airborne organic particles or effluvium. What distinguished Gordon from effluvyists of his time was the inference that the caregivers themselves were the vehicles of transmission, and that they transported the invisible malady to neighboring villages. According to Gordon, the infectious agent was not atmospheric but rather on the carriers' bodies. Thus, the cause of puerperal fever, he concludes, is likely "'a specific contagion, or infection,'" one "'altogether unconnected with a noxious constitution of the atmosphere'" (405). From his direct experience with patients, Dr. Gordon was able to infer (but not prove) the concept of physical contagion.

Other physicians corroborated Gordon's suspicions. Anecdotal evidence lent credibility to the idea that unsuspecting medical professionals carried the infectious agent. The disease, according to some interesting accounts, could be spread through infected clothing. For example, Holmes refers to the story of a nurse who, after washing the linen of a decedent, was implicated in the deaths of a succession of pregnant women for whom she had cared (407). Another anecdote tells of a very ethical obstetrician who, having lost many patients to the fever, voluntarily ceased working and gave the practice over to his associate who did not encounter any fatalities. It is not clear if the original physician blamed the string of deaths on coincidence or if he tried to determine what his associate was doing to safeguard his patients. In 1835, one authority, Dr. Ramsbotham, posited that the disease could be communicated through the clothing of an attendant rather than through the air in the ward (408–09). The evidence, consisting of accumulated cases and of the accounts of local obstetricians over five decades, persuaded Holmes to the view "that the physician and the disease entered, hand in hand, into the chamber of the unsuspecting patient" (410). Holmes alludes to these testimonies because they were the first to appear in the American medical literature, and because their existence had hitherto been ignored.

One of the most revolting citations was that of Dr. Warrington who describes how, after assisting at an autopsy of puerperal peritonitis, "he laded out the contents of the abdominal cavity with his hands," and then set about his normal routine, delivering five healthy women in succession. All of them, not surprisingly, developed some form of the fever, and two died. In a second case, contaminated gloves were implicated. As word got around that Dr. Samuel Jackson's patients were dying after childbirth, women called for other physicians to attend to them, and few died, as a result. As it turned out, his gloves which he had not changed for more than two months were, in Warrington's opinion, "thoroughly imbued with ... effluvia" (414) — that is, with aerosolized particles.

A third example of contagion involves an anonymous physician who experienced several horrible episodes of puerperal fever among his patients, and who recollected that, during this difficult period, he had never changed his coat. To this fact, he attributed a succession of fatalities. However, the series of infections was interrupted when he changed his clothes and, at each visit, washed his hands in chloride of lime (417–18). Recollecting these events in a letter of 1843, he states that, up until 1830, he had not the slightest suspicion that the infection could be communicated from one patient to another by a nurse or midwife. But his sanitary precautions and the preponderance of evidence inclined him to accept that theory. As to what the invisible pathogen was, he and many of his contemporaries had little choice but to consider it to be effluvium or gaseous contaminant.

An astonishing example of how the disease was transmitted through contact appeared in the *London Medical Gazette*, on 10 December 1831. Dr. Campbell of Edinburgh recalls how, in October 1821, he attended an autopsy of a patient who had died of puerperal fever. Campbell helped himself to "the pelvic viscera" for use in the classroom. Not having a proper receptacle, he put the tissue *in his pocket* (italics added)! That evening, he attended to a woman in labor, without having changed his clothes. The woman died. On the very next morning, he delivered a patient with forceps, and she too died, as did three other women (423). Campbell, amazingly, did not connect these fatalities to one another causatively. In June 1823, he again took part in a puerperal-fever autopsy. Unable to wash his hands well "for want of the necessary accommodations" (no soap and water?) or to change his stained clothing, he attended to two female patients at his office shortly thereafter. Both women died of puerperal fever. Campbell, as it turned out, had been an authority against the contagionist theory (423).

Dr. Rigby, a proponent of contagionist theory, stated in the *British and Foreign Medical Review* of January 1842, that to ignore the compelling evidence in favor of this theory was nothing short of criminal. Holmes agreed with Rigby who had written in his *System of Midwifery* that care had to be taken during puerperal autopsies since the tissue of the deceased was contagious (425). Accidents occurring during dissection were of serious concern, as well (426). A sponge used to clean puerperal abscesses, for example, could infect healthy women, whether pregnant or not, a claim repeatedly proven in a Vienna Hospital of the day. On more than one occasion, women who had washed soiled linen of puerperal fever victims in the General Lying-in Hospital developed severe abscesses on their fingers and hands (426–27).

Holmes believed that, if the agent responsible for puerperal fever were eliminated, the number of deaths and miscarriages would be reduced dramatically, and that the elimination of this disease could be achieved through "thorough purification" (421). The mode of purification rather than of contagion was, therefore, Holmes's chief concern: thus, he writes of how antiseptic solutions removed the "virulent atmosphere of an impure lying-in hospital" and "the breath of contagion" (421). It appears that Holmes subscribed to two contagionist theories simultaneously: the miasmatic ("virulent atmosphere") and the effluvyist ("the breath of contagion"). In his discussion of Rigby's findings, however, he implicates the former cause: thus, within lying-in hospitals "there is often generated a miasm[a], palpable as the chlorine used to destroy it, tenacious so as in some cases almost to defy extirpation, deadly in some institutions as the plague; which has killed women in a private hospital of London so fast that they were buried two in one coffin to conceal its horrors" (427).

The miasmatic explanation notwithstanding, Holmes was convinced that contagion was a reality, as one can readily deduce from "this train of cumulative evidence, the multiplied groups of cases clustering about individuals, the deadly result of autopsies, the inoculation by fluids from the living patient, [and] the murderous poison of hospitals" (427). Holmes, it seems, approached the childbed fever problem pragmatically, not theoretically: identifying the disease-causing agent (he reiterates) was not as important as preventing the disease itself through decontamination (421). The evidence, though not definitive, made it highly probable that the disease was transmitted by health-care workers (429).

Accordingly, Holmes outlined public-health precautions: (1) no obstetrician should take part in an autopsy of someone who died of puerperal fever, peritonitis, or erysipelas; (2) if a physician were present at such a procedure, he should "use thorough ablution," change every article of clothing, and then allow twenty-four hours to elapse before attending patients; (3) if a physician were to encounter a single case of puerperal fever, he should stay away from a pregnant patient for some weeks, "to diminish her risk of disease and death"; (4) an obstetrician should suspend his practice if he were to experience two cases of the fever close to each other, and if the disease did not presently exist in the neighborhood; (5) moreover, he should make every effort to free himself of any "noxious influence he may carry about with him"; the occurrence of three or more closely connected cases in a single practice, with no others existing in the neighborhood, and with no other "sufficient cause being alleged for the coincidence," amounts to "*prima facie* evidence that he is the vehicle of contagion" (431); (6) finally, it is the physician's duty to prevent his assistants and nurses from communicating the disease to patients and to warn them "of every suspected danger" (432). The presence of "a private pestilence" in an individual practice can no longer be considered an occupational hazard or misfortune. The physicians' obligations to society are unambiguous; and dereliction, in this regard (as Dr. Rigby had said), is criminal.

Later research corroborated Holmes's thinking on contagion. Before the germ theory of disease was firmly established, physicians like Oliver Wendell Holmes were able to develop a public-health strategy to meet the danger of childbed fever. Holmes based his argument on the growing deposit of circumstantial and of anecdotal evidence, along with the likelihood that cleanliness virtually eliminated the disease. Holmes inferred that the disease was contagious, that medical practitioners were the chief carriers, and that antiseptic practices would help greatly, and he assumed as much without experimental evidence.

Like Holmes and others, Dr. Ignaz Philip Semmelweis (1818–1865), an obstetric assistant at the General Hospital in Vienna, suspected that childbed fever was spread on the hands of doctors who had previously handled corpses infected with the disease. So he established routine, aseptic methods (hand-washing in chlorinated lime) as a way of controlling the invisible pathogens. As a result, mortality in his institution was greatly diminished. Sherwin B. Nuland, M.D., tells Semmelweis' story in *The Doctors' Plague: Germs, Childbed Fever, and the Strange Story of Ignaz Semmelweis.* Amazingly, Semmelweis was dismissed for his efforts because his methods were unorthodox.

I would like to take a close look at Semmelweis's groundbreaking essay, *Lecture on the genesis of puerperal fever* (15 May 1850). In this text, he presents clinical statistics gathered from his work in the General Hospital that showed the value of aseptic methods in obstetrical practice. The General Hospital had two clinics: one was for the instruction of obstetricians, and the other was staffed by midwives. The teaching clinic, surprisingly, had four times as many deaths due to puerperal fever as did the midwives' clinic. Semmelweis concluded that the situation in the first clinic was attributable, not to an epidemic, but to conditions peculiar to it. The problem, which he thought endemic, some thought was due to overcrowding in the wards, to the saturation of the wards through the years "with the miasma of puerperal fever," or to the frequent and crude obstetrical examinations undertaken there. One thing was certain: parturient women brought to this clinic had reason for concern.

Semmelweis rejected possible explanations for the high mortality rate in the physician-staffed clinic because the conditions in both wards were the same, yet the rate of morbidity was lower for the midwives. Semmelweis, like Holmes, did not realize that in the uterus germs entered the system through wounds. Instead of bacteria, he blamed putrescent tissue and blood products for the disease: "the uptake of putrefying organic materials from the uterus" introduced the infection into the mother's bloodstream. Semmelweis compared childbed fever to pyemia, later understood to be a bacterial infection of the blood contracted through wounds that were incurred during the dissection of putrefying corpses. Since the students in the first clinic also did post-mortem examinations, Semmelweis reasoned, they could somehow be transmitting this putrefactive agent to parturient women. Other causes of the transmission of putrefying organic materials, he thought, included decomposing placental tissue or the caregiver's infected hands, contaminated from autopsies (a position aligning him with Gordon, Ramsbotham, and Holmes).

Although Semmelweis was unsure of the offending agent, he inferred that transmission was an unrecognized aspect of everyday practice. Without conducting a trial, he instituted the pragmatic measure of handwashing in chloride of lime after examining a patient. In this measure, he went directly from inference to praxis, since there was less of a need to identify the exact agent of infection than to control the damage it caused. Chloride handwashing, he thought, was sufficient to destroy "any putrefying organic atoms" from the fingers and to remove odor completely.

As it turned out, Semmelweis achieved dramatic success in the first clinic. From 1839 to 1842, he reduced the death rate of the physicians' clinic from 8.3 to 2.3 percent, which was equivalent to what it was in private practice and in other obstetrical clinics. Further proof was that, if assistants worked in the *second* clinic after having examined corpses, healthy women began to contract the disease there, too. Up until 1 May 1847, when chloride-of-lime handwashing was initiated, the childbed fever death rate in both clinics was an unacceptable 5.7 percent. But from 1 May 1847 to April 1850, while handwashing was practiced, the death rate declined to 2.2 percent.

Although Semmelweis conjectured that putrefaction destroyed healthy tissue, he was correct to assume that the disease spread through the body from an entrance site: the problem originated when "an animal-organic substance in the process of putrefying, whether from a sick person or a cadaver, is taken up into the blood of the woman who has just given birth, and causes in her the puerperal (pyemic) disintegration of the blood, with accompanying exudation and metastasis." He was convinced that contaminated hands or instruments communicated these substances to the parturient woman, and that sterilization limited the transmission of the disease in the hospital. The danger still existed if the opening of the uterus were abraded or contused because the infectious material could then be absorbed directly above the inner uterine opening, which was covered by the amniotic membrane during pregnancy. In addition, newborns were at risk from the disease because the uterine cavity was most vulnerable during the first and second deliveries, since examinations occurred most frequently in these areas, and since large amounts of exudation could contact the newborn. This also accounted for the deaths of women whose deliveries were delayed for two or three days.

Semmelweis' great contribution to medicine was his courageous appeal to common sense. He had more than probability to count on: he had quantified results. In this regard, he took Holmes' argument to a higher level and moved from inference directly into praxis. But obdurate conservatives who clung to miasmatic and to anti-contagionist ideas rejected his inspired efforts. In their rejection of the indisputable results, they were no different than ancient pre-conceptualists. As Thomas D. Brock observes, Semmelweis' intelligence and ethical compunction led to his undoing: his colleagues reviled him, and he eventually lost his job (82).

John Snow and Cholera

In the essay, "Mode of Communication of Cholera" (1855), Dr. John Snow (1813–1859) chronicled the history of a cholera outbreak in the Broad Street and Golden Square area of London, which he considered to be the worst to have ever struck Great Britain. He wrote that nearly five hundred cases of cholera were reported in only ten days. Not only was the mortality rate high, but the onset and duration of the disease was acute: people died in a matter of hours. Had the residents of the area not fled in panic, the mortality rate, he had reason to believe, would have been much higher. Since the residents did not know where the disease came from or how it was contracted, they fled in panic. In a short time, the most afflicted streets were virtually uninhabited.

Based on a thorough study of cases, of topography, and of residential interviews, Snow theorized that the epidemic was a contagious disease. The *poison* (as Snow called it) was found in the feces and vomit of its victims, and not in the air; furthermore, its origin was drinking water, contaminated by human excretions. Though he strongly suspected that some microscopic organism in the water was responsible, he had no proof of this but correctly intuited that a deadly toxin was responsible for the illness (it was later learned that the bacteria produced this toxic protein [Wills 113, 116]). At the outset of the investigation, as Christopher Wills correctly observes, Snow proceeded "by *inference*, which grew stronger as the number of cholera cases increased and he could start to make connections" (113; italics added). In 1854, Filippo Pacini was the first to see the microbe, and, in 1884, Robert Koch proved it to be the cause of cholera (Wills 116).

An acute gastrointestinal infection, cholera causes diarrhea, vomiting, and, in half of the cases, death through fluid and electrolyte loss, shock, and metabolic acidosis ("Cholera," WHO). The only host and victim of *V. cholerae* is man. The microbe is transmitted through food and water contaminated with fecal material from carriers or from those with active infections. The signs and symptoms of the disease are particularly alarming: after an incubation period of several hours to five days, profuse diarrhea containing white mucous particles ensues. Intense thirst results because of the excessive fluid loss. The skin becomes wrinkled, the eyes sink in, the muscles cramp, and the bodily systems rapidly fail.

While a physician's apprentice, young Snow came into contact with cholera in 1831, when it first appeared in England (Litsios 181). He sought logical connections between human behavior and susceptibility to infection, noting that miners were frequently afflicted with the disease (181). One characteristic of their daily life, he learned, was that they drank water from underground locations near open latrines; in addition, they had little or no access to washing facilities while underground (181). Thus, as early as the 1830s, Snow had begun to connect polluted water to disease.

In 1849, as a renowned surgeon and personal physician of Queen Victoria, Snow undertook an investigation of the disease during the third cholera pandemic (DeSalle ed., 66), which extended from 1846 to 1863. The British epidemic of 1848–1849 took between 54,000 and 62,000 lives, from autumn 1848 to the end of 1849, and a renewed outbreak, from 1853 to 1854, accounted for an additional 31,000 deaths (Kohn 38).

In the vicinity of Broad and Cambridge Streets, London, nearly five hundred people were sickened, and many died of a disease that caused violent, debilitating diarrhea, and odorless "rice-water stools" (De Salle 66). According to statistics, the pestilence was at its worst between August 31 and September 1. With his 1831 experience in mind, Snow thought that drinking water was contaminated, and that the Broad St. pump was the outlet. When he examined the water, however, he saw no impurities, so he paused. Nonetheless, on the basis of circumstantial evidence, Snow inferred that the water was the source of the contagion, since "no other circumstance or agent" common to the area could be connected to cholera.

Over the next two days, Snow noticed that the water varied in purity. On very close inspection, he saw "small white, flocculent particles." Thus, he concluded that at the commencement of the outbreak the water had been impure. But these speculations were weak. After inspecting the register of cholera deaths during the week ending September 2 for the district in question, he learned that eighty-nine people had died of the disease. Of these, only six had expired in the first four days (i.e., August 27 to August 30), four on August 31, but the remaining seventy-nine in a two-day period (September 1–2). From this information, Snow deduced that the outbreak had officially begun on August 31.

With the suspicion that water-borne cholera was present at Broad St., and with a sense of urgency in view of the sudden increase in deaths, Snow hastened to the scene. All of the deaths on the registry, he learned, occurred in close proximity to the pump. The families of five decedents informed him that the deceased had regularly used the pump for drinking water, actually preferring it over the water from pumps closer to their homes. Two of three deceased children were reported to have drunk the water routinely on their way to school. Furthermore, sixty-one decedents who lived in proximity to the pump used its water either regularly or occasionally. Snow's inquiry demonstrated that no where else in London had there been a sudden increase in the incidence of cholera except in the locality of the Broad St. pump, and, with the exception of twelve cases not conforming to this inference, all those who got cholera had used the Broad St. water-pump. Fortunately, when Snow presented his preliminary findings to the Board of Guardians (the parish of St. James) on the evening of Thursday, September 7, the Board ordered that the pump handle be removed on September 8.

There were other fatalities that had to be added to the record. Snow also learned that, along with the eighty-three deaths at Broad Street, some who had gotten cholera from the very same pump had died in *other locations*, but these deaths had not been registered until the following week. So the epidemic was actually worse than at first thought. On September 1 and 2, one hundred ninety-seven persons had succumbed to cholera. Another part of the complicated puzzle was that some people who were sickened with cholera, but who had claimed not to have drunk the water, may actually have done so without realizing it. For example, a coffee-shop in the neighborhood used the pump, and consequently nine customers died. Further evidence of tainted water was gathered from a local Workhouse situated in the middle of the epidemic zone. Of the five hundred and thirty-five inmates of that establishment, only five died of cholera. They were largely unaffected because they used another pump on the premises, in addition to a supply of water from the Grand Junction Water Works. A Brewery near the Broad Street pump reported that no employees came down with cholera. The proprietor explained to Snow that the seventy men at the Brewery drank malt liquor and water from a deep well on the premises, although he could not be absolutely certain that no one frequented the suspicious pump. Eighteen of the two hundred workers at the percussion-cap manufactory at 37 Broad St. died of cholera: they drank from two tubs of water filled from the Broad St. pump. Considering the virulence of the disease, this locality was worthy of closer scrutiny, but Snow chose not to delve any further into it. Only 10 percent of the employees contracted the disease from Broad St. water, which seemed a rather low percentage. A surgeon, Mr. Marshall, informed Snow that seven workmen employed at a manufactory of dentists' materials at numbers 8 and 9 Broad Street died of cholera while at home. They were in the habit of drinking a half-pint, once or twice a day; two others who lived at the manufactory, but who did not drink the pump-water, only had diarrhea. Perhaps one of the most dramatic anecdotes was of a visiting army officer who dined at Wardour St., drank from the Broad St. pump at dinner, developed cholera, and died in a few hours. Dr. Marshall also furnished Snow with valuable data on the incubation period of the disease. Three cases, in particular, suggested that the disease took about 36 to 48 hours to manifest itself

Circumstantial evidence supported Snow's suspicion that cholera-infected water carried from Broad Street reached Hampstead West End. Once again, Snow benefited from information that medical colleagues contributed to his inquiry. From Dr. Fraser came what Snow thought to be "the most conclusive evidence of all in proving the connection between the Broad Street pump and the outbreak of cholera" (4). The fifty-nine-year-old widow of a percussion-cap maker died from cholera in the space of sixteen agonizing hours. Her son told Snow that she had been in the vicinity of Broad Street, drank the water on August 31 and September 1, returned to Islington (*where no cholera was present*), and rapidly succumbed to the disease (italics added). Snow created a map pinpointing fatalities on and near Broad Street, Golden Square. He acknowledged that the fullest extent of the outbreak really would never be known since death registries were incomplete, and since people carrying the disease felt its impact later on and in distant locations; moreover, it was difficult to track them down. But these variables did not detract from the usefulness of the map. All known cholera fatalities, from August 19 to 30, occurred in subdistricts where the Broad Street pump was regularly used, and statistics for this period were on record. Significantly, deaths were most numerous in proximity to the pump which was located on a wide, much-traveled street.

An unanticipated decline in mortality undermined Snow's hypothesis, which identified the well as the reservoir of the disease: just before the handle was removed, the mortality rate declined sharply, suggesting that the disease was waning naturally. Snow was still convinced, however, that the disease could be stamped out if the handle were removed, even though it was impossible to determine, at that juncture, whether the well still contained active cholera. A sewer passing within a few yards of the well caught Snow's attention. Though nothing appeared to the naked eye, microscopic examination of the water at the time of the epidemic showed organic impurities and "minute oval animacules" that one physician thought to be insignificant. The percussion-cap manufacturer noticed that, after a few days, the water exhibited an offensive odor, which Snow associated with sewage. But most of the people whom Snow interviewed had not observed any change in the quality of the water at the time of the outbreak. The testimony of an eminent ornithologist, Mr. Gould, was that a draft of water from the well, though visibly clear, had a foul odor; his assistant who also drank the water developed cholera but recovered.

The Broad Street pump-water was no doubt suspicious, but whether the pollution derived from the sewers, the drains, or the cesspools, Snow simply could not tell. Another possibility that Snow seriously considered was that the evacuations of cholera patients might actually have been seeping into the drinking water. Since the quantity of morbid matter sufficient to produce cholera was small (as he correctly assumed), this possibility was a reasonable one.

Fortunately, as I said, Snow was able to convince the parish to disable the pump, even though he had only circumstantial evidence on which to base his argument. Snow recognized the importance of finding "oval animacules" in the water, which were macro- and microscopically visible. The offensive odors exuding from the pump water left little doubt that it was necessary to act expeditiously. Whether the particles were disease-causing organisms could not be confirmed, but suspicions grew with each bit of information. Because the majority of deaths were in close proximity to the water source, as the map demonstrated, and because Broad Street had the highest incidence of cholera in London, Snow believed very strongly that the pump was the source. That the outbreak declined precipitously once precautions were enacted indicated, even more convincingly, that the cholera outbreak had its source in Broad Street water, even though the exact reservoir had not yet been identified. The logic of proximity suggested that a nearby sewer contaminated the water, and that the secretions of cholera victims were polluting the water table.

During the time of the fourth epidemic, 1853–1854, the public water sources had become obsolete. At that time, two water companies pumped water directly into households via pipelines. Yet cholera was still a threat. Snow sprang into action, again, interviewing residents, and collecting case studies and statistics; his aim was to correlate these data to households afflicted with the disease (DeSalle 67). It turned out that people whom the Southwark and Vauxhall Companies served were contracting the disease at a high rate because they used a fresh water source *downstream* of raw city sewage which was regularly dumped into the Thames (67; italics added). The second company, Lambeth, had a low rate of cholera infections because their water source was upstream of the sewage. By causally relating contaminated water to the high frequency of disease, Snow revealed a compelling truth.

At the time, Snow's contribution was not appreciated. The third International Sanitary Conference, convened in Constantinople in 1866, officially declared that cholera was a miasmatic rather than aquatic-borne disease, but fortunately this declaration did not affect the revolution in sanitation and sewage disposal being undertaken in both Europe and America at that time (Wills 116).

9. From Etiology to Synergy

Of Greek origin, the word *etiology*, literally meaning *discourse of cause*, was first applied to disease in Bonet's 1684 medical textbook. *The Oxford English Dictionary* defines its current usage as, "that branch of medical science which investigates the causes and origin of diseases," and as "the scientific exposition of the origin of any disease" (*OED* I: 149; "aetiology"). In this chapter, I will survey the emergence of this radically new way of thinking and of writing about disease-causing microbes, one that went far beyond anecdote, observation, and assumption. Etiological thought involves several branches of biology in the pursuit of a common end, namely the discovery of the cause and mechanism of epidemic disease.

Koch, Pasteur and Anthrax

A seminal piece of etiological discourse, Dr. Robert Koch's 1876 paper, "The etiology of anthrax, based on the life history of *Bacillus anthracis*," heralded a new phase of epidemiological thought, and this paper will begin our discussion. Koch (1843–1910), a country physician, proved experimentally that the organism, *Bacillus anthracis*, caused the disease known as anthrax. His method combined observation, hypothesis, and six discrete experiments, each involving observations, corollary proofs, and transitional inferences. With our emphasis on how early biomedical thinkers solved problems, I will demonstrate how Koch painstakingly arrived at this conclusion and, then, how Louis Pasteur applied the new knowledge about anthrax disease to veterinary immunology

Koch's idea that a microbe caused anthrax was not original, belonging as it did to a contemporary, inferential tradition. Other scientists had suspicions that a microbe was responsible for the disease. In 1850, Pierre Rayer (1793–1867) and Casimir-Joseph Davaine (1812–1882) found "small filiform bodies" in the blood of anthrax-infected sheep (Lord 1). Franz Aloys Antoine

Pollender (1800–1879), in 1855, corroborated the observations of Rayer and of Davaine and conjectured that these filamentous structures might be the cause of anthrax (Lord 1). Additionally, Friedrich August Brauell (1803–1882), in 1858, noticed that since healthy animals or those with diseases other than anthrax did *not* carry these bodies in their blood, the presence of these organisms in the bloodstream suggested their close connection to the disease (Lord 1). The circumstantial evidence had, by the mid-1870s, made a strong case for the correlation of the filamentous bodies and anthrax disease. Of course, this was not proof of causation: the "bodies" might just as well have been the effect as the cause. But the stage had been set for Koch.

Using fresh anthrax material in an initial experiment, Koch inoculated a large number of mice at the base of the tail; in each case, the mouse died. The inoculum, it appeared, had produced the disease. He then tried to discover whether or not the microbes in the dead mice were dead or alive. Hypothesizing that they were alive, Koch set out to prove it and thereby to establish causation.

In the second experiment, Koch focused on the effects of the bacilli on live animals. He proceeded to inoculate mice in series from one to another, each time using the spleen of an anthrax-infected carcass. For the twenty mice in series, the results were the same: all of the animals died. Koch gathered more information from dissection and histology (the microscopic study of cells) to learn about the effects of the anthrax microbe on blood and tissue. Examination of the animals revealed that the spleens were swollen, that the organs contained large numbers of similar, transparent rods, and that the rods were immotile and not enclosed in spores. A crucial discovery was that the very same organism was found in the blood of each mouse, with the largest concentration in the spleen. These observations proved that a small number of bacilli, initially introduced through inoculation, multiplied into a large mass of individuals of the same type. These individuals, microscopic analysis revealed, reproduced by doubling in length and then splitting into two individuals. From what he had seen histologically, he postulated that *in vivo* the structure of the bacilli remained consistent, even after a prolonged series of inoculations.

Having established that the organisms were definitely alive, grew in the body, spread into the bloodstream, and appeared to remain physiologically constant from generation to generation, Koch had then to isolate the bacilli for further study. Embarking on a third experiment, he placed on a glass slide a drop of fresh beef serum or bovine, aqueous humor, removed anthrax-infected spleen tissue from an animal, placed the tissue in the medium, and covered the slide with glass. After placing the slide in a moist chamber to prevent evaporation, he incubated it for 15 to 20 hours, at 35–37 degrees C. After 20 hours, Koch noticed, in the middle of the preparation and between the tissue cells, a small number of unaltered microbes. At a distance from the animal tissue in the fluid, he could see organisms that were three to eight times longer than the unaltered ones previously mentioned; the larger organisms had shallow bends and curvatures. Many of these long filaments had lost their uniform structure, their contents appearing finely granulated and light refractive. At the edge of the cover glass where the gas exchange with the nutrient fluid was richest, the organisms developed extensively. Strung along the filaments at regular intervals were ovular, light-refractive spores. Small, free clusters of spores that had broken off could be seen between the filaments.

On the basis of these detailed observations, Koch experienced the breakthrough he had anticipated. The fourth hypothesis in the series was that, if the preparation was favorable and if the experiment went along normally, the growth stages of the anthrax bacillus—from short rods, to spore-forming filaments, to free spores—could be seen and documented. Definitive proof that the spores arose from filaments was in sight.

Patient observation brought the truth to light. Inspecting the slide carefully at ten- to twenty-minute intervals, Koch observed that the bacilli were thick and swollen, hardly showing any change in the first two hours. But they began to grow after three or four hours, lengthening ten to twenty times beyond their original size, curving, pushing against or crossing each other, and making a network. After a few more hours, long individual filaments appeared. Observing the free end of a filament continuously for fifteen to twenty minutes, one could actually witness its lengthening. It was therefore possible to obtain visual evidence of the further development of these filaments. After ten to fifteen minutes passed, the contents of the most luxuriant filaments showed fine granules, which separated from the vine at regular sequences. These segments enlarged over several more hours into ovular spores. Eventually, the filaments fragmented at the ends, and the spores were freed, remaining loose and immotile for weeks.

Koch wondered if the bacilli emerged directly from the spores. To answer this question, he had to establish conditions conducive to this end, to observe and record the outcome, and, if successful with the foregoing experiment, to replicate the findings before his peers. One problem he encountered at the outset of the fifth experiment was finding the appropriate medium through which the transformation might be observed. Placing spores in either distilled or well-water failed. Although bacilli developed in serum or aqueous humor, the number of filaments in either medium was too small for him actually to see the spores yielding germs. Needing a pure culture, he collected free spore-masses, air-dried them on a cover glass, dropped aqueous humor on the specimens, and covered the spore-mass to keep it wet. The purpose was to isolate the spores and to promote and visually record their possible transformation into free microbes. Placing these preparations in a moist chamber, incubated at 35 degrees C., Koch recognized that, after one-half hour, the remains of the filament began to disintegrate; and, after one and one-half to two hours, they disappeared altogether. After three to four hours, the spores drifted freely on the slide. At high magnification, each was an oval imbedded in a round transparent mass; the round mass appeared as a light ring surrounding the spore. According to Koch's description, *new filaments arose from spores* (italics added). If one were to roll a spore in various positions, the spherical ring became visible, and the material gradually lost its spherical shape, lengthened itself on one side in the direction of the long axis of the spore, and became ovular. The spore remained fixed in one of the poles of the cylindrical body, and the transparent covering became longer and filamentous. At some point in the process, the spore lost its heat-resistant characteristics, became pale, smaller, detached, and completely disappeared. The spore mass, before Koch's very eyes, gradually transformed into filaments, and a second generation of spore-containing filaments appeared.

From microscopic observations, Koch inferred that in the bloodstream of a sensitive animal anthrax spores bore a new generation of microbes. Yet another experiment, the sixth in the sequence, was needed to prove the hypothesis that the blood-borne spores had actually become bacilli. To this end, he inoculated mice with tissue either rich in spores or sparsely contaminated with them. The higher concentration killed mice in twenty-four hours; the lower concentration, in three to four days. He repeated the trial several times, air-drying sporiferous tissue, moistening it with water, and injecting it into healthy mice. When he did so with spores from pure *in vitro* cultures, all of the animals died. Thus, Koch once again had demonstrated that anthrax bacilli form filaments which, in turn, produce budding spores, and that free spores turn into a new generation of bacilli. As for the destructive activities of the microbe, they were apparent from dissection and histology; the organism multiplied in the infected body and in the culture dish; and if injected into test animals, individually or in series, it had lethal results.

Koch had proven what the renowned bacteriologist, Ferdinand Cohn, had already suspected. In "Studies on the biology of the bacilli" (1876), Cohn remarked that understanding the growth cycle of the anthrax bacillus was essential to understanding the pathology it presumably caused (54–5). On the basis of his work on spores in 1875, Cohn anticipated that the rods of anthrax would form spores, and that these would infect the bloodstream. When Koch told Cohn that he had discovered the complete life-cycle of *B. anthracis* and was willing to replicate the experiment at

Cohn's laboratory, the latter invited Koch to Breslau where, from April 30 to May 3, 1876, he successfully repeated the anthrax experiments on frogs, mice, and rabbits. In this way, Cohn confirmed Koch's findings.

In the March 24, 1882 paper, "The Etiology of Tuberculosis," read before the Physiological Society in Berlin, Koch outlined a method establishing causation between bacteria and disease. His "perfect proof" required four sequential activities: (1) the isolation of the foreign substance from the diseased organism; (2) the culturing and introduction of the microbe into a new animal host; (3) the identification of the microbe in the blood and tissue of the animal stricken with the disease in question so as to prove the hypothesis that the micro-organism transmitted the disease (blood and tissue samples, in turn, would reveal the organism); and (4) the reintroduction of the disease into healthy animals through the inoculation of small quantities of diseased blood.

Jean Antoine Villemin and Robert Koch had isolated the bacillus in 1882, and the latter applied his methodology to tuberculosis: the aim was to determine if the microbe (now known as *Mycobacterium tuberculosis*) was responsible for the illness. Koch's initial task was to show that a "foreign parasitic structure" in the body was "the causal agent" of tuberculosis. Using a sophisticated staining method, he identified "characteristic" organisms in tubercular organs (109). The staining method tinted the structures of animal tissues brown and the tubercular bacilli blue, making visual differentiation easy. The bacillus in question had distinct characteristics, allowing Koch to establish its taxonomy. Since they were rod-shaped, they belonged to the group *Bacilli*. In 1872, Cohn had divided bacteria into six groups or Tribes: the ball or egg-shaped (*Micrococcus*); the short, rod-like (*Bacterium*); the straight, fiber-like (*Bacillus*); the wavy, curl-like (*Vibrio*); the short, screwlike (*Spirillium*); and the long, flexible spiral (*Spirochaete*). He revised the sixfold nomenclature to four in the 1875 paper, "Studies on bacteria." In this text, Tribe I is Spherical (with *Micrococcus* a genus); Tribe II is Rod bacteria or *Microbacteria* (with a subtype); Tribe III is Filamentous bacteria or *Desmobacteria* (with two subtypes, *Vibrio* having been demoted to a genus); and Tribe IV is Cork-screw bacteria or *Spirobacteria* (with two subtypes, including *Spirillium* and *Spirochaete*) ([1872] 16; [1875] 214).

Koch put Cohn's classificatory system to good use in his tuberculosis experiment. The organisms he saw were very thin and only one-fourth to one-half the diameter of the red blood cell. In form and size, moreover, they resembled the leprosy bacillus, the cause of Hansen's disease. The presence of abundant organisms was also suggestive of causality. Other observations supported this assumption. The microbes formed small groups of cells and pressed together in bundles, and they were discovered frequently both inside and outside of cells. When the tubercular eruption reached its peak and passed, the bacilli declined in number (110). Moreover, bacilli of lighter hue or those barely visible either were dying or already dead (110–11).

Despite these observations, Koch recognized as he had with anthrax that the coextension of tuberculosis disease and of the bacilli was not definitive proof that the latter caused the former. Nevertheless, he wrote these extraordinary words: "a high degree of probability for this causal relationship might be inferred from the observation that the bacilli were present most frequently *when* the tubercul[ar] process is developing or progressing, and that they *disappear* when the disease becomes quiescent" (111; italics added). To move from high probability to unequivocal certainty, one had to show that the bacilli penetrated the body to cause parasitic disease, and that the propagation of these germs brought on the illness. To begin the process of discovery, one had to remove the suspicious germs from the body, to culture them in a pure or uncontaminated medium, and to differentiate the organisms from the by-products of organic disease in the body. Once the bacilli were isolated and free of other material, the investigator could transfer the isolated germs to healthy animals in the expectation of inducing tuberculosis. Needing a reliable solid medium, Koch placed serum from cow or sheep blood in cotton-plugged test tubes and heated the tubes every day for six days, one hour per day at 58 degrees C. As a result, it was possible to sterilize the blood products. Further heating at 65 degrees C. solidified the medium (111).

Once the investigator had sterile solid media, he needed to procure tubercular material, ideally lung tissue, from an animal that had died of the disease. Tubercular masses, in Koch's experience, appeared as particles about the size of millet seeds. Using a flamed platinum wire, he transferred this material to test tubes and then to the surface of the solidified serum, and he recommended that five to ten tubes be transferred to the media this way. In the second week after seeding, scaly dots appeared to the naked eye. Low magnification (at 30–40 power) revealed colonies by the end of the first week. After several weeks, the colony ceased growing.

To identify the inoculum with the naturally-occurring organism, Koch compared two animal infection-sites to each other. One was in the lungs, usually heavily involved in a case of spontaneous tuberculosis. The physiological effects in this case were easy to distinguish from tuberculosis induced through abdominal inoculation. In the latter case, successful inoculation caused swelling. Since the concentration of bacilli in culture was greater than what would normally be present in natural contagion, the induced infection progressed quickly. Spleen and liver biopsies showed that the abdominal inoculation had caused obvious changes, leading Koch strongly to suspect that the development of tuberculosis in an experimental animal was indeed due to the activity of inoculated culture. Koch demonstrated this idea using a number of guinea pigs: he inoculated the animals with microbial culture (at the same time and with the same material), segregated the group from other animals, and, in a short period of time, brought on tuberculosis symptoms in them all. The results of this experiment were uniform: in all animals inoculated with fresh masses containing tubercle bacilli, the inoculation sites coalesced on the next day, remained constant for about eight days, became nodular, and then flattened into dry abscesses (113). He also learned that bacilli-containing material produced extensive infection with tuberculosis after four weeks. The disease process was the same in bovine, in simian, and in human trials (114).

On the basis of these experiments, Koch established that "a characteristic bacillus is always associated with tuberculosis, and that these bacilli can be obtained from tubercular organs and isolated in pure culture" (114). The most difficult hurdle was to prove that *the isolated bacilli* were able to bring about "the typical tuberculosis disease process when inoculated again into animals" (114; italics added). Koch met the challenge by injecting a large number of animals in different ways. With only one exception, all tests induced tuberculosis, whether the inoculation was in the abdomen, in the eye, through the skin, or directly into the bloodstream (114–15). Koch concluded that, "All these facts, taken together, justify the statement that *the bacilli present in tuberculous substances are not only coincidental ... but are the cause of the process*, and that we have in the bacilli the real tuberculous virus [i.e., microbe]" (Pinners' translation [1932], 404; italics added).

Equipped with a pure culture technique, Pasteur went to work in the spring of 1881 on anthrax-immunization trials (Dubos 107–08). In this pursuit, he was working in the inferential tradition of Edward Jenner and of the latter's precursors who had conducted rudimentary tests to prove the efficacy of vaccine against smallpox. Pasteur was reasonably certain (in light of Jean-Joseph Henri Toussaint's recent work in the area) that Jenner's method could be applied to anthrax.

Pasteur's findings were published on June 13, 1881, under the title, "Summary Report of the Experiments Conducted at Pouilly-le-Fort, Near Melun, on the Anthrax Vaccination." Pasteur reminded his audience that, in February 1881, he had undertaken the project "to discover a method for preparation of attenuated anthrax." This weakened strain would function as a vaccine, the recipient of which would suffer only a "benign variety of the disease" (59).

Controlling anthrax could save millions of animals each year in France and have a profound effect on agriculture and on the economy. In April of 1880, Pasteur recalls how he and the president of the Agriculture Society of

Melun had planned a pivotal experiment to immunize livestock against this disease. The plan called for Pasteur to have at his disposal sixty sheep, ten of which would not undergo any treatment. Of the remaining fifty, twenty-five were to receive two vaccinations of unequally attenuated anthrax, administered at intervals of twelve to fifteen days, presumably to build up their immunity in stages. After a third interval of twelve to fifteen days, the twenty-five treated sheep and the twenty-five untreated ones were to receive a very virulent strain of anthrax, the hope being that the untreated twenty-five would die while the immunized group would resist the more dangerous exposure; the two groups would be distinguished from one another by a hole punched in the ear, and the fifty were to be intermingled in one cattle shed. The sheep that died of anthrax would then be buried in designated pits in a secure enclosure to preclude soil contamination. The plan was then to place twenty-five additional sheep in the contaminated enclosure to test Pasteur's supposition that microbes could strike animals at any time, as worms reputedly brought the organism to the surface. To demonstrate that the disease could be contracted from contaminated soil, and that uncontaminated soil was harmless, they decided to herd twenty-five more sheep a few meters away from the infected area where no anthrax carcass had ever been buried (60). The vaccination experiments were extended to include cows: among a group of ten, six were inoculated and four were not. As had the fifty immunized sheep, the six inoculated cows were to receive the virulent strain to test their resistance. Pasteur expressed confidence that all would go as predicted.

On May 5, at a farm located in the commune of Pouilly-le-Fort, near Melun, the experiment commenced, involving two goats, fifty-eight sheep of different ages, sexes, and breeds, eight cows, one ox, and one bull. At the outset, they inoculated twenty-four sheep, one goat, and six cows, each with five drops of attenuated anthrax, using the methods developed by Jean-Joseph Henry Toussaint. On May 17, they revaccinated the twenty-four sheep, the goat, and the six cows with more virulent anthrax. And, on May 31, they introduced the most virulent strain generated from spores that had been stored in Pasteur's laboratory since March 21, 1877. How the test animals reacted to the third inoculation would determine the efficacy of the inoculations given between May 5 and May 17. Altogether, twenty-nine vaccinated animals received the virulent strain, the group consisting of twenty-four sheep, one goat, and four cows. Since none of these animals had received inoculum, they were not expected to survive. The observers and the scientific team decided to meet again on Thursday June 2, forty-eight hours after the introduction of the virulent microbe (60).

According to Pasteur, the results were astounding. On June 2, they found the inoculated animals healthy, whereas the twenty-one sheep and the goat that had not been inoculated were all dead; two unvaccinated sheep died before their eyes, while another died on June 3. Unvaccinated cows did not die, although they showed extensive swelling at the injection sites, along with increases in temperature. The vaccinated cows when exposed to the aggressive strain were unaffected. Pasteur concluded that although cows, unlike sheep, were less likely to die from anthrax, the differences in symptoms between the two groups of cows inclined him to believe that the vaccinations had a protective effect (61).

Pasteur believed that they indeed had a vaccine for anthrax capable of saving animals from the disease, and he claimed that the vaccine, consisting of live cultures "prepared and controlled" in the laboratory, was never lethal. Based on the conditions described in the experiment, he asserts that his anthrax vaccine "constitutes significant progress" beyond that attained by Jenner's vaccine, which had not been tested under rigid experimental conditions (62).

Pasteur's claims did not go unchallenged. Robert Koch wrote an acrimonious refutation of Pasteur's claims in an 1882 essay, "On the Anthrax Inoculation," the gist of which was that Pasteur's methods were sloppy. Koch questioned Pasteur's conclusions from several perspectives, notably that the Pouilly-le-Fort experiment was not corroborated microscopically and that the workers allegedly used impure substances, along with unsuitable test animals (2). These defaults, thought Koch, subverted the experiment entirely. Moreover, Koch wondered how Pasteur, a chemist, could make sound judgments about pathology and symptomology, which only a physician or veterinarian was trained to make. Furthermore, Koch took issue with Pasteur's secrecy: that he deliberately refrained from publishing his methods for attenuating anthrax so that others might not be able to replicate the experiment. Above all, Koch resented Pasteur's reputed claim to have discovered the etiology of anthrax which Koch's 1876 work had already clearly demonstrated. Other Pasteurian claims, with which Koch took issue, were that birds were immune to anthrax, that earthworms brought live spores to the surface soil, and that animals contracted the disease through oral wounds caused by prickly fodder. The most concentrated source of anthrax spores and the means through which most animals picked up the disease, Koch pointed out, was through ingestion: the spores need not enter the bloodstream through cuts; rather, they were regularly ingested, since the microbe existed naturally in rotted vegetation; therefore, animals most commonly contracted an intestinal infection.

Koch charged that Pasteur habitually jumped to conclusions. Pasteur's success with a chicken-cholera vaccine and his limited results with sheep, for example, had inspired him to make grandiose claims, one of which was that *all* animals could be made immune through anthrax vaccinations (italics added). Koch upbraids Pasteur for not being familiar with the precedent-setting work of Friedrich Löffler who proved that through natural exposure an individual could become immune to certain bacterial infections, and that certain species of animals, such as horses, "did not become immune to anthrax" through experimental inoculations (3). Thus, (according to Koch) Pasteur wrongly assumed that a universal law of immunity could be obtained through anthrax inoculations. To make matters worse (in Koch's judgment), the latter's imprecision about the vaccine — i.e., method of preparation, time of inoculation, and the measurement of virulence levels— was flagrantly evident (4). Koch asserted that the original culture, from which the attenuated versions were made, was impure and contained bacterial species other than anthrax, a claim that, if true, would invalidate the experiment entirely. Tests using Pasteur' vaccines, Koch alleged, were inconsistent: those conducted in Turin, Italy, and elsewhere showed that a significant number of sheep had withstood the second vaccine but then died upon receiving the virulent strain. A participant at the June 8, 1881, meeting of a prestigious veterinarian society suggested that this inconsistency could be attributed to the attenuation of the original culture: because the vaccine was weak, the animals did not have sufficient immunity to withstand the virulent strain (5). One conclusion was obvious: the process of attenuation was much more complicated than Pasteur believed it to be. To explain the attenuation process, one had to consider vaccine temperature, the operation of chemical agents, and other variables, some of which were not yet understood. The most critical charge that Koch levied against Pasteur was that he ignored these failures and, when pressed about them in professional circles, tried to circumvent the evidence (6). Koch's *Pasteur*, if you will, is depicted as an unethical man who communicated "only favorable aspects of his experiments," and who ignored "decisive unfavorable results."

On January 20, 1883, Pasteur wrote a lengthy vindication of his methods, entitled "The Anthrax Vaccination: Reply of M. Pasteur to a paper of M. Koch (Extract from the *Scientific Review*, Paris)." Rejecting Koch's claim that he had not acknowledged the former's great breakthrough of 1876, Pasteur thought the charge groundless since, on April 3, 1877, he had praised Koch's work. Turning the tables, Pasteur accused Koch of ignoring his own work on spore-forming bacteria that afflicted silk worms, a discovery integrally related to the understanding of anthrax spore formation. According to Pasteur, Koch purposefully ignored this work so that he would not have to credit Pasteur, while he (Koch) was in the process of conducting the etiological experimentation. To counter Koch's charge of using impure cultures, Pasteur reminded him of his work, from 1856 to 1876, on fermentation and on the search for the responsible microbes. Since Koch's serious work on bacteria *began* in 1876, Pasteur reminds his German colleague of all that he (Koch) owed to predecessors, namely to Davaine (1863), Chauveau (1868), Obermeier (1868), and Klebs (1872), whose earlier efforts formed the groundwork of his discovery. In light of Pasteur's work on fermentation, and although he acknowledged that he was not trained in medicine, no one could rightfully dismiss his contributions to microbial etiology. As to the preparation of anthrax cultures, Pasteur noted that he used methods similar to those successfully employed in his fermentation experiments, and that he was able to maintain purity, then and now, when growing microbes in solution.

Pasteur refuted the charge that losses of vaccinated animals were higher than he cared to admit. On the contrary, Koch's interpretations of test results at Beauchery and at other test sites (countered Pasteur) were flawed because the former misread the statistics; for example, Koch states that, at Beauchery, two hundred ninety-six animals were in the vaccination trial, whereas the real count (as Pasteur has it) was six hundred seventy-two. Pasteur cites experiments proving that small animals could indeed be inoculated against anthrax, contrary to Koch's opinion. Pasteur challenged Koch's notion that natural anthrax infection was more dangerous to the sheep than anthrax infection caused by laboratory cultures. Experiments that Pasteur conducted in 1878 proved the opposite was true: inoculated cultures are 100 percent lethal, while spore-contaminated meal killed animals 33 percent of the time. Koch's vituperative language, Pasteur proclaimed, would not impede the success of the inoculative method which was aiding humanity in the struggle against refractory diseases.

Despite the acrimony between Koch and Pasteur over anthrax, which has been attributed to causes such as international competition, their work displays common features and goals. In terms of man's relation to infectious disease, these scientists had no pre-conceptual inclinations. The minds of antiquity understandably created systems and constructs to account for the phenomenon of infectious disease. Faced with unanswered questions as well, germ theorists such as Koch and Pasteur developed methods by which pathogens could be removed from the natural environment, contained in artificial ones, and cultured for microscopic study. Although, at the time, the mechanism of immunity was not understood physiologically, smallpox immunization had become commonplace by virtue of its protective effect, even though the method of immunization ran risks that today would be considered as unacceptable. Koch's work on the etiology of anthrax definitively linked the organism with the disease, and Pasteur's use of laboratory grown bacilli to immunize animals (the question of methodological accuracy notwithstanding) were complementary achievements instrumental to the control of anthrax. Despite the wrangling and the turf wars, biomedical researchers of the later nineteenth century were engaged in worthwhile endeavors. In the hands of Pasteur, of Koch, and of many others, biomedical science was working for the betterment of mankind. The most outstanding aspect of Pasteur's work was to have successfully applied Koch's method to immunization.

The incisive records of the Koch-Pasteur debate have a number of distinguishing rhetorical features as well. These essays are directed by reasonable hypotheses, based on precedent, and formed within a tradition of inquiry; they are concerned with differentiating causes from effects; in addition, they establish that certain micro-organisms produced adverse physiological effects; their experiments are systematic, and the reports describe step-by-step laboratory procedures, such as removing infected tissue from dead animals, dissecting carcasses, culturing samples (with emphases placed on temperature, time, and medium), examining colonies in detail, recording transformations, extracting culture samples for *in vivo* trials to test the effects of the sample on animals (e.g., whether the microbe proliferated *in vivo* and whether it could be communicated in series to other animals). The experiments were so complex that any omission or the slightest error could skew the findings.

Other rhetorical modalities come into play in these texts: classification and division, to understand the taxonomy of pathogens and the diseases they cause; and the comparison of one disease process to another leading to new therapies. Clarity and exactness, which we find in the prose of both Koch and Pasteur, are essential to etiological writing: statistical and descriptive elements must accurately communicate the experimental findings and the logic of a systematic procedure.

Pasteur on Puerperal Fever and on Rabies

Pasteur also contributed significantly to the research on puerperal fever. Because his contribution in this area is etiological rather than inferential in nature, I have included his work in this chapter. The paper exemplifying his views on the disease, *On the Extension of the Germ Theory to the Etiology of Certain Common Diseases*, was delivered before the French Academy of Sciences, on May 3, 1880. Pasteur analyzed cases of infected patients with the acumen of Hippocrates; but unlike "the father of medicine," he drew conclusions from these case studies.

Each hospital *observation* or casestudy involved a particular female patient stricken with the disease. The first, whom Pasteur observed on

March 12, 1878, became seriously ill during the post-partum period. He understood that the degree of infection could be ascertained through physical examination, since micro-organisms could spread to remote sites in the body. Whereas, in the first case, physical examination and specimens disclosed an abundance of different micro-organisms, a blood sample taken under sterile conditions was clear of bacteria, a fact determined after the blood was sown in chicken bouillon. But, on the next day, with the patient's condition worsening, a blood culture showed bacterial growth. On March 15th, eighteen hours before death, a blood culture taken from the foot was abundantly fertile, and the patient expired on March 16, the blood having been affected for three days. As the micro-organisms increased in number and dissemination, the patient precipitously declined.

Not only did Pasteur attain laboratory results corresponding to the patient's rapid decline, but he was also able to differentiate visually between micro-organisms that he found under the light microscope. Two were found: one that was common to furuncles (bacterial infections of hair follicles or skin glands, resulting in abscesses), and another, differing from it configuratively, that formed long chains tangling into packets like "strings of pearls" (123). More information was compiled from the autopsy. Pus was found in the stomach cavity, and blood from the basilic and femoral veins was sown and culled from other areas (i.e., from the mucous surface of the uterus, from the fallopian tubes, and from the lymphatic structures in the uterine wall). All samples yielded the new organism (the long chains), and no other organism could be identified except in the stomach pus (123–24). Persuasive biomedical information was bridging the gap between symptoms and the inferred cause. Though clinical observations, laboratory cultures, and bacteriology furnished Pasteur with a wealth of information, he had not yet arrived at a convincing diagnosis. Under the heading *Interpretation of the disease and of the death*, he incorrectly surmised that the parasite impeded the resorption of pus, and that this somehow was responsible for the fatality (124).

In the cases that followed, Pasteur removed infected excretions to use in animal experiments for the purpose of determining if animals could be infected. The second observation, on March 14, was of a deceased woman who had just succumbed to the disease. Pus and blood samples taken from various parts of the body, notably from the peritoneal cavity, corresponded precisely to the previous findings: the long-chain organism appeared in culture, along with a smaller organism, a pyogenic (pus-inducing) vibrio (an organism, rigid, motile, and S-shaped).

The third observation, on May 17, 1879, was of a woman who had given birth on May 15. Both she and her nursing infant were ill. The lochia or vaginal discharges were positive for two species of troublesome bacteria. When specimens were cultured, both organisms appeared; in her breast milk was found the ominous, long-chain bacteria, implicated as one cause of puerperal fever. The mother died and was not autopsied. On May 28th, with the help of attending physicians, Pasteur inoculated a rabbit under the skin of the abdomen with five drops of the vibrio culture associated with the skin lesions. In one day, the rabbit developed huge, hard abscesses, and on June 8 the lesions opened spontaneously to exude "cheesy pus." The abscesses enlarged but continued to drain until finally, in July, the lesion closed and the rabbit was well (124–25). Pasteur's experiments revealed how damaging the organism could be to the post-partum woman if it got into the bloodstream. The vibrio (which appeared in pairs under the microscope), in Pasteur's opinion, was much more dangerous than the unidentified long-chain organism. Since both organisms lived naturally on "the mucous surfaces of the genital tract," and since both threatened the mother's health, Pasteur realized that more than one microbe could be responsible for puerperal fever.

Laboratory results of a post-partum woman who had died on June 14 were revealing. Cultured pus taken from an arm abscess was filled with the long-chain organism, while a cultured blood sample was sterile. During the autopsy on June 16, additional specimens were drawn: blood from an arm vein, along with pus from the uterine walls and from the synovial sac of the knee. All three cultures contained long-chain bacteria. Apparently, the uterus had been injured during confinement, producing pus; and this wound "gave a lodging place for the germs of the long chains of granules," which probably passed through the lymphatic system, to the joints, and to other sites; in this way, the infection spread to remote sites and abscesses developed and eventually caused death (126). Despite the outcome, Pasteur had completed the picture.

On June 17, Pasteur learned that the blood of a newborn whose mother had had "febrile symptoms with chills" prior to birth was positive for pyogenic vibrio. Yet blood taken from the mother on the morning of her death (on June 18), along with subsequent specimens, was negative. The June 19 autopsy of the mother was normal, except for the liver which contained metastatic abscesses; notably, pus cultured from the liver showed the presence of vibrio. Pasteur interpreted the findings to mean that the vibrio, which was found naturally in the uterus, or which may already have been in the mother's body before birth, had spread from that site to the liver, inducing a purulent and fatal infection (126).

A sixth case followed a predictable course. A post-partum woman was reported ill on June 18, 1879. On June 20, blood taken from her finger was found to be sterile. On July 15, the blood was cultured and again found to be sterile. Yet the woman was dangerously ill, even though no organism was "distinctly recognizable in the lochia" (126). She died on July 18. An autopsy revealed significant infection in the pleura, the membranes separating the lungs. Pus nodules were also discovered on the external surface of the uterus, as well as in the shoulder. Even though the blood was sterile, long-chain bacteria were found in three distinct areas: the pleura, the shoulders, and the uterine lymphatics. Pasteur interpreted this to mean that *an infection, beginning in the uterus, had spread to distant sites, causing death* (127; italics added).

The seventh observation, dated June 18, involved a woman who had undergone an embryotomy, and whose post-operative condition had raised some concerns. The lochia specimen sown on the June 18 was negative for bacterial growth, so Pasteur assumed that she would recover, and she did. The pus forming at the surgical site also dissipated.

Pasteur's clinical, histological, and serological studies greatly illuminated the obscure world of infectious disease. He concludes that puerperal fever is a class of related diseases and the result of the growth of "common organisms," naturally existing on the skin and mucous surfaces, and that these organisms "infect the pus naturally formed on injured surfaces and then spread, by the blood and lymphatics, to various localities in the body," eventually inducing "morbid changes varying with the condition of the parts, the nature of the parasite, and the general constitution of the subject" (128). Pasteur did not realize that pus, liquid plasma accumulating in the immune response, contained phagocytes that engulfed bacteria, along with decomposed body tissues, infectious microbes, and other blood products. It was obvious to Pasteur that, if antiseptics such as carbolic and boric acid had been used during confinement, infection could have been prevented. He proposed that sterilized boric-acid compresses be made available for use before and after delivery (129). So the problem of localized infection in the uterus, which Semmelweis and Holmes did not address, was finally solved.

Pasteur's development of rabies immunization is one of the greatest examples of inferentiality in the history of medicine, made all the more amazing because the existence of the pathogen was known only through its dreadful, convulsive effects (de Kruif 167–68). While developing the rabies vaccine, Pasteur learned that the culturing techniques perfected by Koch for the study of bacteria would not work for microscopically-invisible organisms that were so minute as to pass through the finest filter. At the outset, Pasteur proceeded on the assumption that the cause of rabies was a bacterium but discovered otherwise when he was unable to grow any organism in conventional media (109). At this juncture, he conceived of the idea of using "susceptible tissues of experimental animals, instead of sterile nutrient solutions" as a way of growing and of storing the pathogen (110). In "Prevention of Rabies: A Method by which the Development of Rabies after a Bite May Be Prevented" (1885), Pasteur used intracranial inoculations to infect dogs with rabies and, in the process, to make them immune to the virus.

Pasteur sought a valid animal model that would lead the way to human treatment. Of all laboratory animals, he determined that the neurological tissue of rabbits was the most efficient medium in which to grow, and from which to harvest, live virus. His experimentation began in November 1882 and continued into 1885. His method was to dissect the dead rabbits, to preserve the infected spinal cords as viral media, and to inject the infected tissue into dogs in order to induce immunity to the virus gradually. He insisted on precision. In a letter of July 19, 1883, for example, he urged his young assistant, Louis Thuillier, to pay attention to important details: only specific breeds of dogs "considered as safe and sure" are to be used, and he reminds his colleague, Pierre Paul Emile Roux, to instruct the lab technician "as to the trepanation of the rabbits and the extraction of brains from rabid rabbits, so that the rabbit series will not be interrupted" (*Correspondence* 217).

Each day, Pasteur and his colleagues suspended in flasks morsels of fresh, infected spinal cord from a rabbit that had died of rabies after a seven-day incubation period; the air in the flask was kept dry by placing fragments of potash at the bottom. As a daily routine, Pasteur then inoculated a dog under the skin with a syringe-full of sterilized broth in which small fragments of one or more spinal cords had been broken up. He commenced the series with a spinal cord that was old (its dates ascertained by previous experiments) and determined to be invirulent (the older the cord, the lower the virulence). On the succeeding days, he conducted the same operation with newer cords, separated from each other by forty-eight hour intervals, until he was ready to use the most virulent cord that had been in the flask for two days, a relatively brief period of time. This method never failed. As a result, Pasteur gradually induced 100 percent immunity in fifty dogs, an extraordinary achievement. Yet a gulf existed at this point between the canine trials and the practice of using a vaccine in human beings. Pasteur inferred that an anti-rabies vaccine would work for human beings but, as things stood, he could not prove this experimentally.

At this eventful moment, and as if preordained, three desperate people from Alsace, Germany, unexpectedly arrived at Pasteur's lab. The date was Monday, July 6, 1885. One was Mr. Theodore Vone, a grocer of Meissengott, a town near Schlestadt, Germany. He had been attacked, although not bitten, by his own dog which had contracted rabies. Nine-year-old Joseph Meister, accompanied by his mother, was not as fortunate. On July 4, at 8 A.M., the child had been knocked to the ground, mauled, bitten *fourteen times*, and found covered with blood and foamy saliva. His wounds were cauterized at 8 P.M. and disinfected with phenic acid, but the physician, Dr. Weber, knew that the boy was doomed; the dog, it had been determined, was indeed rabid and had been ingesting wood, straw, and hay. Pasteur and his colleagues assured Vone that, since he had not been bitten, he was safe (although coming into close contact with such an animal nowadays could warrant treatment). Pasteur realized that Meister had but one chance: the untried vaccine. Though tedious, the animal trials had worked. But would the vaccine work on human beings? The inference had to be tried out, and the opportunity to put it into praxis was before him in the person of young Joseph Meister.

On July 6, at the weekly meeting of the Académie des Sciences, Pasteur who was a biochemist discussed the case with his medical associates. They agreed that, in view of the number of bites the child had suffered, he was almost certain to die of rabies. Pasteur explained the new results of his work on rabies, updating them on research reported at an 1884 meeting in Copenhagen. Pasteur recalled how he then decided, "not without lively and sore anxiety," to apply his method to the boy. The fifty laboratory dogs that he had immunized were inoculated with the laboratory-grown virus, but none of them had contracted the disease naturally through a bite. Though he had had some success with bitten dogs, the efficacy of his treatment in the case of bites could only be inferred since he had not conducted extensive trials. But there was no time.

On July 6, 1885, at 8 P.M., sixty hours after Meister had been attacked, Pasteur in the presence of his colleagues inoculated the boy using one-half of a Pravaz' syringe containing the spinal cord of a rabbit that had died of rabies on June 2; the cord, hanging in a flask of dry air, had been preserved from June 2 to July 6 and contained dead organisms. Over a ten-day period, the boy received a series of fresh inoculations composed of prepared rabbit spinal cord: from day one to five (i.e., on July 6, 7, 8, 9, and 10, respectively), he received dead virus; from day six to ten (on July 11, 12, [13 is omitted], 14, 15, and 16, respectively), he received live virus in progressively higher concentrations and virulence. The uninfected rabbits inoculated on July 15 contracted rabies after a seven-day incubation period. Those of July 12 and 14 developed the disease after eight days, and those of July 11 developed the disease after fifteen days.

For the tenth inoculation, Pasteur utilized an extremely virulent serum, one that had produced rabies after seven days' incubation in rabbits and after eight or ten days in dogs. When the condition of immunity had theoretically been reached, Meister was to receive, and was expected to tolerate, the most virulent strain; the final stage of the treatment was done to ensure immunity.

Joseph Meister survived, thanks to his immune system's response to a rabies strain more lethal than that normally found in dogs. There was a tense waiting period after the final inoculation. For Pasteur knew that, if immunity had not been secured, this strain would manifest itself faster than one incurred from a bite. Fifteen weeks after the incident, on October 25, Joseph Meister was declared cured. Pasteur replicated his treatment for many others (Wills 228).

Pasteur was jubilant but realized soberly that his new method preventing rabies after bites required further experimentation in order eventually to adopt "the best of the various possible interpretations" (34). Pasteur was chiefly concerned about predictability with respect to the attenuation of the lethal viruses and the method of achieving prophylaxis. These essential factors, hinging on relatively commonplace factors such as air temperature in flasks, had to be precisely defined.

More than a decade after his successful application of Jenner's techniques to the etiology of rabies, scientists were able to isolate subcellular organisms or what we know today as *viruses*. In 1898 Friedrich Löffler and Paul Frosch in Germany discovered that whatever caused foot-and-mouth disease in cattle passed through porcelain filters and, if inoculated into healthy cattle, induced the disease (149–53). Löffler and Frosch inferred from this result that, if "a minute living being" were indeed responsible for foot-and-mouth disease, other elusive pathogens (smallpox and others) "may also belong to this smallest group of organisms" (152). Dimitri Ivanovski, in 1892, and Martinus Beijerinck, in 1899, showed that the organism responsible for tobacco mosaic disease could pass through the minuscule pores of the Pasteur-Chamberland filter without becoming inactive; the filtrate, they found, contained a virulent property that could induce the disease in tobacco plants (Oldstone 13–14). Beijerinck concluded, in his paper "A *contagium vivum fluidum* as the cause of the mosaic disease of tobacco leaves," that a small amount of virus could infect a large number of leaves, and that the virus exists outside the tobacco plant but cannot reproduce unless introduced or combined with the "living protoplasm of the host plant" (155–56).

An amazing recent medical report rekindles the excitement that must have been felt in July 1885 with the cure of Joseph Meister. In October 2004, the CDC reported that on September 12 a young woman in Fond du Lac, Wisconsin, contracted rabies from a bat that had bitten her at a church service. Because the bite was small and seemed like a scratch, there was no medical evaluation. On October 18, however, she developed symptoms of rabies: slurred speech, fluctuating consciousness, and other symptoms. Once symptoms appear, however, it is too late to administer Pasteur's vaccine. Doctors, equipped with medicine and inspired by a hunch (an inference), decided to induce a coma and, as a last-ditch measure, to give her four anti-viral medications, the identities of which were not disclosed, pending publication of the event in a medical journal. She recovered. The rigors of scientific investigation require that the treatment be duplicated in order to determine which of the four drugs, alone or in combination, was responsible for the cure. Her case has rightly been called historic: she is "the first human ever to survive rabies without vaccination" (Rosenthal A28).

3. Yersin, Kitasato, Simond and the Bubonic Plague

The gram-negative bacillus, *Yersinia pestis*, is the cause of bubonic plague (McGovern and Friedlander 480–81; "Plague," CDC). The disease is transmitted from animals to man (thus, it is an *enzootic* disease), most commonly from a variety of rodents to which the disease is endemic. If the disease erupts amidst a rodent population, it is called an *epizootic*. As the rats die off, the parasites then seek a suitable food source, whether buffalo, cat, or man. Their blood-feeding causes them to regurgitate micro-organisms into the bodies of their hosts; in this manner, the disease is spread to mammals. Responsible for three great pandemics (in the sixth, in the fourteenth, and in the late nineteenth and early twentieth century, respectively), the disease causes a high fever and painful lymph-node swellings. When the infection reaches the bloodstream from the initial flea bite/regurgitation, the host suffers from septicemic plague. The most dangerous form of the disease, however, is plague pneumonia or pneumonic plague. A secondary form, it is usually the result of human-to-human contact: one can inhale infected droplets from a coughing patient; thus, the disease can spread like influenza.

The historical focus of our discussion is the third pandemic. In 1894 a plague outbreak in China spread throughout the world, as a result of maritime commerce and international travel (Kohn, 268–69; Snodgrass 293–94). That year, Alexandre Emile Jean Yersin (1863–1943), a Swiss bacteriologist, discovered the bacillus, which he called *Pasteurella pestis* (in honor of Louis Pasteur), and he prepared a serum against it. While Yersin used Koch's postulates as a means of proving that the bacillus caused the disease, he was unaware that rats were the enzootic reservoir of the pathogen, and that fleas transmitted the microbe through bites. These facts came to light through the work of Paul-Louis Simond (1858–1947) who discovered that the flea ingested the infected blood from the rat (the primary host) and disgorged it into the human body (its secondary host). The reason why fleas leave rats for human beings is that, during the epizootic, rodents die in great numbers, and the fleas which will not feed on carcasses must find other mammalian blood sources (e.g., livestock, domestic animals, and human beings) (Chin 382). According to one authority, "naturally-acquired plague in people occurs as a result of human intrusion into the zoonotic (also termed sylvatic or rural) cycle during or following an epizootic" (Chin 382). In other words, man stumbles into the plague cycle.

According to the CDC's outline of the plague's natural history, in 1894 the independent work of Alexandre Yersin and of Shibasaburo Kitasato (1852–1931), a Japanese bacteriologist who developed tetanus antitoxin and anthrax serum, led to the discovery of the bacillus ("Plague," CDC). Their efforts in Hong Kong made it possible for later researchers to find out how the disease spread. Both Kitasato and Yersin described the presence of bipolar organisms in the lymph nodes, in the blood, and in the organs of decedents. They drew cultures from these tissue specimens, inoculated these substances into laboratory animals such as mice, and the animals exhibited characteristic symptoms, dying rapidly. The investigation was brought full circle when dissections showed that the injected animals contained the bacillus originally found in human cadavers.

Neither Yersin nor Kitasato understood how the disease was transmitted. In 1898, Simond recognized that persons contracting the disease need not have been in close proximity to someone already infected. He inferred that rats were connected with the epidemic when he learned that Chinese in Yunnan Province ran away from their homes if dead rats appeared. Formosans recognized that handling rats increased the risk of plague, even though they were unaware that the flea was the vector. Observations of human behavior and of the environment (notably that widespread rat deaths preceded human outbreaks) led Simond to suspect that the flea was an "intermediary factor" in the epidemic. Once again, popular observations stimulated biomedical inference and experimentation.

Four classic texts (paraphrased and analyzed below) will occupy our attention in this section. Yersin's, "La Peste Bubonique à Hong-Kong" (1894), Kitasato's, "The Bacillus of Bubonic Plague" (1894), and Simond's, "La propagation de la peste," (1898) and "Comment fut mis en évidence le rôle de la puce dans la transmission de la peste" (1936) describe how researchers entered forbidden plague worlds, tested their hunches systematically, and, with astounding courage, struggled with one of the most terrifying diseases that has ever afflicted mankind.

In early May 1894, Yersin recounts that a deadly outbreak of bubonic plague erupted in Hong Kong. The epidemic raged for a long time on the high plateaus of Yunnan and intermittently recurred near the French Indo-Chinese possessions in Mong-Tze, Long-Tcheow and Pakhoi. The substantial commerce existing between Canton, Hong Kong, and Tonkin (Viet Nam), along with the difficulty of establishing effective quarantines on the coastlines of these countries, convinced the French government that Indo-China would not escape the epidemic. Thus, the Minister of the colonies ordered Yersin to Hong Kong to study the nature of the outbreak and the conditions under which it spread. Furthermore, he was commissioned to discover the most effective way of preventing it from reaching the French colonies. Thus, Yersin was to undertake etiological and epidemiological work in the field.

By the time Yersin arrived in Hong Kong on June 15, 1894, more than three hundred Chinese had already died of plague. His team hastily constructed temporary barracks, since the colonial hospital was no longer able to shelter the sick. With the authorization of the British government, Yersin set himself up with his laboratory equipment in a makeshift straw hut within the courtyard of the hospital.

In his paper, Yersin summarizes the history of the disease. Widespread exclusively in the Chinese quarters of the village, the current outbreak exhibited clinical characteristics of the bubonic plague that, in past ages, had decimated areas from Western Europe to the Levant. This terrible disease, quiescent since the end of the second pandemic in the fourteenth century, had flared up repeatedly in London from the sixteenth to seventeenth century and notoriously in Marseilles, in 1720, an episode that happened to be the last on record to afflict France. Up to 1894, the disease had been mostly confined to limited foci in Persia, in Arabia, and in the Chinese province of Yunnan.

Describing the well-known clinical aspects of the disease encountered in the field, Yersin writes that, after an incubation period of up to six days, the infection causes acute fatigue, prostration, high fever, and delirium. During the first day, widespread and egg-size lymph-node swellings appear, 75 percent of which are in the groin, 10 percent in the armpit, but rarely any in the neck or in other regions of the upper body. Death ensues in about forty-eight hours and frequently much sooner. When life is prolonged five or six days, the prognosis improves. By that time, supple nodes can be drained of pus. Yersin observes that despite this bit of hope, the mortality rate, even in the hospital, was an astonishing 95 percent.

Yersin's team tried to track down the cause of the disease. The correlation between environmental conditions (i.e., insanitation, polluted water, and stench) and the presence of contagious disease was foremost in his mind. Observing that, in the infected quarter, decomposing rat carcasses were strewn about in the sun, they initially suspected that a sewer system might have been implicated in the outbreak, for in the sector of the village where the epidemic erupted and was most virulent a new drainage system had been installed. The narrow conduits of the system were separated at intervals by decantation basins that were virtually impossible to clean. As a consequence, the system was thought to be a focus of disease, especially by those who connected the plague outbreak to sewage. Yersin's colleagues conjectured that the inoperative sewers were responsible for plague, but we now know that unsanitary conditions such as these, though certainly conducive to an array of water-borne diseases (e.g., dysentery, cholera, typhoid), contributed only indirectly to the plague epidemic by providing a supportive habitat for disease-carrying rodents.

Pursuing the public-works issue because it was a flagrant health concern, Yersin explains that there were two kinds of drainage systems in Hong Kong: a large, functional one conducting rainwater runoff; and another line, obstructed with contaminants, used for household waste water (including human waste) and for domestic garbage. To mitigate these conditions, the city installed mobile latrines that could be cleaned and replaced everyday; human waste, thereafter, was used to fertilize flower gardens bordering the Canton River, opposite the island of Hong Kong. Yersin did not say if the outbreak diminished after these measures had been taken (the likelihood is that it had not).

The next area of investigation was that part of the village the epidemic had not yet reached. Yersin and his inspectors were shocked to see how the Chinese peasants lived. One could not enter their hovels because of the crowded, unsanitary conditions. Many huts lacked windows and were situated directly beneath the sun. Yersin shuddered to think what would happen if the plague were to reach this locality, inasmuch as it would be difficult, if not impossible, to control there. The only prophylactic remedy was to evacuate the people and to burn down the village; apparently, this tactic had been proposed before Yersin's investigation, but, for some reason, it had not been carried out. At this point in time, Yersin's workers continued to associate unsanitary conditions with plague.

The upscale European quarter was another area of investigation. At that time, few Europeans had been stricken by the disease, probably because they lived in areas distant from current infection-sites, and because their living conditions were better than those of the indigenous Chinese. Their homes, it turned out, were not absolutely safe: European residents were finding dead rats, suggesting that plague was not far away. Although Yersin did not yet understand the intricacies of the plague cycle (i.e., its three phases of transmission: rodent-to-flea. flea-to human, and human-to-human), he was right to suspect that the dead rats were ominous. The local Chinese physicians who had observed the epidemics of Pakhoi and of Lien-Chu, in Canton Province, along with Monsieur Rocher, consul de France to Mong-Tze, had already remarked that, before the plague struck human beings, it broke out with great intensity among mice, rats, buffalo, and pigs, among other mammals. As they had been for Edward Jenner, common sense observations proved vital to the understanding of how this disease progressed. For Yersin, this was a unique opportunity to investigate the plague process and to uncover the connection between rodents and man. The susceptibility of certain animals to the disease provided him with favorable conditions under which he could conduct an experimental study.

The research up to 1894, Yersin was well aware, showed that a microbe existed in the blood of the sick and in the tissues of the lymph nodes. In all cases, the pulp of the lymph nodes was filled with a thick and well-rounded purée of microbes, easily tinted with aniline stain. The extremities of the bacillus, Yersin reported, were more deeply colored at the two poles than at the center (hence, the organism's bipolarity), so that a clear space appeared at the middle of the organism. One could easily retrieve large quantities of this purée from aspirated nodes and ganglia. The blood Yersin assayed sometimes contained the organism (indicating septicemia) but in less abundance than in the nodal sites. Significantly, Yersin found that the organism was more abundant in the blood of severe cases, which strengthened the argument for the causative relation between the organism and the disease. Gradually, the etiological reality was materializing.

Nodal pulp from human cadavers, if sowed on gelatin, generated undeveloped white, transparent colonies that, when illuminated, had iridescent borders. In a bouillon medium, the bacillus looked like a strain of streptococcus: its colonies, appearing as lumpy deposits, adhered to the length of the wall and to the bottom of the test tube, but the medium remained clear. Under the microscope, Yersin found that these cultures displayed short bacillus chains with large spherical bulges. If one examined this material carefully under the highest possible magnification, one could see the bacilli form slender filaments; eventually, he saw rod-shaped microbes uniting laterally into long chains.

The most difficult phase of the study was to determine if the *in vitro* culture was the lethal germ. When Yersin injected the lymph-node pulp into mice, rats, and guinea pigs, the laboratory animals died. Thus, the infectious cycle was being clarified gradually: (1) histology showed that a specific organism was present along with the disease; (2) the organism could be grown in a dish; and, (3) after it was injected into uninfected lab animals, the same disease developed. The penultimate phase of the experiment came when (4) the animals were dissected: the tissues of all species involved in the experiment exhibited lesions characteristic of the plague. A number of bacilli were (5) extracted from the animals' nodes, spleens, and blood, cultured separately, and then inoculated into other animals, to be incubated *in vivo* and at a different rate for each species; as a result, (6) guinea pigs died between two and five days; the mouse, in one to five days. Analyses of blood and tissue of the second group of animals, along with clinical observations, elicited important information; (7) the animals' immune systems were fighting the pathogen (leucocytes were apparent in the blood and had enveloped the germs); and several hours after inoculation with plague culture, a guinea pig developed a noticeable area of swelling at the injection site, and nearby ganglia became palpable. In twenty-four hours, the fur became bristly, the animal stopped eating, and then suddenly fell on its side, convulsed, and died. If one dissected the guinea pig immediately, one found swelling at the inoculation site, along with hemorrhage around the nearby ganglia which were engorged with bacteria. Red blood was in the intestines, the suprarenal capsules were congested, the kidneys were purplish-blue, and the liver was enlarged and red, all of which suggested internal bleeding. In addition, the swollen spleen frequently presented with a specific kind of eruption of the small tubercles. Yersin also discovered infected sera in the pleura and peritoneum, and rat livers were very rich in microbes.

Yersin noted anomalies. Human-to-guinea pig transferences, interestingly, did not work. To ascertain if the infection was contagious *between* non-human mammalian species, Yersin injected rat lymphatic pulp or blood into guinea pigs. Death arrived quickly after these infectious transferences. The investigators successfully recultured the original microbial strain in another medium, and new colonies developing abundantly from the original pulp. When healthy lab animals were inoculated with the newer cultures, the disease recurred but with diminished intensity. Over a very long period of time, a new possibility arose: (8) successive generations of the original bacilli appeared to have become attenuated, for samples no longer killed guinea pigs but did kill white mice. Yersin speculated, on the basis of these observations, that the less virulent colonies developed rapidly and tended to smother the others, and that successive cultures also lost their virulence very quickly. Mice and most rats died after being injected either with spleen or liver fragments from animals that had died of the plague. Dissections found bacteria in the blood, in the liver, in the spleen, and in the lymphatic system.

Dead rats retrieved from the houses and streets almost always contained a high concentration of microbes in their organs, especially in the nodes. At this point, Yersin continued to pursue the question of how the disease was communicated from animal to animal. So he placed healthy mice in the same bottle with plague mice, an experiment foreshadowing Simond's, four years later. The infected mice died first; but, on the very next day, one after another of the healthy mice died, and plague microbes showed up in their organs. How did this happen in the closed environment of the bottle? Yersin was unable to answer this crucial question definitively, although he speculated on modes of transmission. Though Yersin inferred that rats played a part in the contagion cycle (an idea borrowed from Chinese physicians), in this paper no further progress is made.

What is overlooked in the historical literature is Yersin's suspicion that insects carried the disease. This was an original idea. While in Formosa, the Japanese bacteriologist, Masanori Ogata, replicated Yersin's work in 1896, isolated the plague bacillus, and suggested in 1897 that insects played a role in the transmission of plague (Snodgrass 236). But Yersin deserves acclaim for having observed a critical anomaly in 1894: an unusual number of dead flies were scattered around tables and in cages where dead animals were housed. Suspecting that plague killed the flies, too, Yersin gathered them up, removed the legs, wings, and heads, ground the bodies up into a bouillon, and inoculated this material into a guinea pig. The fly broth, it turned out, contained a large quantity of bacilli identical to those of the plague, and the guinea pig injected with the fly-slurry exhibited characteristic plague lesions and was dead in forty-eight hours. Two possibilities could account for this chain of events: either the flies contracted the bacilli from the excrement of lab animals or, if they were biting species (the crux of the issue), they contracted it from blood-feeding. In the context of the paper, however, Yersin failed to identify the species of dead fly that he had discovered and whether or not it was a blood-feeder (as are females of the *Tabanidae* family, for instance). On the threshold of a momentous discovery — that is, of finding a vector linking rats to man in the infective process— Yersin's inquiry concluded.

Yersin's ability to isolate the pathogen contributed to the development of an anti-plague vaccine. From cultures sown from blood or from plague-infected nodes, Yersin isolated a variety of pathogens with differing levels of virulence in animals, and he concluded from this procedure that certain colonies had become innocuous in guinea pigs. In fact, he obtained several colonies absolutely devoid of virulence for mice. The mechanism of attenuation, however, remained a mystery. Human-to-animal contagion was established when Yersin extracted virulent microbes from a patient who had recovered fifteen days earlier from septicemia. Blood serum drawn from the septicemic patient retained its virulence when injected into mice and guinea pigs. Yersin knew that serum could carry immunizing properties, so he wondered if plague serum could confer immunity against the disease. In the heritage of Jenner, and even though he was dealing with a bacillus, Yersin inferred that blood products exposed to the plague might actually stimulate immunity. The Russian physician, Waldemar M. W. Haffkine (1860–1930), while working in India in 1897 would create the first plague vaccine which consisted of killed whole cells (McGovern and Friedlander 498). And, in 1914, William Bacot (1866–1922) and Charles James Martin (1866–1955), staff members at the Lister Institute, London, determined the plague's exact mechanism of infection (Parish 86).

Guided by Koch's postulates, Yersin began his groundbreaking work with the reasonable assumption that dead rats were involved in the infectious process. Whether they were the reservoir of some disease or collateral victims was not immediately clear. Macroscopic examination of human sera cultured *in vitro* showed abundant bacterial growth, and microscopic study revealed what is today described as a gram-negative, inert, nonsporiferous bacillus (initially called *Pasteurella pestis* and renamed *Yersinia pestis* after Yersin himself) ("Plague," CDC) that made filaments and chains. These minute organisms, if injected into laboratory animals, were lethal. When the dead animals were dissected, the researchers found pathology corresponding to that found in rats and in humans. *In vitro* cultures infected different species, thus confirming that the disease was not confined to humans. An *in vivo* experiment, in which infected and healthy rats were housed together, was positive for transmission, although it is not clear from Yersin's paper if the healthy rat was bitten by the sick one. Though the mode of initial transmission of the disease (i.e., from infected flea to man) had yet to be established, Yersin strongly suspected that insects were involved in the process, as he identified flies as a vector and even tested this hypothesis briefly, achieving positive results. Yersin's interdisciplinary approach (e.g., bacteriology, clinical practice, human and veterinary pathology, entomology, and epidemiology) moved the world closer to a comprehensive understanding of the etiology and prevention of bubonic plague.

Written on July 7, 1894 and published on August 25, 1894, Kitasato's paper exemplifies the etiological mode and can profitably be compared to Yersin's paper. Working independently of Yersin, Kitasato writes that, from May to August 25, 1894, bubonic plague had spread widely in southern China, from Canton to Hong Kong. In response, the Japanese government sent a commission to Hong Kong to study the plague's bacteriological and pathological characteristics. Kitasato was the resident bacteriologist, and Professor Aoyama was the medical expert. The expedition left Japan on June 5 and arrived in Hong Kong on June 12. The Acting Superintendent of the Government Civil Hospital, Dr. Lowson, conducted them to the

Kennedy Town Hospital, the only institution in the colony specializing in the treatment of plague. At this institution, they began work on June 14. Hong Kong authorities knew that the plague had arrived via maritime traffic from Yunnan province where it was endemic.

The medical content of Kitasato's paper is more substantive than Yersin's. Aoyama's post-mortem findings revealed that plague decedents had enlarged inguinal nodes and bacilli in the heart, lungs, liver, and spleen; unfortunately, since post-mortem examinations were done eleven hour after death, their reliability was compromised. Nonetheless, he reported that the lymph-node sites were swollen, black to red in color, and oozed gelatinous material; in addition, the spleen was often enlarged. The period of incubation appeared to be three to five or as long as eight days. Lymph-node swelling, a prominent symptom, could have antedated, coincided with, or even followed, the onset of fever and severe pain. The femoral chain of lymph nodes was affected initially, followed by the inguinal, axillary, and cervical chains; the tongue was often furry, grayish-white or dark brown in color; headaches, delirium, and cardiovascular symptoms occurred, occasionally vomiting and diarrhea as well, which were often forerunners of fever. Survivors generally had temperatures for one week and convalesced slowly; the gender and age of a patient appeared irrelevant. The examination of blood usually disclosed bacilli. Of thirty patients, twenty-five were positive for septicemia, two were negative, and two were negative for plague (one was unaccounted for). Kitasato acknowledged that, with the techniques then available, it was difficult to detect bacilli in the blood.

While Aoyama was at work on autopsies, Kitasato was conducting microbiological studies in accordance with Koch's postulates. Unlike Yersin, Kitasato had ample facilities and equipment, and his bacteriological description is more detailed than Yersin's, in the 1894 paper. Kitasato easily replicated Yersin's first transmissive procedure: that is, to inoculate lab mice with sera from the spleens of human plague victims. Observing strict precautions, he also took fingertip blood from a sick patient who had enlarged nodes in the upper body and a temperature of 40.5 degrees C. Under the microscope, Kitasato found encapsulated bacilli that stained more deeply at the poles than in the middle. The inert germs were rod-like and rounded at the ends, and those incubated in beef solution clouded the mixture. The growth of the bacilli was greatest in the blood. At normal temperature in the human body (98.6 degrees F. / 34 degrees C.), the culture grew luxuriantly in agar-agar jelly or in glyerine agar, was moist in consistency, was yellowish-gray to the eye, and did not liquefy in the serum. Under the microscope, the microbes had a whitish-gray color and a bluish appearance in reflected light. The organisms congregated in moist, rounded patches with uneven edges and were piled up everywhere like glass wool and appeared to have large, dense centers. Significantly, had Kitasato used agar-agar jelly and then stained the colony, he no doubt would have viewed long threads of bacilli.

Puncture cultivations in jelly medium performed at ordinary temperature were also productive, yielding in only a few days the growth of bacilli in the form of fine dust around the puncture. Using potato-slice cultures at 28 to 30 degrees C., he found no growth after ten days' observation. But, at 37 degrees C., bacilli developed sparingly in a few days and in the form of whitish gray and dry clumps. It became clear that the bacilli grew best from 36 to 39 degrees C. (i.e., at human body temperature), but at how low a temperature growth began was not known. He was certain, based upon these observations, that the organism did not form spores.

On June 15, all sera cultivations taken from cadaver organs and from the fingertips of living patients showed the growth of micro-organisms. The organisms in both cases looked identical to one another, except that the post-mortem cultures produced organisms that were longer and that stained more easily than those taken from the blood of living patients. Kitasato inoculated mice, guinea pigs, rabbits, and pigeons with the sera. The mice inoculated with autopsied spleen tissue and fingertip blood died in two days. Post-mortem examinations of the mice revealed edema at the inoculation sites and the very same bacilli in the blood and in the internal organs. With the exception of the pigeons, all laboratory animals died in one to four days (at rates in direct proportion to body size), and all showed the same pathological signs. In effect, Kitasato had duplicated Yersin's experiment and compiled valuable physiological information on the effects of the disease.

The Japanese team carefully examined patients in an effort to isolate the pathogen. Blood samples revealed the presence of the bacilli described above (i.e., the bi-polar ovoid) and in varying concentrations. The most important conclusion was that, *at every post-mortem examination*, they found the same bacilli concentrated in the lymph nodes, spleen, lungs, liver, and blood, as well as in the heart, brain, intestines, and, without exception, in all internal organs (italics added). Every cultivation engendered from a particle of infected tissue invariably produced the same bacilli. For instance, if one simply rubbed a piece of spleen on a cover-glass, stained the cover-glass with methyl blue, and then examined the slide under the microscope, one found the same organism on both the slide and in the pure colony. The deduction that he drew was incontrovertible: *the pathogenic organisms proliferating in the human body were identical to those grown in isolation* (italics added).

In the human splenetic tissue under examination, bacilli aggregated in heaps. Kitasato reasserted that any cultivation produced the same form of bacilli. Pure cultivations of tissue and of blood proved, beyond doubt, that the organism and the disease were intimately connected. If one inoculated mice, rats, guinea pigs, or rabbits with pure cultivations, with infected blood from a plague patient, with lymph-node contents, or with organ or intestinal tissue, the laboratory animals contracted the disease in one to two days. Their eyes became watery, and they became lethargic, avoided food, hid in their cages, developed temperatures of 41.5 degrees C., convulsed, and died in two to five days. The size of the animal, as noted above, was a significant factor in this process insofar as the rapidity of the infection was concerned. Experiments on large animals showed that life could be prolonged. The laboratory animals uniformly presented with a reddish exudation infiltrating the site of inoculation, enlarged spleens, swollen lymph nodes, and bacilli in all organs. Kitasato's team also observed that, in Hong Kong, many rats and mice died spontaneously, and mice, in particular, harbored the microbe in internal organs.

Whereas Yersin initially focused on sanitation as a way of preventing plague, Kitasato tested disinfectants. To determine if the plague organism could resist chemical agents, the Japanese scientist wiped the contents of infected lymph nodes over cover-glasses that had been heated and alcohol-cleansed to remove other organisms. The cover-glasses were then air-dried at 28 to 30 degrees C.; other samples were exposed to sunlight (for one, two, and three hours, respectively, for up to six days). He removed culture material from dishes, placed the specimen in beef-tea, and then incubated each of the samples. Those that had been in the room more than four days showed no growth, even after one week's incubation. After three to four hours, colonies exposed to direct sunlight were all destroyed. Those in beef-tea, heated for thirty minutes in an 80 degrees C. water bath, were entirely destroyed, and those placed in a vapor apparatus heated to 100 degrees C. were destroyed in minutes. It was clear, therefore, that *mild heat* destroyed the plague bacillus (italics added).

In carbolic acid and quicklime, authorities had an effective disinfectant for wide-scale use in villages. To test the effectiveness of chemical disinfectants further, Kitasato gradually added measured quantities of the acid to culture media: to every ten cubic centimeters of growing beef-tea cultivation standing in an incubator for two to three days, he poured acid in three strengths (one-half, three-quarters, and one percent of the whole, respectively); he did this to ascertain the effectiveness of each concentration. The mixed samples were left at room temperature. From each of these cultivations, Kitasato took a few drops and placed them into sterilized beef-tea containers. The mixtures were left to incubate for one, two, and three hours, respectively. After having stood at room temperature for one hour, the plague cultivations with one-half percent and with three-quarters percent carbolic acid grew in the incubator after two days; the one-percent cultivations, having stood for one hour, did not grow after one week in the incubator; and the one-half percent acid solution, having stood for two hours, showed no growth, a condition persisting for one week in the incubator. Cultivations with one-percent acid strength destroyed the microbe completely. Quicklime was also bactericidal, more so than carbolic acid. Beef-tea cultivations of one-half percent quicklime grew sparingly after two hours, while one-percent concentrations stopped the bacilli entirely. Whereas carbolic acid at one-half percent failed to kill the plague over a two-day trial period, quicklime did so in only three hours.

Though Kitasato was able to diagnose bubonic plague from the examination of blood, technically this was no easy task. By 1894, scientists had found only two micro-organisms in blood: the microbe that caused anthrax and that which caused relapsing fever, respectively. The blood of plague victims had a bacillus that had never been seen before; it was abundantly present in lymph material, in the blood, and in internal organs. In animals, after injection of infected tissue, it was possible to produce effects identical to those in human beings. Thus, Kitasato concluded unequivocally that the bacillus under investigation caused bubonic plague.

In the final analysis, neither Yersin nor Kitasato determined how the bacillus entered the body. Kitasato's group posited that the disease could be spread either through respiration, external wounds, or ingestion (some laboratory animals, he thought, developed the disease through feeding). To test these postulates, the Kitasato team, like Yersin's contingent, began fieldwork among the Chinese. The former concentrated on Tai Ping Shan village, one of many hardest hit during the epidemic. They observed that these dwellings were filthy and unfit for human habitation. Although the connection between unsanitary living conditions and the plague was not explicit, common sense dictated that preventive measures, such as general hygiene, good drainage, cleanliness in the houses and streets (especially removal of animal and human feces), and purification of the water supply, had to have a mollifying effect. Yersin was thinking along these lines, too. In addition, it became policy in Tai Ping Shan and in similar locales that, when the epidemic broke out, the sick had to be isolated from the healthy. Thanks to Kitasato's work on disinfectants, household dwellings were cleansed effectively, not with the minimum strength of one-percent carbolic acid, but rather with two-percent solutions of the acid or with quicklime.

Reminiscent of civic measures instituted in Pistoia, Italy, nearly five hundred and fifty years earlier, the Kitasato team made a number of recommendations: wearing apparel, linen, and bedding were to be steam-disinfected for one hour at 100 degrees C. or sun-dried for hours as an alternative; articles unfit for use were to be burned; corpses had to be cremated or interred (in the latter case, the corpse had to be covered with quicklime and buried at three meters' depth); mice and rats that died spontaneously of plague had to be disposed of cautiously; and patients who recovered were to be isolated for one month. The team realized that, for three to four weeks after symptoms ceased, bacilli still persisted in the convalescent's blood, so there remained a risk of contagion, the exact modality of which was as yet unknown. Isolation was essential: individuals were advised to keep away from plague houses and from patients. On the possibility of naturally-acquired immunity, a theory to which Yersin subscribed and one that he would subsequently explore, Kitasato had no opinion, at least not in this paper.

The third scientist to contribute significantly to our understanding of plague etiology is the medical missionary, Paul-Louis Simond. He discovered that rat-fleas communicated the bubonic plague, and he published his findings in the 1898 paper "La Propagation de la Peste." Simond recapitulated the circumstances of his experiment in a 1936 paper, "Comment fut mis en évidence le rôle de la puce dans la transmission de la peste."

Simond recollects that, in 1898, the scientific missions of England, of Germany, and of Italy were preoccupied with the plague outbreak in Bombay, India. From conversations with European colleagues, he learned that three theories had been propounded to explain plague transmission: (1) the agent was spread through excrement, both human and animal; (2) it was inhaled when mixed in with dust and spread as particulates (contagion via particulates could also occur through excoriated skin and through mucous membranes); (3) and it could be ingested in contaminated food (as suggested by an intestinal form of plague). European medical professionals came to these conclusions on the basis of observations made in Bombay, one of which was that impoverished villagers who habitually walked barefoot in contaminated dirt probably contracted the disease through cuts in their feet. The findings of Yersin and of Kitasato, apparently, had not impressed the Bombay researchers. For example, the investigators in India, after having conducted redundant experiments in 1898, came to the following conclusions: (1) plague bacillus was not viable outdoors; (2) the microbe died in moderate heat; and, (3) unlike anthrax bacillus, it did not form spores. These findings replicated Kitasato's 1894 work.

Simond was skeptical about the popular theories, but it is not clear if the work of Yersin and of Kitasato influenced his thinking. Observations and common sense did serve Simond well. The rapidity with which the plague spread perplexed him. He tried to make sense of the facts at hand: for example, sometimes a person caught the plague while in close proximity to a sick person, but sometimes not, since cases were found more than a kilometer from infected villages (the possibility that a person might contract the plague in one place and then travel to another was not raised). New cases neither dwelled in the infected village nor had any suspicious contacts before the appearance of the plague in their area. So how were they exposed? At this point, Simond was inclined to agree with his European colleagues who thought the disease had been transported atmospherically. For one thing, that theory explained away geographical anomalies. Eventually, however, he came to agree with Yersin and others, inferring that the rat epizootic, rather than a plague cloud, was the source of the disease; but, unlike them, he transformed this inference into a hypothesis.

It was common knowledge that the plague killed rats before it struck people, and that this had happened in Bombay. Even though the epizootic and the epidemic were consecutive events, Simond realized that did not mean the former was causally related to the latter. To make the transition from inference to etiology, he learned all he could about local opinion on rat-to-human contagion. One anecdote stood out in his mind: in many cases, when someone threw a dead plague rat out of a home, usually by the end of the tail, the thrower developed symptoms of the plague in two or three days. It was plausible, he thought, that prolonged contact with dead rats had something to do with transmission of the disease. In a local food warehouse, Simond examined native workers employed to clear the facility. The workers regularly collected and disposed of dead rats. Many of the men who swept the place while barefoot, and those who threw out dead rats and excrement using dust pans (even if careful not to touch anything), manifested plague symptoms in just four days. These observations bolstered the theory of European investigators that plague entered the body via inhaled dust or through the skin; in this sense, they were likening the plague microbe to anthrax or to another spore-forming microbe (we now know that certain viruses, such as hanta, can be inhaled via dry rodent excreta). In the late 1890s, the question of absorption remained unanswered: did rats and other mammals absorb the infectious agent through the skin and mucous membranes, through respiration, or through ingestion? The researchers of 1894 had made a breakthrough in definitively showing that the plague bacillus was a frail creature if exposed to the elements, precisely because it did not have the ability to form protective spores.

Simond was dissatisfied with the theory of absorption, for he suspected that rats played a crucial and unrecognized role in the cycle of disease. Anomalies related to contagion had yet to be explained; for example, at times, a rather insignificant contact with dead rats was sufficient to transmit the plague, whereas, at other times, prolonged contact with dead rats had no effect; at times a short trip to a plague locale where there were dead rats brought on the disease, even if there were no contact with the carcasses of these animals. Despite these questions, he was virtually certain that the mode of transmission involved infected rat carcasses and *not* the atmosphere (italics added).

The mystery was solved when Simond examined plague patients. An inconspicuous symptom held the answer. In a few patients who, early on in the illness, had developed bubonic enlargements requiring hospitalization, Simond spotted tiny vesicles or pustules, lesions smaller than the head of a pin and bordered by small roseate areoles. Each ordinary-looking blister was usually located on an arm or leg and in proximity to the enlarged lymph node. Since the base of the lesion, the vascular lymphatic tracts, and the node itself corresponded to each other anatomically, Simond suspected a causal relationship between them and the infective process. One could find nothing else that was unusual in any other part of the body of a patient who had been infected at this early stage. On rare occasions, an affected node itself could become as large as a walnut, but ordinarily it grew a little bigger than a lentil. No prognosis could be based on the size or shape of the node, inasmuch as patients at that early stage had an even chance of survival.

The nodes furnished Simond with a concentrated source of bacilli, as they had for Yersin and Kitasato who harvested micro-organisms from animal carcasses and human cadavers in order to grow cultures. The real breakthrough for Simond was finding plague germs in *both* the blisters *and* in the nodes, a coincidence strongly suggesting causality (italics added). Moreover, drops of serum from scattered blisters contained the microbe and produced pure plague cultures *in vitro*. Early in this phase of the research, Simond entertained the thought that the blisters and the early onset of the disease, especially in its febrile stage, were coincidental rather than causative. The idea that the blister was the source or entry-point of infection became more plausible, however, when he encountered plague victims who had been bitten by infected rats: in the latter case, the rat bite, like the suspicious blister, *was in anatomical proximity to enlarged nodes* (italics added). Thinking comparatively, Simond conjectured that the blister was a point of entry into the body, analogous in this way to a rat bite. Approaching the possibility of insect transmission with utmost care, he noted that, in patients with early-stage bubonic plague, both blisters and enlarged nodes were present on the lower extremities, but excoriated skin was *not* found on the feet: therefore, the blisters as opposed to broken skin on the soles were probably how the disease entered the body. He noted, as well, that blisters were discovered not on rough calloused soles but on the soft, fine, and undamaged skin of the legs and lower torso — on regions, that is, where one would expect to find an insect bite. Observations of this kind, and the resemblance between skin lesions on plague victims and the typical flea bite, led Simond to hypothesize that fleas carried and transmitted the microbe. If the flea transmits "the Yersin microbe," Simond posits, it can infect either rat or man with the plague, while biting extremities and ingesting blood.

Just as Yersin's contemporary, Kitasato, was working on plague etiology independently, Simond's efforts were paralleled by those of Dr. Masanori Ogata, a professor of the Hygiene Institute of Tokyo, who was active during the Indian epidemic in 1897. Ogata wrote these prescient words: "one should pay attention to insects like fleas for, as the rat becomes cold after death, they leave their host and may transmit the plague ... to man" (*Science Odyssey*, P.B.S.).

To demonstrate the flea's role in the process, Simond needed to isolate the germ in the intestinal tract of the insect, a technical impossibility in 1898. At this juncture in the inquiry, he was remiss in his research. Although he had not read Yersin's 1894 paper which suggested that flies carrying the bacilli could be easily puréed for inoculation into laboratory animals, Simond decided independently to purée fleas and then to use the slurry as inoculum. Mashing live contaminated fleas, however, was not a routine procedure (Yersin had a much easier time collecting dead flies). So Simond had to figure out how to kill or to immobilize the fleas for puréeing. Observing reasonable precautions, he tried to remove the parasites from live animals, but, since his team did not have the capacity to tranquilize the rats, this procedure was much too awkward and dangerous. A possible solution occurred to him. He recalls that, while washing a dog with soapy water, he found between its paws a number of engorged and immobilized fleas. which might have been carriers (e.g., the dog flea, *Ctenophalus canis*, carries plague). He decided to employ this method in order to gather insects from rats. In the initial phase of the research, he used experimental rats that had died of plague through natural exposure. At the last possible moment before the rats died (so that the fleas would still be active in the animals' fur), he pulled the dying animals out of the cage with pincers and let them fall immediately into a sealed paper bag. The bag was then submerged in a receptacle filled with soapy water. Using shears, he snipped holes in the bag to allow the carcasses to soak. After a moment of immersion, it was possible for him to remove live, infected, soap-immobilized fleas from the dead animal's fur.

Simond traveled to Saigon briefly on February 22, 1898, in the search of better facilities for his flea experiments. While in the process of doing so, he was urgently requested to return to Bombay and to Kurachi. The plague had recurred rather dramatically in the form of a terrifying epizootic, littering the streets and homes with dead and dying rodents. It was common knowledge that, where plague was endemic, dead rats were a harbinger of a coming epidemic. Simond returned to the Indian cities to find that both captured live rats and carcasses were so badly infested with fleas that they could not be safely examined. To preclude the danger of spreading contaminated fleas in his quarters and laboratory, he placed into a glass jar each rat that had been inoculated with laboratory-grown plague; then he covered the jar with a metallic sheet, overlain with a linen cloth secured around the receptacle. With infected rats contained and clearly observable, he proceeded with his experiment: to prove that the flea got the microbe from the rat, and that the flea, in turn, spread the disease to man and animal.

On his return to Kutch, Western India, Simond brought with him material necessary for the construction of a simple experimental apparatus: one large glass and a high-neck glass beaker, the bottom of which was covered with a layer of sand to absorb animal urine. The top of the bottle was secured by a metallic lid and a fabric which were fastened at the mouth of the bottle. For this experiment, Simond needed a plague rat, a healthy laboratory rat, and a supply of fleas. He managed to capture an infected rat from a village home and a supply of fleas (using the soap method). The hypothesis was that the fleas would feed on the dying animal at the bottom of the jar and abandon the plague rat when it died. With an abundance of plague organisms in the foregut, the fleas would then hop onto the healthy rat in the cage above, feed on its blood, and, in the process, regurgitate bacilli into the wound and bloodstream of the healthy animal. In twenty-four hours, just as predicted, the infected animal rolled up in a ball, became immobile, its fur bristled, and it appeared to be in agony. Simond then lowered into the jar, just above the dead rat, a small cage containing the perfectly healthy young rat that had been captured in Bombay two weeks before, and that had been kept in captivity, free of contamination. He suspended the cage against the wall of the jar several centimeters above the sand layer at the bottom. Thus, the enclosed healthy animal would have no direct physical contact with the infected animal at the bottom of the jar, with the inside of the jar, or with the fecal- and urine-contaminated sand.

On the following day, the infected rat was dead, and the blood and organs were found to contain an abundance of Yersin's bacilli. Over the next four days, the rat imprisoned in the suspended cage continued to feed normally. Nearing the fifth day, however, it seemed to have trouble moving around. On the sixth day, it was dead. The autopsy showed enlarged inguinal and axillary lymph nodes. The liver and spleen were swollen and congested, the plague bacillus having infiltrated the organs and blood. That very day, June 2, 1898, Simond proved that fleas carried the plague germs.

The parasites, after leaving the dead animal, found a new host in the healthy, encaged rat that had been suspended above it.

Simond's ingenious work stimulated discussion in scientific circles. Among the doctors who were familiar with the bubonic plague, however, arose many who expressed incredulity. Simond concluded, from this resistance, that the medical establishment was not yet prepared to include insect vectors in the field of epidemiology.

Charles Nicolle et al. and Typhus Fever

The word *typhus* comes from the Greek word for smoke, vapor, conceit, vanity, and stupor (*OED* XVII: 559; "typhus"). The stupor and prostration caused by the disease is likely to have suggested the use of the word to De Sauvages, who had employed it in 1759 as a medical descriptor. Before the application of the word to the disease, typhus was known by a number of epithets (for example, "Putrid Fever" as well as "Camp," "Jail," "Hospital," or "Ship Fever"). Robert's medical handbook of 1877 attributes the cause of typhus to "a specific poison" that was highly contagious. Bristowe remarks, in 1878, that patients were best treated in "large, airy, well-ventilated chambers," the conventional wisdom being that the contagious poison was in the atmosphere and would eventually dissipate. According to the etymological history of the word, from 1759 to 1877, typhus had been described in terms of its physiological effects and of the localities in which it appeared. Obviously, a comprehensive understanding of the disease could not have been built on the basis of such disjointed observations, but this was a beginning.

The vague descriptions noted above contrast with what is now known of the disease, a body of knowledge comprising clinical, historical, epidemiological, entomological, zoological, and ecological information. An infectious disease, typhus is caused by a microorganism, called *rickettsia*. According to the CDC, rickettsias live in vertebrates and are transmitted by bloodsucking parasites, particularly fleas, lice, and ticks. The organism was named after the American pathologist, Harold Tylor Ricketts (1871–1910), who confirmed its existence, but who died of typhus while in Mexico. The microbes themselves, which are gram-negative and rod-shaped, pose a challenge for laboratory study. Unlike bacteria, rickettsiae cannot be cultured outside living hosts. Usually, the organisms live and multiply in the gastrointestinal tract of an arthropod carrier such as the louse, and the disease is transmitted to mammals through bites or in contagious feces.

The CDC Report, to which I am here referring, enumerates eight forms of the disease. *Rickettsia prowazekii* which is carried from person to person by two species of lice causes a virulent form of typhus. The body louse, *Pediculus humanus corporis*, picks up the infection by feeding on the blood of a patient who has acute typhus fever. Infected lice then excrete rickettsiae on the skin as they feed on blood; the excreta are then rubbed into a skin abrasion or into a bite when the patient scratches. Other infections result when dusty excreta are inhaled. A second type, *R. mooseri*, is transmitted from rodents to persons by infected fleas. This occurs when infectious rat fleas, usually *Xenopsylla cheopis* (which also carry plague), defecate rickettsiae while sucking blood. Opossums, cats, and dogs and other wild or domestic animals transport infective fleas (e.g., *Ctenocephalides felis*) to humans. A third type, *R. quintana* or trench fever, notorious for epidemics in World War I, is transmitted via the flea from rats to persons or from person to person. *R. akari*, the fourth type, causes rickettsialpox, a mite-borne infection transmitted from house mice to people. Scrub typhus (*tsutsugamushi* fever), a fifth type, is a mite-borne infection ascribed to *R. tsutsugamushi*, which is found in Japan and Southeast Asia. *Coxiella burnetii*, the sixth type, which can live outside of a host, is blamed for Q fever. This infection can be transmitted by the inhalation of contaminated organic materials from livestock. Usually the organisms grow in cells lining blood and lymph vessels, causing rash, fever, and flu-like symptoms. All rickettsial diseases respond to antibiotics (e.g., tetracycline and chloramphenicol). Most cause high fevers, rash, and headache. The most virulent form of the disease, responsible for many historic outbreaks, is *R. prowazeki* which is also transmitted by the feces of body lice.

It is incorrect to assume that, as late as the mid-nineteenth century, little was known about typhus. On the contrary, the history of typhus research leading up to the contributions of Dr. Charles Nicolle, though discontinuous, can be traced back as far as the sixteenth century. Girolamo Fracastoro described the disease in 1546 (1–3). At some time between 1505 and 1528, he writes, typhus first appeared in Italy but was known previously on Cyprus and on neighboring islands. It was popularly called *lenticulae* or *puncticulae* because lentil-size spots appeared on the skin. Fracastoro correctly assumed it to be a contagious disease: travelers from Italy where the disease was present died of it in countries where it had not previously existed. As a contagious disease, it did not infect by fomites or inanimate material, or at a distance, "but only from the actual handling of the sick." Fracastoro's observation would be essential to Charles Nicolle's discovery nearly three centuries later: tactile contact with the sick spread the disease. But the question still needed to be answered: how was the disease-causing element transferred from patient to health-care worker?

This pivotal question regarding the mode of contagion was answered incrementally. The American physician, William Wood Gerhard, in the paper "On the Typhus Fever ... Philadelphia ... 1836," began his inquiry by trying to define the nature of the disease. He not only distinguished typhoid from typhus, which had been confused with other, but also identified the malady commonly known as British typhus as being one and the same with ship fever, jail fever, camp fever, or petechial or spotted fever (4–26). His work evoked a series of interconnected questions: what did all of these localities have in common? Did they promote typhus in some way? Was Fracastoro's tactility premise the common denominator?

Clinical practice and the assessment of common symptoms sharpened the focus considerably. On the basis of experience with more than two hundred patients in Philadelphia during the outbreak of 1836, Gerhard drew conclusions with respect to: (1) the social classes of individuals affected, (2) the mode of propagation, (3) the age of the patients, (4) their genders, (5) their residences, (6) their lifestyles and habits, (7) their use of alcohol, (8) the morbidity rate and time of year, (9) their occupations, (10) their ethnicities, (11) their ages, and (12) pathological anatomy.

For Gerhard, the mode of propagation was an especially interesting area of study, but he made little headway. His most substantive contribution, as outlined above, was his assessment of typhus patients during the epidemic of 1836. He discovered that the disease attacked the poor, intemperate, and huddled masses, foremost, and at miles distant from an original focus of infection. From this information, he deduced (1) that the disease had, "a general cause, which extended its influence throughout the vicinity of Philadelphia"; and (2) that the fever seems to have been propagated in the great number of patients "by direct contagion" (precisely as Fracastoro had suspected three hundred years earlier). Evidence of contagion at the Philadelphia hospital where Gerhard practiced was "direct and conclusive." Fever patients and attendants were equally afflicted. Gerhard, however, could go no further since he subscribed to the atmospheric theory of contagion and had no idea that arthropods spread the microbe: "the matter of the contagion ... was generally mingled with the air, but sometimes seemed to be combined with the pungent hot sweat of the patients. In some cases the contagion was evidently from body to body" (14).

R. L. Thomas, M.D., in *The Eclectic Practice of Medicine* (1907), summarizes the conventional knowledge of the typhous-group of diseases at the turn of the century. A highly contagious disorder, it was associated with great masses of people congregating in small areas and lacking proper sanitation (as per Fracastoro and Gerhard). As late as 1907, according to Thomas's summary, researchers did not know that ticks spread the disease. Thomas describes the clinical manifestations accurately: the sudden onset of high fever, a distinctive rash, and neurological effects lasting some twelve to sixteen days. Its predisposing causes undoubtedly are "filth, poverty, and overcrowding, without due regard to cleanliness in regard to the removal and destruction of human excreta" (as per Gerhard). A related factor is "intemperance," which weakens the system (as per Gerhard). Poor diets contribute to making people more susceptible to the toxins in the bloodstream (as per Roberts). Thomas acknowledges that the specific cause had yet to be isolated. But according to the annals of public health, it is likely that "it" (i.e., the infectious agent) enters the system of one who was "susceptible to the poison or germ"; from that point on, it multiplies and produces "the original toxin."

Doctors and nurses who came into close contact with an infected patient, argues Thomas, were at greatest risk of contracting the disease (an important clue and an anomaly for Charles Nicolle). The disease process had three early phases: exposure, incubation from three to twelve days (suggesting the presence of living organisms in the bloodstream), and invasion. Early symptoms, such as fever, languor, and loss of appetite, intensified as the disease moved from the incubational to the invasive phase. For want of a better term, Thomas describes "it" as "an unwelcome guest," the bringer of high fever, pain, prostration, heart problems, and often death. In its earliest stage, as the disease stupefied its victim, a characteristic rash appeared, along with bright red macules, subcutaneous hemorrhages, and petechia; urine retention and delirium succeeded this phase of the disease; from the seventh to fourteenth day, convulsions were a danger. After the fourteenth day, stupor gave way to lethargy, and, if the patient survived, a period of dramatic discharges of bloody and putrid material occurred.

It is interesting to note that Thomas's treatment regimen relied on herbal and on chemical remedies, several of which are quite startling. For instance, to stimulate a comatose patient, he prescribed belladonna or deadly nightshade, a poisonous plant containing atropine, scopolamine, and hyoscyamine, all of which depress the parasympathetic nervous system; for restless and sleepless patients, he encouraged the use of hycoscyamine especially. Echinacea (popular nowadays), which comes from the stems and roots of certain plants, reputedly alleviates the dusky hue and furred tongue brought on by the disease; in truth, echinachea stimulates the immune system in the short term (Fetrow and Avila 190–1). Thomas even advocated the use of diluted hydrochloric acid as an oral antiseptic!

In 1910, Ricketts and a volunteer assistant, Russell M. Wilder, while studying typhus in Mexico, discovered a bacillus-like organism in the blood of typhus patients and in the intestines of infected lice. They were circumspect about what they found, realizing as had Koch and many others that the presence of the organism in man and in ticks did not constitute sufficient grounds "for claiming an etiologic role on the part of the organism described" (46); however, they noted that "the conditions under which [the organisms] are found, together with the theoretical argument presented [in the paper], appear to demand that they be taken somewhat seriously, and subjected to further study in their relationship to typhus" (46). Despite the optative mood, Ricketts believed, on the basis of probability and inference, that the typhus pathogen had to be investigated further. Dr. H. da Rocha-Lima, in 1916, continued the work of Ricketts. Da Rocha-Lima studied the physiology of the vector, describing the agent of typhus fever in infected lice and how it proliferated in the louse's stomach. This work established, beyond a doubt, "the causative relation between the micro-organism found in infected lice and epidemic typhus fever" (74).

Charles Jules Henry Nicolle, M.D. (1866–1936), in 1903, proved definitively that typhus fever was transmitted by the body louse, and his work helped later investigators to distinguish between louse-borne epidemic typhus and murine or rat-flea typhus. In Nicolle's work, the investigative process reached the etiological phase. He collaborated with Dr. Roux in Paris, was director of the Pasteur Institute in Tunis from 1903, and professor at the Collège de France from 1932. For his breakthrough on typhus, he was awarded the Nobel Prize in Physiology or Medicine in 1928. In Tunis he established a center for bacteriological research, where he produced sera to combat a number of infectious diseases.

Nicolle's 1928 Presentation Speech for the Nobel Prize, "Investigations on typhus," a seminal piece of etiological writing, recounts his great discovery. When he arrived in Tunisia at the beginning of January 1903, he encountered native cases of typhus fever in the suburbs. At that time, the disease was not an epidemic. The last Tunisian epidemic which was in 1868 had killed at least 5,000 people in the capitol city of Tunis (Kohn 348). According to Kohn et al., the outbreak of 1868 owed its severity to predisposing conditions: dirty, crowded domiciles and food shortages in 1867. Worsening these conditions was frigid weather and human and animal cadavers in the streets. Lice that carried rickettsiae flourished under these ideal conditions. After mid-February 1868, typhus cases began to appear. Since the Tunisian government did not treat the outbreak seriously, a European sanitary council had to intervene by imposing public-health regulations with respect to the disposal of cadavers, the isolation of typhus patients, and the disinfection of prisons and army barracks. At the time, it was not known that the body louse was the main carrier of the disease, but disinfection inadvertently killed the lice responsible for the disease. Some had speculated that as many as 50,000 people died in Tunis, especially in places where quarantines were not in effect. Apparently, the disease remained endemic in Tunisia at the time of Nicolle's arrival, flaring up each winter in the rural districts and, from there, spreading to makeshift houses, to the prisons, and to the outskirts of towns. The disease, usually subsiding in June, was found in remote country districts, and it did not resurface until the end of 1903.

Although Nicolle realized that inconclusive experimental findings did not prove that the disease spread from person to person and via the bloodstream, he inferred as much. So, in June 1903, he undertook preliminary studies. At the time, typhus was active in a native prison, 80 kilometers south of Tunis, in Djouggar. Because Nicolle was indisposed at the time, he was unable to accompany the local physician on his weekly rounds at the prison. He therefore sent his colleague, Dr. Motheau, in his place. After spending only one night in Djouggar, Motheau and his servant died of typhus. In fact, most of the Tunisian administrators who were in the country districts contracted the disease, and as many as one third of them died. Nicolle's early experiences while in contact with infected patients shaped his intuitive sense of how the disease spread.

The story of how Nicolle's idea of transmission developed is fascinating and recapitulates some of Fracastoro's insights that had been enunciated three centuries earlier. In the native hospital in Tunis, the focal point of his research, Nicolle noticed that he had to walk over prostrate typhus patients in order to enter the hospital. In itself, this was not unusual. But an irregular phenomenon caught his attention. Typhus patients were customarily accommodated in open wards, probably in the belief that the infection was spread by noxious contaminants in closed hospital wards. However, even before they reached these wards and while outside in the fresh air, the patients infected their families and hospital personnel — anyone, that is, who came into close physical contact with them (as per Fracastoro). Especially prone to infection were those who disrobed the patients upon admittance, and those who laundered their clothing. Yet, when the patients entered the ward *after being disrobed*, incidents of contagion virtually disappeared (italics added). What happened in the interval between the pre-admission and admission of patients that increased the possibility of contagion? The answer, quite obviously, is that the sick patient "was stripped of his clothes and linen, shaved and washed." From this simple realization, Nicolle hypothesizes that, "The contagious agent was therefore something attached to his skin and clothing, something which soap and water could remove. It could only be the louse. It was the louse."

Of course, Nicolle realized that the idea of louse-borne transmission was unprecedented, so he undertook an experiment. Failing to transmit typhus to laboratory animals, including small monkeys, he procured a chimpanzee, thinking that he might be able to induce the disease in man's closest relative. He inoculated the chimpanzee with typhus-infected blood drawn from a patient at the Rabta hospital. The second benchmark of his remarkable work, initiated by astute observations, was about to be made: the animal developed typhus fever. Then Nicolle inoculated a monkey of the genus Macaca (species unknown) with the chimpanzee's blood, and the monkey, too, came down with the fever. The turning point had come. Nicolle then placed lice on the monkey to see if these parasites would pick up the infectious agent through blood-feeding, although it is not clear from the Nobel Prize address how Nicolle was certain that the experimental lice were free of rickettsia *before* they were placed onto the monkey. This was an important consideration: had the lice been infected prior to the experiment, the procedure would have been invalidated. In any event, when Nicolle transported lice from the typhus-infected monkey to healthy ones, the latter developed the disease. In the process, he discovered that the infected monkeys' bouts with the disease gave the animals a degree of immunity to typhus which was demonstrated by their resistance to a subsequent inoculation of the organism. Nicolle's success with primates reinforced the idea that a typhus vaccine could be made.

In June 1909, Nicolle successfully reproduced typhus in the chimpanzee, demonstrated in August 1909 the role played by the louse, and published these results in September. Along with Charles Comte and Ernest Conseil, he undertook in the following years more detailed experiments on the disease and on the conditions of its transmission. As long as a sufficient quantity of the microbe was inoculated through the peritoneum, all species of monkey could be infected. From 1909 to 1911, he conducted experiments on man-to-monkey and on monkey-to-monkey transmissibility during seasonal expansions of the disease. When he found out that the guinea pig was also susceptible to the infection, he was then able, in 1912, to preserve the pathogen in this animal; thus, in the time between seasonal eruptions of the disease, he had at his disposal a natural reservoir of infectious organisms that was cheap to maintain and easy to use (a problem Pasteur had grappled with while developing a rabies vaccine). The most significant step forward was the discovery that guinea pigs, as well as primates, could be used experimentally.

Infection could be induced in animals five days or more after inoculation. The laboratory animals experienced febrile symptoms similar to those in man, except that the former's were less pronounced and of shorter duration. The monkeys, especially, exhibited hypothermia after the fever diminished, a symptom less pronounced in the guinea pig. If it were not for the fever, the presence of the infection in guinea pigs would have remained undetectable, a state Nicolle called *unapparent* (or without symptoms); in monkeys, minor general symptoms were always detectable. The inconsistent reactions some animals had to experimental inoculation were unexpected, so Nicolle tried to find an answer. He observed that when blood was used for transferring the disease between individuals in a group of guinea pigs, each of which had received an equal dosage of infected blood, some of the animals showed no signs of fever. Positing that susceptible animals reacted differently, on a graduated scale from grave to unapparent reactions, Nicolle concluded either that a benign form of the disease existed or that certain animals were more resistant to the disease than others. In 1911, he definitively proved that unapparent infections were caused by administering low levels of infectious material to laboratory animals, insufficient to induce fever.

Nicolle had still to establish that the guinea pigs lacking symptoms were carriers of the disease. To prove this, he inoculated healthy guinea pigs with blood drawn from unapparent ones. If a healthy guinea pig received enough infectious material from an unapparent animal, the former would develop observable symptoms, including fever. The appearance of fever in the second group of animals proved that the asymptomatic ones were indeed carriers of typhus. Additionally, Nicolle discovered that more could be learned about typhus from the latest batch of guinea pigs which now had symptomatic disease. Once these animals recovered from induced bouts with the malady, Nicolle re-inoculated them with infectious material, but now they showed no symptoms even though they definitely had the pathogen in their bloodstreams. Unapparent primary typhus, as it turned out, was rare in guinea pigs but often the case with laboratory rats and mice. The disease which could be transmitted from one rat to another was asymptomatic, had an incubation period during which the blood was virulent, and conferred a degree of immunity on the animal, demonstrable after subsequent reinoculations. On two occasions, Nicolle and his colleagues produced twelve such transmissions. At the twelfth transmission, the brain tissue of the last rat in the sequence, after being dissected and injected into guinea pigs, induced febrile typhus.

Applying this new knowledge to measles and to other infections, Nicolle inaugurated a new field of study which he labeled *sub-pathology*. It was now known that, in human beings, primary typhus infection conferred lifelong immunity to the disease, and Nicolle was able to establish that laboratory animals acquired the same immunity, though of a shorter duration.

The next phase in the exploration of typhus was to develop an immunizing serum from convalescent typhus patients. Lucien Raynaud, an Algerian, and E. Legraini of Bougie (a northern Algerian town now called Bejara) had used serum from convalescents to treat typhus, but Nicolle and Conseil demonstrated that this approach was ineffective. They found that serum derived from both human convalescents and from recovered animals had limited protective properties. Although Nicolle states that the serum provides "sure protection to persons in contact with typhus patients, as well as to doctors and nurses," the word "sure" does not imply permanence, for the effect of the serum was temporary, and additional inoculations had to be administered when necessary. The knowledge gained from this method was not lost: it encouraged Nicolle and Conseil to apply this method to the treatment of measles: thus, they took serum from children cured of measles and inoculated it into non-immune patients to stimulate immunity. They demonstrated the same flexibility that Pasteur had shown when he applied Jenner's method to the creation of a rabies vaccine.

Although Nicolle worked assiduously on the problem of immunization, immediate success was not forthcoming. He was able to vaccinate a number of people by injecting them with a sequence of small doses of infectious material (brain tissue from guinea pigs had the best results); however, this method was both unreliable and risky. Moreover, since there was a limit to the amount of serum that could be drawn from convalescents, the obvious challenge was to find a reliable and plentiful source. If it were possible to produce effective serum in large animals, he hypothesized, the supply would be unlimited. The germ could be preserved in guinea pigs and cultivated in large mammals whenever the serum was needed. Animals could therefore be used as serological factories.

The search for a suitable species began. Repeated inoculations of virulent typhus into a donkey evidenced no preventive properties in the blood. To find out why this was so, Nicolle had to ascertain, in the first place, if the donkey was resistant to typhus or whether it could harbor an unapparent form of the disease; the latter proved to be the case: the donkey had an asymptomatic case of the disease. While trying to induce symptoms in donkeys using intracerebral inoculations of typhus, he raised a fever but only inconstantly. Serum from the donkey that had been cured of febrile typhus did possess preventive capabilities, but, beyond this point, Nicolle's immunological research did not extend.

After Nicolle established that the body louse was the typhus vector, he was able to describe how the disease was transmitted. When a patient contracted the disease, he or she was contagious while febrile for the two or three days before typhus appeared and for two or three days after the temperature had fallen. During this period, the louse could contract the organism from the patient that it had bitten. After the seventh day following the bite of an infected louse, the infection was not immediately present. By the ninth and tenth days, however, the bite produced a virulent infection. A necessary condition for transmission was for the virus to multiply within the louse, at which point the vector was hazardous. Nicolle observed, in 1910, that the organism proliferated in the gastrointestinal tract of the louse, its feces becoming virulent at the same time as did the bite. In 1914, Nicolle and George Blanc developed a method for locating the infectious organism in the louse's intestine, and an Algerian, Edmond Sergent, was the first to describe these inclusion bodies, later called rickettsiae.

Nicolle also had to prove that lice excrement carried the germ and was also a means of contagion. When the native was infected, it was supposed that he scratched the bite, which was also where the feces had been deposited. Teeming with microbes, fecal matter then got into the bite or skin abrasion; the disease could even be transmitted to the eyes where the organism was readily absorbed.

After 1914, these findings formed the basis of typhus prophylaxis. Conseil, Director of the Bureau of Public Health in Tunis, eradicated typhus there in three years. Owing to the joint efforts of medical administrators, typhus was eliminated from the mines and prisons and restricted to remote rural districts, where it remained until finally wiped out. From Tunisia, this method would be applied world-wide.

A distinctive feature of etiological investigation is its interdisciplinary approach to disease. The examples I have presented in this chapter exhibit this feature unquestionably. Koch who began his work on anthrax in the 1850s eventually demonstrated that *B. anthracis* was the probable cause of the disease. The arduous route he traversed required familiarity with veterinary medicine (he was a country physician), and with several inchoate disciplines: human and veterinary pathology (especially in serology [a term coined in 1911] and histology [coined in 1844–46]), microbiology (coined in 1888), and bacteriology (coined in 1884). An interdisciplinary approach allowed him to formulate a method for establishing the causality of other bacterial pathogens, such as anthrax and tuberculosis. Pasteur's research on puerperal fever, similarly, demanded knowledge of obstetrical medicine, of pathology, of bacteriology, and of histology; and, most importantly, it required collaboration with medical colleagues who guided him in his investigation. The discovery of the rabies vaccine, an accomplishment in the heritage of Edward Jenner, demanded competency in veterinary medicine and experience in the areas of animal and of human immunology. Yersin's work on the plague, foreshadowing the rigors of modern epidemiological fieldwork, combined the geographical and casestudy methods of Snow with the laboratory methodology of Koch. While engaged in field work, Yersin et al. (undoubtedly, his team included medical doctors) described and evaluated clinical symptoms, mortality rates, and environmental conditions (e.g., housing, sanitation, animal-human contact, and broader ecological concerns). Yersin and his team recognized the importance of morbidity and of mortality rates among various species of indigenous animals that, they believed, had an undefined role in the cycle of contagion, and he speculated on the theory of insect vectors. Dissections and biopsies furnished bacterial specimens to be used in laboratory trials on animals. Clearly, Yersin's pioneering work involved a number of interrelated disciplines.

Kitasato's concurrent investigation of plague replicated Yersin's findings. The Japanese bacteriologist, however, had a marked advantage over Yersin in terms of material and of professional support. Although Kitasato was ostensibly concerned with the bacillus of plague, his group was involved in much more: clinical description, autopsy/dissection, histology/serology, fieldwork, and sanitary/aseptic measures. While Simond's experiment proved, definitively, that the rat flea carried plague from one animal to another, as well as to man, the catalyst of his work was clinical examination: the anatomical proximity of insect bites and of infected lymph nodes in plague sufferers suggested that bites, either from rat or flea, transmitted the pathogen. Finally, while working in a fertile tradition of experimentation and of field studies on the cause of typhus, Charles Nicolle proved that body lice carried the disease, and he speculated that an immunizing serum could someday be cultivated in animal reservoirs. Nicolle's breakthrough, like Simond's, arose from a spontaneous observation, the noticing of an anomaly. When health-care workers contracted typhus from sick patients in the open air, Nicolle realized that dressing and washing them somehow made workers susceptible. The obvious answer was that lice on the patients' bodies and contaminated clothing bit the workers and spread the disease.

Synergy and Legionellosis

The investigation of epidemic disease in the late nineteenth century, exemplified by the work of Koch, Pasteur, Yersin, Kitasato, Simond, Nicolle, and many others, bears a unifying characteristic: the importance of interdisciplinary and collaborative efforts. Microbiology was essential to the understanding of causality, but the facts revealed on a microscopic level would have remained there had they not been applied to veterinary medicine and to the formulation of vaccines. To the comprehensive understanding of plague, clinical and epidemiological observations were imperative. But, without a broader scope encompassing zoology and parasitic entomology, the effects of the disease would never have been tracked to the cause, and the cycles of contagion within which man had become a vulnerable component would never have come to light.

The word *synergy* describes the activities of agents or of medicines that, when taken concertedly, enhance each other's effectiveness (*OED* XVI: 381–82; "synergy"; *Random House*, 1333). I will employ the term here to characterize the interdisciplinary work of today's biomedical professionals. This section highlights the comprehensive response of the biomedical community to the 1976 Legionnaires' disease (LD) epidemic in Philadelphia. Work on this disease has inspired important studies in every dimension of this pathogen's natural history. The struggle against Legionnaires' disease shows that the control of epidemic pathogens depends on the cooperative efforts of front-line physicians, research specialists, technicians, statisticians, civil authorities and many others. Together, their work is synergistic: the success of the whole depends upon, yet is greater than, the contribution of each individual.

An epidemic broke out in July 1976, afflicting persons who attended an American Legion State convention at the Bellevue-Stratford Hotel in Philadelphia (Kohn et al. 260–61). One of the chief investigators of the event, Dr. Joseph E. McDade, Deputy Director of the National Center for Infectious Diseases at the Centers for Disease Control, recounts the event in, "The Ecology of Outbreaks: Discovery of *Legionella pneumophila*." McDade recalls that the convention had been going along normally when a number of attendees developed fever, coughs, and pneumonia. The Pennsylvania Department of Health reported that similar illnesses were occurring around the State, involving persons who had attended the convention. For this reason, the press labeled the disorder *Legionnaires'* disease, since the initial cases involved military veterans (135).

Local public health authorities and the CDC dispatched personnel to the scene to gather available information. In a short time, they registered the numbers of afflicted and of deceased, determined their locations and activities, and tried to track down their contacts. From this preliminary information, they were able to deduce that none of those in contact with the sick persons developed the illness. This suggested that there was a localized source of infection, likely an airborne pathogen, since the sick veterans had been congregating in the lobby of the hotel and on the sidewalk in front of the building. Although observations and deductions were made, without definitive laboratory results, the inquiry could proceed no further. The preliminary findings alluded to above were published in the *New England Journal of Medicine*, in the issue of December 1, 1977. D. W. Fraser et al. reports that 29 out of 182 cases were fatal, that the spread of the bacterium appeared to be airborne, and that, although its source was as yet unknown, investigators inferred that "exposure may have occurred in the lobby of the headquarters hotel or in the area immediately surrounding the hotel." Since hotel employees appear to have been immune, the investigators infer that the agent "may have been present in the vicinity, perhaps intermittently, for two or more years."

McDade was assigned the task of determining if the mysterious infection was Q fever, a disease causing mild pneumonia and afflicting domestic livestock workers and meat-packers. He ruled this possibility out after he inoculated guinea pigs with lung tissue from decedents. The laboratory animals became ill, but he was unable to culture the Q fever pathogen (a type of *rickettsiae*). In the process of the Q fever search, McDade did find a suspicious anomaly: a rare, rod-shaped bacterium. Since he could not cultivate this microbe on synthetic medium, he did not follow up on it, assuming instead that it was a contaminant. By December, with the Philadelphia outbreak still a mystery, he began to wonder about that anomalous bacterium.

That winter, McDade and his co-workers adopted a new approach to the isolation of the LD organism. Retrieving a suspension of the infected guinea pig tissue, he inoculated it into hens' eggs containing live embryo, a favorable environment for bacterial growth. The embryos died a few days later. He repeated the isolation procedure, this time by injecting the embryonic yolk-sacs with tissue samples taken from human decedents. When he recovered the anomalous bacterium from the embryos injected with guinea-pig suspension *and* from those with the human specimens, it became clear that the anomalous bacterium was not a contaminant. This breakthrough, however, did not prove that the microbe was the cause of the infection since the bacterium could still have been an "experimental artifact" (136).

McDade and his co-workers published their findings in the paper "Legionnaires' Disease: Isolation of a Bacterium and Demonstration of Its Role in Other Respiratory Disease" (December 1, 1977). According to the paper, tissue samples from the lungs of four of six patients produced a gram-negative bacillus in guinea pigs, and the bacillus was then transferred to yolk-sac cultures of embryonated eggs to isolate its antigen for further study. Specimens taken from 101 to 111 patients, when compared to controls, showed increases in antibody levels meeting the clinical criteria of Legionnaires' disease. Significant antibody levels were also detected in 54 percent of sporadic cases of severe pneumonia. On the basis of these findings, they suggested that a gram-negative bacterium "*may be responsible* for widespread infection" (italics added). Twenty-two years later, McDade could state with certainty that, in 1977 they had indeed "found the cause of the Legionnaires' disease outbreak" (136).

Several CDC scientists took the initiative in 1977 and consulted their archives to see if there were records of unsolved epidemics resembling LD (136–37). They recalled having worked on earlier outbreaks of pneumonia and of other respiratory illnesses, specifically in Washington, D.C. (1965), and in Pontiac, Michigan (1968); the causes of these epidemics were unknown. Fortunately, for future study, serum specimens of patients from these outbreaks had been stored in CDC freezers. McDade and others tested them and found that most had high levels of antibodies *to the LD bacterium* which proved that the suspicious microbe had caused the epidemics of 1965 and of 1968 (italics added). Archival studies continued to reveal that LD had a long history in the United States. In "A 1957 Outbreak of Legionnaires' Disease Associated with a Meat-Packing Plant" (1983), for example, Osterholm et al. demonstrate that a 1957 pneumonia outbreak in Austin, Minnesota, was actually LD. Serological data, along with 1957 clinical and epidemiological observations, support the hypothesis that the Austin epidemic, which struck 78 persons (46 of whom worked at a local plant), was "the earliest documented outbreak of Legionnaires' disease" (Osterholm et al.).

How *L. pneumophila*, the organism the causes LD, survives and spreads to human beings was of vital concern. One hypothesis was that the bacterium existed naturally in the environment. Laboratory studies showed that it could survive for more than one year in tap water. After the Philadelphia outbreak, scientists began to test this hypothesis. It turned out that *L. pneumophila* was indeed an aquatic pathogen with a long natural history, and it was this agent that had developed in the air-conditioning cooling tower of the Bellevue-Stratford Hotel. The organism traveled in sprayed droplets of water that cooled off condensers. These minute droplets, coating machinery and pipes, contained the infectious agent; the microbes eventually became airborne, and victims inhaled the bacteria. Subsequent studies have traced LD outbreaks to spas, to plumbing, to decorative fountains, to air conditioners, to whirlpool baths, and even to unsterilized respiratory-care equipment in hospitals. A spate of post-1977 studies has implicated devices such as these. Two studies are representative. In 1980, Dondero et al. implicated the air-conditioning cooling tower in an August-September 1978 outbreak of LD in Memphis, Tennessee. Forty-four cases correlated with the use of a hospital's auxiliary air-conditioning cooling tower. *L. pneumophila* was found in two water samples. Ventilating air contaminated with the microbe affected patients whose rooms were cooled by the auxiliary tower. According to the report, tracer-smoke studies made it clear that contaminated aerosols could reach the air-intakes to the hospital, as well as the sidewalk (four pedestrians had also come down with the disease during this specific time period). D. B. Jernigan et al., in the 1996 edition of the *Lancet*, writes of an LD outbreak onboard a cruise ship which was traced to whirlpool spas.

Not everyone exposed to the microbe contracts the disease. Studies have shown that epidemics occur only if virulent strains of the bacteria are involved, if aerosolized droplets enter the air, and if susceptible persons, such as the elderly, smokers, pulmonary disease patients, or immuno-compromised patients, are exposed (McDade 138; "Legionellosis," CDC).

The conquest of Legionellosis began when the first clinicians encountered patients stricken with pneumonia of unknown origin. The circle of inquiry, centering on the study of LD, gradually expanded to include the endeavors of pulmonologists, epidemiologists, molecular biologists, bacteriologists, geneticists, and even air-conditioning technicians. The history of LD research exemplifies the concept of synergy, the apex of the investigative modality.

10. THE DEMOCRACY OF AFFLICTION

Modern Eyewitness Reporting

When the Union newspaper reporter, John McElroy, was captured by the Confederate Army in the spring of 1864 during a military operation, he was interned in the infamous prisoner of war camp at Andersonville, south-western Georgia. Tens of thousands of Union soldiers were confined there during the Civil War, more than 12,000 of whom died under the Camp's horrendous conditions. McElroy's detailed autobiographical account of his time in the camp, entitled *This Was Andersonville*, tells of their struggle against a variety of pestilential diseases, and it is representative of the eyewitness report.

In the tradition of Thucydides, McElroy paid close attention to the environmental conditions of the camp. Upon his arrival, there were 35,000 prisoners occupying 12.5 to 13.0 acres of arid land (53); each inmate, therefore, had 12.5 square feet to himself, nothing greater than a three-by-four foot rectangle and barely enough room in which to lie down. A Confederate medical officer, Dr. Joseph Jones, testified that the stockade, built to hold 10,000 men, by August 1864 housed 39,899; each man was allotted 35.7 square feet of ground (a six-by-six foot box) (293–95). Although Dr. Jones claims for each man three times more space than did McElroy, even the Confederate officer admitted that the Camp was dangerously overcrowded and that these conditions set the stage for epidemics. McElroy, on the other hand, had no doubt that his quarters amounted to the space within which he stood.

In the middle of the grounds ran a creek that was "a seething mass of corruption" and human waste (53). On May 15, 1864, 2,000 new men arrived, and they were followed by General Benjamin Franklin Butler's army of 40,000, defeated at Drewery's Bluff by Confederate General Beauregard (55). Though the estimates might be somewhat inflated, it was clear that the camp was well over capacity. The captors ordered the prisoners to strip down to shirts and pants and to proceed to the eastern side of the swamp, where sewage from the upper part of the camp flowed down to them. In addition, the heat was intense, and the men had to stand on burning sand without shelter. Sun exposure was severe. Even more men were packed into the camp, when an army from Plymouth arrived in May. Most would die that summer.

McElroy's interest in demographic and in topographical details indicates that he understood the connection between these factors and disease. Four pathological conditions were rampant in the camp. Two of them, typhus and dysentery, are communicable diseases. Two others, scurvy and gangrene, result from inadequate nutrition, from unsanitary conditions, and from the lack of medical care, especially for wound management. Since the relationship between bacteria and disease had been suspected by at least 1840, though it had not yet fully established (Pasteur had been doing groundbreaking work in 1861), neither McElroy nor the medical establishments of the North or the South at that time understood that lice spread typhus or that contaminated drinking water (Snow's work in 1854 notwithstanding) could be responsible for dysentery and cholera. Dr. Joseph Lister (1827–1912), the great British surgeon, would make extraordinary strides in the management of infections with the use of carbolic acid in 1867, but in 1864, under the conditions McElroy describes, little could be done to control infections caused by war wounds, malnutrition, or parasites.

Although McElroy recorded with graphic accuracy the extent of lice infestation in the camp, he did not link this phenomenon to typhus. Some background on the history of lice is in order. The word *louse* is a common name, first used in c. A.D. 700 to describe two orders of wingless, parasitic, disease-bearing insects (*OED* IX: 461–62; "louse"). Lice are small, flat, and adapted for clinging to a host ("Pediculosis," CDC). The lice of the order *Anoplura* feed off the bodies of mammals by piercing the skin and sucking blood. The group *Pediculus humanus* includes head lice and *Phthius pubis*, the crablike pubic louse. The females, each of which can lay three hundred eggs, glue them to hair and clothing. Infestations are routinely found in overcrowded conditions, where clothes are rarely changed or washed. As we recall from our discussion of Nicolle's discovery, body lice transmit rickettsial diseases. The microbe lives and breeds in the intestinal tract of the immune insect; through the arthropods' mouthparts or feces, the germ gets into the system of the vertebrate host. None of this was known in 1864. Writing retrospectively, in 1879, however, McElroy betrays his familiarity with the works of the germ theorists, Pasteur, Koch, and others. A textual comment, dated 1866, shows that he had been keeping abreast of contemporary microbiology and understood the power of invisible germs. Of his fellow prisoners' dire condition, he remarks: "If one of them survived, the germ theory of disease is a hallucination" (55).

The experience at Andersonville in the spring of 1864 was no hallucination. Without clean clothing and boiling water, the captives found it virtually impossible to keep the lice down to a manageable level: that is, to one "spoonful" per man (38). When a man became sick or was unable to help himself, the insect volume swelled rapidly into the millions, with a man bearing pints or quarts of insects; dead men where found to be infested with more than a gallon (i.e., eight pounds) of lice. Even when a man was besieged by uninfected insects, the health consequences were severe because of irritation, blood loss, and secondary infections.

Despite these horrendous conditions, the men managed to work together. De-lousing one's clothing could be done simply by turning a garment inside-out and by placing it above a fire, just high enough to be singed. The burning lice swelled up and "burst like popcorn" (38). The practice of popping lice became a sport and a diversion. However, as the weather became warmer and the number of detainees grew considerably, the lice became unendurable. McElroy recalls how, "They filled the hot sand under our feet, and voracious Troops would climb up on one like streams of ants, swarming up a tree" (38). At that time, writes McElroy, they had full comprehension of the third plague of Exodus inflicted on the Egyptians (38). McElroy is alluding to *Exodus* 8:15–18, when Aaron, at the Lord's behest, struck the dust with a stick, turning it into lice, which spread "throughout all the land of Egypt" (verse 17). The ironic reversal, of course, is that the pediculosis plague in the Bible was sent against the Egyptian captors to free the Israelites. In Andersonville, the reverse was happening, as the plague beset the captives. By April, 576 men had died (about nineteen per day). Losses at Andersonville due to lice infestation and to related disease exceeded those incurred in combat by 11 percent (38).

McElroy mentions as a primary cause of death "malignant typhus," an illness characterized by fever, rash, and headache (53). Since no one knew that lice and fleas carried what we now know to be *typhus*, it is difficult to state with any certainty if the disorder in question was lice-borne or had been confused with another illness. Since vector-borne disease was not yet understood, the general consensus was that the disease was an air-borne effluvium. Despite McElroy's familiarity with the germ theory of disease (as a reporter, he undoubtedly was aware of the latest scientific theories), he subscribed to the long-standing miasmatic theory. His conclusion was in keeping with this theory: the warm weather and the seething swamp produced blood-poisoning effluvium, a toxic vapor originating from human exhalations and putrid waste.

Confederate doctors had much to explain after the war was over. Dr.

R. Randolph Stevenson, M.D., Chief Surgeon of the Confederate States Military Prison at Andersonville, disagreed with McElroy's descriptions (292–93). The former testified at his war crimes trial that, despite the crowding and filthy conditions, "contagious fevers were rare." As for typhus fever, still believed to be an atmospheric constituent, Dr. Stevenson testified that it was unknown in the camp, even though conditions were conducive to the disease. The reason for its absence, he claimed, was that noxious fumes from the Hospital and Stockade (according to the miasmatic theory) simply drifted away from the localities of the prisoners.

A second disorder rampant in Andersonville was scurvy, a deficiency disorder resulting from the lack of vitamin C in the diet. The first disease to be associated with dietary deficiency, scurvy weakens capillaries, causes bleeding, loosens teeth, and leads to hemorrhages, debility, and death (Goebel and Driscoll). Since fresh fruit and vegetables were unheard of at Andersonville, vitamin-C deficiency compounded the medical crisis for Federal detainees. McElroy records the first deaths from the disease: two Norwegian-born POWs, John Emerson and John Stiggall, wasted away to skeletons (64–5). The graphic description suggests that McElroy witnessed their decline firsthand. One sufferer had fetid breath and swollen gums; and, when he bit hard corn bread, his gums and teeth literally broke into fragments. Since scurvy causes the breakdown of the skin and of the immune system, one soldier developed frightful ulcers on his body, which soon filled with swarming maggots. Characteristically, scurvy swelled the lower parts of the leg to the size of the thigh, and the flesh became colorless and transparent. If the swelling reached the ankle joint, the foot became useless, at which point there was little hope of recovery. The mortality rate due to scurvy was high (3,574 died of scurvy, that is, 10 percent of the camp population). As a remedy, Confederate surgeons offered a measly handful of berries (66). McElroy also developed a case of severe scurvy, but he survived (147). How he did so is not explained.

Dysentery and gangrene claimed the most lives. The former is caused most commonly by bacterial or amoebic infection, and the unsanitary conditions in the camp, especially the polluted water, can be blamed as a primary source of infection ("Epidemic Dysentery," WHO; "Gangrene," MayoClinic). With no knowledge of the disease-causing properties of certain microbes, McElroy attributed epidemic dysentery to a lack of proper food and to the diet of coarse corn meal (39). He also blamed the infection on the consumption of great quantities of water, and he attributed his freedom from disease to abstention from water drinking (67). The paradox, of course, was that the drinking of polluted water produced the disease. But diarrhea depleted the body's water to the point that one had to drink copious amounts of polluted water or become dehydrated. McElroy does not explain how he avoided the foul creek or if he had an alternative water source. Aid for dysentery patients was unavailable. Those debilitated with diarrhea were hospitalized, but three-quarters of them died.

Gangrene, which has two forms, is the local death of bodily tissue ("Gangrene," MayoClinic). Dry gangrene results if the blood supply to tissue is interrupted, and it can be caused by scurvy. Moist or gas gangrene occurs when toxin-producing bacteria invade the body. Any wound, even the slightest cut, made an inmate susceptible to gangrene. So many soldiers developed this condition that the medical staff of the camp was forced to isolate them in special wards. McElroy writes of the excoriating horrors he saw in the ward: "Horrible sores, spreading almost visibly from hour to hour, devoured men's limbs and bodies" (147–48). He recalls the terrible condition of one soldier, whose "ulcerations appeared to be altogether in the back, where they ate out the tissue between the skin and the ribs." Confederate medicine made matters worse: "The attendant seemed trying to arrest the progress of the sloughing by drenching the sores with a solution of blue vitriol [a metallic sulfate, possibly sulfuric acid!]. This was "exquisitely painful," caused "agonizing screams," and sometimes killed a man in one week.

Minor wounds, as I said, meant a horrible death since there was no disinfectant, and the unwashed skin was overgrown with infectious bacteria. McElroy recounts the instance of a man who was cut by the corner of a corn-bread box which he had been lifting from a supply wagon. The author relates how "gangrene set in immediately and he died four days after" (148). The activity of bacteria in open wounds was an unusual sight. McElroy uses the word *cancer*, another loosely used term, to describe a common, fast-moving bacterial infection. It usually began as "an ulcer at one corner of the mouth" and would eventually eat "the whole side of the face out." The sufferer could neither eat nor drink, so whittled wooden tubes were used for a straw (147). The "mouth cancer," as McElroy calls it, seemed contagious, so no one allowed the afflicted man to use cooking utensils.

The camp's doctors resorted to mass amputations in gangrene cases, and McElroy recalls two-hour "limb-chopping" sessions every morning (148). The chief limb-chopper, Confederate surgeon, R. Randolph Stevenson, M.D., testified at his war crimes hearing that hospital gangrene of the extremities and of the intestines caused cardiovascular clots, a primary cause of death. Having no understanding of infectious disease or of bacteriology, Stevenson conjectures that gangrene is essentially "a species of inflammation ... in which the fibrinous element and coagulability of the blood are increased" (292–93). In calling gangrene an inflammation with an unspecified cause, the doctor was not perjuring himself, since the linkage between these factors and disease was still being debated, despite what was known and suspected about cholera, puerperal fever, and smallpox. In regard to the origin of gangrene, Stevenson alludes vaguely to "poisonous matter" and to "various external noxious influences" (293). Yet Stevenson does not deny that the environment and physical constitution predisposed one to severe infection which was brought on rapidly because of poor diet, and by the "neglect of personal cleanliness" (293). The doctor refers, quite interestingly, to an internal form of the disorder, possibly the moist form of gangrene, that "attacked [the] intestinal canal of patients with bowel ulceration." The exact diagnosis of these disorders, as far as one can see from McElroy's account, is a matter of guesswork.

Of the 3,709 Union soldiers hospitalized by August 1864, 1,189 died, a rate increasing up until liberation (147). McElroy realized that the generally inhospitable conditions opened the way for a succession of crippling diseases: "Fever, rheumatism and lung diseases and despair ... came to complete the work begun by scurvy, dysentery and gangrene.... Hundreds, weary of the long struggle, and hoping against hope, laid themselves down and yielded to their fate" (216).

McElroy deplored the inadequacy of Andersonville's medical department. There was neither medicine nor food, just some root decoctions and an overcrowded hospital one was advised to avoid. At the morning roll call, doctors made "some pretense of affording medical relief" (145). There was an outdoor hospital area, five acres bordering the polluted creek. The area was reasonably clean, and some improvement in food is noted, with the addition of rice (to help the dysenteric) and of soup made from the pods of the okra plant (to help scorbutic patients), but these improvements had little nutritional value. Passing for medicine was a "rank, fetid species of ... spirits," distilled from sorghum seed and mixed with water (some sorghum produced a sugary syrup used for fodder) (147). Without soap and clean water baths and without hair cutting, the hospital area itself was infested with lice. Thus, writes McElroy, "If a man recovered, he did it almost in spite of fate" (147).

Other than Confederate Doctor Isaiah White, the Chief Surgeon of the prison who seemed "of fair ability," the other doctors were "illiterate quacks" who subscribed to superstitious cures. To cure convulsions, for example, they reputedly killed a black cat in the dark of the moon, cut it open, and bound the carcass upon the naked chest of the patient (148). A transcript from the Official Records of the prosecution's case against the camp's commandant, Captain Henri Wirz (November 1865), charges that he ordered prisoners to be inoculated with "poisonous vaccine matter." One eyewitness testified that he witnessed the results of forced inoculation on Union soldiers: large sores the size of a man's hand on the arms and underneath the armpit that left holes under the arms (303). The witness, Union soldier Oliver B. Fairbanks, was vaccinated against his will. Wirz put a gun to his head, and asked why he disobeyed his order. Fairbanks told Wirz that the vaccination matter was poisonous to which Wirz replied that the sooner Fairbanks died, the sooner he could get rid of him. After being placed in chains for two weeks, Fairbanks finally consented. It seems that Wirz had ordered his doctors to vaccinate everyone because smallpox was rumored; it is unclear as to whether the Confederates were inoculated as well. After inoculation, however, hospital gangrene set in. McElroy knew enough about vaccination to realize that sanitary practice was essential, and that the use of "genuine virus [not in the modern sense of the term]" never led to such high mortality (306). He refers explicitly to "variola vaccination." Although few cases of death by smallpox occurred at the Stockade, the chief surgeons, White and Stevenson, along with Captain Wirz, appeared to have exposed the soldiers to contaminated vaccine, which demonstrated their "heartless and implacable cruelty" in compelling prisoners of war to be vaccinated (306).

Although McElroy does not tell his readers how he and many others survived the ravages of disease at Andersonville, his book remains an important contribution to the corpus of epidemiological literature. An eyewitness, compelled to preserve the terrible experience for posterity, McElroy includes statistics, horrific descriptions, along with topographical and demographic details, that convey the moral obscenity of Andersonville. *This Was Andersonville* belongs to the heritage of Thucydides.

In an epidemic world, captivity can become a haven. Precisely such an inversion of expectations is found in Jack London's (1876–1916) South Pacific travelogue, *The Voyage of the Snark* (1911). Accompanied by his wife, Charmian, and by two crew members, London left San Francisco in 1906 on a custom-made 55-foot boat, *The Snark*. Their visit to the leper colony on the island of Molokai, Hawaii, literally transformed his thinking about disease and human behavior.

Leprosy or Hansen's disease is actually a chronic, mildly infectious illness that today can be treated successfully, but treatment must begin early and, for many, can last for as long as five years ("Hansen's Disease," CDC). The Norwegian physician, G. Armauer Hansen (1841–1912), identified the microbe in 1874 as a rod-shaped organism, *Mycobacterium leprae*. According to the CDC, the bacteria affects the skin and peripheral nerves and produces two forms of disease: the first, *paucibacillary* Hansen's disease, is a mild form that causes "hypo-pigmented skin macules"; and the second, more severe form is *multi-bacillary* disease. The latter is extremely destructive and leads to a number of skin lesions (nodules, plaques, thickening of skin and involvement of the nose). Even though the microbe grows very slowly, researchers have been unable to cultivate it in the laboratory (though it has been grown on "mouse foot pads"). Nor have they been able to determine how it is spreads, although they speculate that person-to-person infection through respiration is the likely route.

The accommodations and amenities Jack London found on Molokai contrast sharply with conditions found in turn-of-the century leprasaria. In *The Recrudescence of Leprosy and Its Causation* (1893), for example, William Tebb, M.D., during his inspection of the lazaretto on Robben Island, South Africa, reports of typical substandard conditions. The male ward, according to Tebb, was atmospherically foreboding, and the lepers looked like the living dead. The air was heavy "with the evil effluvia of decaying living bodies—death-in-life—supplemented by the odor of influenza." Tebb compares the scene to a field of battle, littered with "hand-less, footless, ulcerated, feature-swollen, and distorted patients." Leprosy, he observes, is a hopeless condition, one of protracted suffering. Along with this "repulsive" disease, syphillis was rampant. The belief was that leprosy and syphillis were contracted from contaminated smallpox inoculations, with Hansen's disease appearing as late as two years after inoculation. Both the conflation of maladies and the poor living condition evidenced the need for scientific research and for more appropriate facilities (though a new and more spacious hospital with fifty beds had just been opened, a fact Tebb found encouraging). Though the authorities were unable to support a research program, they had been trying to ameliorate hospital conditions, but this was a work in progress.

Tebb objected to the practice of housing the emotionally ill with the lepers. In his opinion, the island should be used for lepers, and those suffering from other maladies should receive appropriate medical care and separate housing. Some lepers whose disease was not severe worked as shoe-makers and tailors, but employment was difficult to find, and for most there was little desire or incentive to work. Some suffered terribly and had to rely on missionaries for their everyday needs.

One of the worst features of South African policy towards lepers was forcible deportation, a policy that was unevenly enforced since the rich could evade it and the poor could not. The Leprosy Repression Act enforced in Cape Colony, instead of focusing on laboratory work, called for the sys-tematic hunting down of lepers, a policy which resulted in the separation of parents from children, of husbands from wives, and so on. Tebb remarks that, while a considerable number of lepers lived successfully in conceal-ment, the well-to-do were left unmolested. In addition to this inequity, poor lepers were stigmatized by the medieval association of the disease with moral impurity (Watts 72). Robben Island, Cape Colony, was typical of the late nineteenth-century leper colony. Segregation, poor living conditions, inadequate medical care, moral, social, and religious stigmatization, along with racial prejudice, made for an abject lifestyle.

When London uses the phrases "[t]he pit of hell" and "the most cursed place on earth" to express his feelings about Molokai, he is being ironic; in fact, the travelogue functions as a corrective to popular exaggerations and to misconceptions about leprosy. Thus, he writes ebulliently of having had "a disgracefully good time along with eight hundred of the lepers who were likewise having a good time" (91). He recalls the excitement of horse and donkey racing and that the participants and the jubilant crowd consisted of lepers of every nationality and their guests (91–2). The races illustrate London's realization that the so-called "horrors of Molokai" did not exist (94). Sensationalism had victimized the Settlement; one example is of a particular newspaper writer who unjustly describes the beautiful serenading of leper bands and glee clubs as "wailing" (94–5).

In his efforts to rehabilitate the public image of the lepers on Molokai, London avoids hyperbole and strikes a balance between the medical reality and the need to uphold human dignity. On the one hand, the fear associated with the disease was exaggerated. There is no need, for instance, to wear "long gauntleted gloves and keep apart from the lepers"; rather, London and his wife reputedly intermingled with them freely. On the other hand, sensible precautions had to be observed since the disease was definitely contagious. To prevent contagion, physicians and superintendents "merely wash their faces and hands with mildly antiseptic soap and change their coats" (95). London reminds his readers, however, that the lepers were "unclean": they carried contagious disease, and they had to be segregated to control its spread. Mindful of this, he reiterates that: "the awful horror with which the leper has been regarded in the past and the frightful treatment he has received have been unnecessary and cruel" (95).

In his efforts to demythologize the disease, London tells of his participation in festivities. Like the Fourth of July horse race, the activities of the Kalaupapa Rifle Club demonstrate that those afflicted with the disease could pursue active lives. London's visit to the shooting event was his first experience of "the democracy of affliction and alleviation that obtains" (96). The Club consisted of people with and without the disease and who hailed from every ethnic and socio-economic class. Even the physicians participated. To London's amazement, "lepers and non-lepers used the same guns, and all were rubbing shoulders in the confined space" (96). To top it off, London and his wife Charmian watched a baseball game; the players, of mixed nationalities, were both leprous and non-leprous, but these distinctions meant nothing to the participants. Only an outsider noted these irrelevant distinctions (96–7).

The sporting nature of the islanders, London remarks, contrasts profoundly with the historical misconceptions surrounding Hansen's disease. It was theorized that the Crusaders carried the disease to Europe, where it slowly spread and affected many people. Europeans of the twelfth century thought that the disease was spread by contact, and that contagion could be controlled if the afflicted were segregated. But this tactic was carried to an inhumane extreme. As London points out, the medieval leper was considered to be legally and politically dead. He or she was even placed in a funeral procession, was led to church, and then endured a burial service read by a clergyman, hence the leprous epithet death-in-life. To symbolize his or her living death, earth was symbolically thrown on the unfortunate person's chest (97).

Admittedly awful and dehumanizing, lepraphobia actually helped to control the rate of infection: ostracized lepers were, in effect, under quarantine. London's point is that historically the *means* of segregation and not its practice has been repugnant. Ever since lepers had been segregated on Molokai, he observes, the disease had been decreasing (97). London understood that segregation need not have been "the horrible nightmare" that sensationalistic writers had contrived (97). Instead of the leprous suspect being arrested and forcibly removed from his or her family, he or she was "invited by the Board of Health to come to the Kalihi receiving station at Honolulu" in order to undergo medical tests to determine if *bacillus leprae* was present (97–8). If the test was positive, the person was "declared" a leper, and the Board of Health sent the person to Molokai (98). There was no evading the medical reality: the person had to be isolated to keep the disease in check (98).

The difference between Molokai and places like Robben Island was that, during the evaluation of the case, the afflicted person in Hawaii had the right "to be represented by a physician whom he can select and employ for himself" (98). Furthermore, the leper was not rushed off into isolation but was allotted sufficient time to remain at Kalihi and to make business arrangements. This also meant that the leper, though segregated, could remain economically self-sufficient (98). Unimpeachable rules obtained, nonetheless: although business agents and relatives could visit the segregated, they were not permitted to eat and sleep in the lepers' house. Specially maintained visitors' houses were provided for that purpose (98).

The Settlement of Molokai, contrary to popular belief, was not a shanty town. The climate and scenery of the island surpassed Honolulu in beauty. Mountain valleys and green pastures made the scene idyllic. Hundreds of horses owned by lepers roamed the grasslands; the residents had carts, rigs, and wagons, along with fishing and steam boats; their seafaring, however, was restricted (perhaps to proscribe illegal departures or visitations). The lepers had many occupations: fishing, farming, carpentry, small business, and whoever was unable to earn a livelihood received food, shelter, clothes, and medical care (101). The Board of Health developed agriculture, stock-raising, and dairying, and employment was available at fair wages. And, for the young, the elderly, and the infirm, homes and hospitals were provided at no cost (101). Clearly, the Honolulu authorities realized that a solvent local economy was necessary if leprous society was to remain self-sufficient.

Many of the residents implored London to write the truth about Molokai and to stop the "chamber-of-horrors rot" (101). Morally obliged to do so, he avowed that, despite their disease, the one thousand residents of Molokai lived in "a happy colony," comprising two villages, numerous country and seaside homes, six churches, several assembly halls, a racetrack, a baseball field, firing ranges, and band stand, and the people belong to an athletic club, glee clubs, and two brass bands (101). To silence those who might accuse him of exaggeration, London contends that people who were misdiagnosed as having the disease and threatened with deportation actually "fought against being sent *away* from Molokai" (italics added); many were lucky enough to find useful jobs on the island and were allowed to remain (103).

London's revelation upon visiting Molokai concerns the corrosive nature of fear. He is right in saying that: "the chief horror of leprosy obtains in the minds of those who have never seen a leper and who do not know anything about the disease" (104). The author's experience on Molokai illustrates the axiom that ignorance fosters fear and hatred. On the mainland of the United States at that time, the treatment of lepers reflected the impulses of fear and ignorance. London learned that the segregation of mainland lepers was loosely enforced, for they were left to wander the streets without support services. Though leprosy is a terrible disease, the institutions of Molokai far surpassed the hospital for the poor, the tuberculosis sanitaria, or the overcrowded and confined environments of urban American (105). The lepers of Molokai lived as freely as possible. Their society was the product of two interdependent mandates: the safeguarding of public health in the greater Hawaiian community and the upholding of human dignity on Molokai, despite the isolation of its residents.

The nature of Hansen's disease, London's experience makes evident, required a medical infrastructure suited to its victims. He recognized that, because leprosy is a chronic disease, usually progressing from an acute phase to an indeterminate period of dormancy, good health could last for as long as a decade, when the disease could re-erupt. The patient suffering with the initial onset of the disease or the "ravages" would not experience remission without medical care. Because the first attack can destroy a limb and threaten life, a leper living in seclusion will suffer and perhaps even die of complications. On Molokai, on the other hand, surgeons operated on ulcerous tissue and arrested "that particular ravage of the disease" with skill born of experience. Intermittent treatments allowed the patient to resume regular activities, for there was no reason to hide in shame or to fear recriminations and the loathing of an ignorant public.

The irony of London's Molokai description is that "the leper is rigidly segregated" yet "humanely treated" (108). Rigid segregation was justified since the disease remained "the same awful and profound misery." The best that bacteriologists had been able to do at the time of London's visit was to isolate the microbe, but they knew nothing of how it was transmitted to a healthy person (108–09); research in this area had been inconclusive (110).

The narratives of McElroy and of London share a common viewpoint on disease. Each author, standing at one remove from the epidemic zone, wrote objectively about the environment's impact on human beings. McElroy's distancing, of course, came with time (he published his book more than a decade later), for in the confines of Andersonville he had all to do just to survive. Nonetheless, he wrote with the acuity of a modern epidemiologist perceiving the intrinsic relationship between disease and ecology. In the perverted ecology of Andersonville, we find human beings becoming the staple of parasites. London's distancing was both circumstantial and geographical: a visitor to an epidemic world, he surveyed the life of Molokai objectively, and he wrote a humane testimony. He soon realized that Molokai had become a viable society: the people, though stricken to various degrees with a common disorder and isolated by law, received excellent care. Moreover, on Molokai, unlike in Andersonville, isolation did not subvert the community. It was in the interest of the Hawaiian government to support the colony and, most important, to help its residents to help themselves. At the turn of the century, lepers in Hawaii came from every walk of life, so it was a logical decision not to sever them from the past — that is, from their interests, vocations, and families. In Andersonville, on the other hand, the Confederate overseers, who were unable to support the prisoners, realized that liberating them meant the POWs would fight again (the Union thought likewise of Confederate POWs). Short of mass execution, they allowed Andersonville to become a concentration camp. In this densely-populated location, the mass executioners were the elements, malnutrition, and parasitic disease.

Primo Levi at Auschwitz

On January 11, 1945, Primo Levi, a chemist of Italian-Jewish descent who had been deported to Auschwitz, developed scarlet fever and was sent to Ka-Be, an infirmary the Germans called *Infektionsabteilung* (151). The tiny fifteen-square-foot room held ten bunks on two levels, a wardrobe, and three stools. Levi was the thirteenth prisoner to be sent there. Of the twelve already there, four had scarlet fever (two were Hungarian Jews; two were French political prisoners), three had diphtheria, two had typhus, one had a facial infection, and two others had several unidentified illnesses and were severely wasted. Levi who had a high fever managed to find a bunk for himself. He knew that he was permitted forty days' of isolation and rest since he was a laborer and therefore temporarily useful to the Germans.

Levi's long experience of camp life had made him resourceful and creative. His personal belongings consisted of a belt of interlaced electric wire, a knife-spoon, needles, five buttons, and eighteen flints stolen from the camp laboratory; the flints were especially valuable since one could start a fire with them. Days one to four were peaceful. Although it was snowing and quite cold, Levi was in a heated room. And although he was very sick and unable to eat, he was being treated with large dosages of sulfa drugs which hastened his recovery (151–52).

The two Frenchmen with scarlet fever had entered the camp only a few days earlier. The older man was Arthur and his bed-ridden companion, a thirty-two-year-old school teacher, was Charles. On the fifth day, the barber revealed that they were all going to be transported westward, a foreboding revelation. Levi relates that, by this time, he could no longer feel pain, joy, or fear (152). Though emotionally numb, he understood how dangerous such an evacuation could be since the Russians were driving towards Auschwitz from the south, and since the Germans were becoming desperate. A twelve-mile march in the dead of winter for an ambulatory patient like Levi was not promising (153). Upon hearing of these plans, some patients panicked and tried to escape, but the SS (*Schutzstaffel*) killed them (154). Healthy prisoners began to leave on the night of January 18, 1945. As many as twenty thousand inmates undertook the terrible journey that night, but Levi remained bed-ridden, helpless, and in the hands of fate (155). At that moment, the remaining inmates of Ka-Be were alone with their illnesses. All together, eight hundred prisoners were left behind in the infirmary camp, with thirteen in Levi's room. For them, an eventful ten-day period began, "outside of both world and time" (156).

On the night of the evacuation, Levi and his coinhabitants surveyed the environment with the intention of improving conditions (155).

Although the central heating plant had been abandoned, and although the scantily clad inmates faced an outside temperature of 5 degrees F., they were able to determine that the kitchens still functioned. Some SS officers remained in the camp, and some of the guard towers were still occupied, so Levi and his companions had to be careful. At midday, January 18, a touring SS officer appointed a chief in each of the barracks who would divide Jews from non–Jews, another frightening development. Meanwhile, Levi's group had managed to get extra bread rations, and they found blankets that, though contaminated with dysentery, were essential to their survival in the freezing weather. Without working clocks, they lost track of time, but around 11 P.M., on January 18, Auschwitz came under Russian bombardment, as did the outlying infirmary camp. Huts and makeshift barracks were blown to pieces, and many prisoners were forced outside to escape the shelling and the fires. Despite the danger and the chaos, Levi likened the Russian bombardment to the racial memory of biblical salvation, which passed like a wind through his mind (157). This spiritual reverie was short-lived. Levi realized that what they had scavenged from the kitchen was only the beginning of their reconstructive work. With the last of the Germans fleeing for their lives, the stranded inmates had to recreate a civilization in the midst of a shattered world and to do so while burdened with infectious illnesses of several kinds (157). With the help of Arthur and Charles, they set about the immediate task of securing the infirmary and of making it livable. At the outset, they needed to close the broken windows and find food and a stove.

On January 19, up at dawn and outside, they discovered that the Lager had begun to disintegrate: there was no water or electricity, and the ground was littered with loose iron sheets. The most startling sight was that of the "ragged, decrepit skeleton-like patients," who dragged themselves in the frozen soil, "like an invasion of worms" (158). The group ransacked empty huts looking for food and wood and even entered forbidden German quarters. Levi observed that hundreds of dysenteric patients were fouling the snow, the only source of fresh water. This was a critical issue, for as the temperature rose to melt the snow all of the surface water would be undrinkable and water-borne diseases would infect everyone. Realizing that the needs of the moment had to be met, they returned to Ka-Be with a supply of potatoes, a heavy cast iron stove, wood, coal, and with material to repair broken windows (159). The recivilizing process had commenced: they had food, water, and heat.

At this point in the narrative, heat, sustenance, and the absence of the Germans allowed for relaxation, and Levi's emotional obduracy began to soften (159). A twenty-three-year-old Franco-Pole named Tomarowski, who was suffering from typhus, proposed to the other Ka-Be inmates that, for their hard work, they reward Levi, Arthur, and Charles with a slice of bread for each (160). This expression of gratitude impressed Levi. He reflected upon how markedly the gesture contradicted the law of the Lager (i.e., to eat your own bread and what you can steal from your neighbor) which, at that moment, had become obsolete. To Levi, "that moment can be dated as the beginning of [their]" rehumanization (160).

Caring for one's neighbor was an important aspect of the rehumanizing process in that tiny room. Practical tasks had to be undertaken. Arthur was to maintain the stove, to cook potatoes, to clean the rooms, and to help the other patients. Charles and Levi scrounged outside of the infirmary. They found a tin of yeast and a pint of spirits that had been thrown in the snow; the yeast provided a good source of B vitamins and was apportioned to each man. When darkness fell, the population outside, numbering nearly eight hundred, learned of the stove. Many tried to gain entrance, but Charles barred the door and drove them away. Had he not done so, the ward would have been looted.

The stove and the environment it had created also united the thirteen men of the *Infektionsabteilung*. Levi's spiritual reflection is ironic: "In the middle of the endless plain, frozen and full of war, in the small dark room swarming with germs, we felt at peace with ourselves and with the world. We were broken by the tiredness, but we seemed to have finally accomplished something useful perhaps like God after the first day of creation" (161). If not for scarlet fever, Levi probably would have been deported with the other able-bodied prisoners. Ironically, his rebirth, if you will, was owed directly to a life-threatening illness and to isolation. The infirmary, a microcosm of infectious disease, had become a momentary safe haven.

On the morning of January 20, the recivilizing process was resumed in earnest. Though weak from the effects of scarlet fever, Levi used his flints and spirit-soaked paper to light the stove and to set up the fire (160). Exploring the decaying camp further, Charles and Levi acquired a two-day supply of food and secured a snow-covered area as a fresh-water source. The sight of ragged, starving prisoners disturbed them, but nothing could be done for so many, given the meager resources (160). The image of two Yiddish-speaking skeletal men squabbling over putrid potatoes symbolized the desperation that had gripped the prisoners outside (161). To this ravaged scene, Levi contrasts his systematic foraging, which uncovered potatoes, turnips, and cabbage. They even found a charged battery to power the lights in the domicile (161).

Despite the good feelings, the morbid atmosphere of the camp continued to weigh heavily on Levi. On January 21, he writes of how, at one time, he wanted to stay in bed under the blankets and to abandon himself to exhaustion. A creeping indifference had gripped his consciousness, but he was roused from his depression when Charles lit the stove to start the day. Work relieved their abjectness as they industriously emptied excrement buckets, searched for wood, gathered clean snow, and mobilized the other patients in their room to peel potatoes (162). While Charles and Levi sought a suitable location in their barrack for a working kitchen, the camp latrines in the adjacent ward began to overflow and human waste saturated the ground. More than one hundred dysentery patients in the adjoining room had fouled every corner of their domicile and had even used ration buckets and pots for defecation. Despite this difficult situation, Levi and his group indefatigably set up parameters for their survival. They searched for and found a small area of floor not excessively soiled to make a laundry area. They lit a fire in the area and disinfected their hands with a chlorine solution. And they created a sanitary site in this manner. When they cooked vegetable soup, the aroma drew a throng of starving, half-dead individuals whom Charles had no choice but to turn away (163). Indeed, civilization needed security. It also required commerce and trade. For example, a Parisian tailor who was an outsider manufactured clothes for Charles and Levi out of blankets (jackets, trousers, and other garments), which he traded for two pints of vegetable soup (163). With the sound of Russian artillery in the air, Levi ironically reflects that life outside of the camp and of the depressed confines of the mind was once again beautiful. They began to talk of returning home.

Work had to be done if this dream were to come true (165). The companions drew up a protocol for the group, a code of behavior: each person had to look after his own bowl and spoon; no one was to offer his soup to another; one was not to climb down from the bunk unless going to the latrine; if anyone needed anything, he was to ask Levi, Arthur or Charles; and Arthur would be responsible for supervising discipline and hygiene; and lastly one should not wash utensils or bowls since they could be contaminated by water. The logic behind these simple rules was obvious and quite astute: each inmate was to police himself and need not fear his fellow prisoner. In addition, Levi and his friends established order, under which the cooperation and welfare of each individual was subsumed: they had a government.

With the rudiments of civilization encoded, the group once again explored the SS camp outside the electric fence, earlier a zone of certain death. They successfully raided the SS stores and returned to the infirmary with frozen soup, beer, and other valuables, which they entrusted to Arthur's care to prevent pilfering and to ensure equitable rationing. The raid was more daring and dangerous than Levi realized at the time. One-half hour after their return to the infirmary, eighteen French prisoners tried to replicate the feat. Unfortunately, a party of fleeing SS men discovered them and left their bodies in the snow.

The safe room that Levi and company had created was in close proximity to the worst squalor imaginable (166). Behind the wooden wall were dysentery patients, dying and dead, and lying on the floor amidst frozen waste. When they smelled Levi's soup kitchen, they implored him for help, and this time he spared a small portion. The men of the infirmary had their hands full with the sick patients among them. Even with their meager resources, they helped each other. In the bunk below Levi was a seventeen-year-old Dutch Jew, named Lakmaker. He had been bedridden for three months with typhus, scarlet fever, and cardiac problems. To make matters worse, he had bedsores and was so infirm that he could not speak. He consumed more soup than he could handle, becoming more ill. Rather than to abandon him next door among the dying, Levi's society treated him with dignity. Charles lit a lamp to ascertain the youth's condition: his bed and the floor were soiled, the odor was overwhelming, and there were neither blankets nor straw to spare; moreover, as a typhus victim, Lakmaker was also a source of infection. So, for the benefit of the group and the individual, Charles lifted Lakmaker tenderly from the ground, cleaned him with mattress straw, remade his bed as best he could, and proceeded to disinfect the area with a tin plate containing diluted chloramine (a pungent liquid derived from ammonia), which they had found in the infirmary (167).

On January 23, Charles and Levi once again embarked on a foraging expedition. By this time, it seemed, the SS were gone for good. Levi recollects that, for the first time since his arrest, he found himself genuinely free, without armed guards and barbed-wire fences separating him not only from home but from *himself* (167–68; italics added). His sense of dignity and of the importance of his friends was revived by the evaporation of German tyranny and also by the newly-found food, a treasure trove of potatoes unearthed 400 yards from camp. On January 24, they experienced true liberty as they breached the wire fence, forever free of German brutality. Yet the sudden departure of the Germans, paradoxically, left the camp in a state of anarchy. Though the SS were gone, "all around lay destruction and death" (167). Piles of corpses were everywhere, everyone remained weak, and there was little hope for tuberculosis patients and for others with acute diarrhea. Their spirits were lifted when, during an excursion, they met British POWs who gave them much needed supplies which they brought back to Ka-Be.

Industry and commerce, though rudimentary, continued to transform Ka-Be into a small civilization (170). Levi fumigated the hut with candles made out of cardboard molds, beeswax, and wicks soaked in boric acid. On January 25, he was able to reflect on the past and on the effect the Lager had had on the human mind generally. Not only did the concentration camp prisoner give up hope, but one also loses the very ability to think logically and to solve problems. In a concentration camp like Auschwitz, moreover, it was futile to think because events were unpredictable. By contrast, in the shelter of Ka- Be, it was possible to speak freely and to become enthusiastic and nostalgic, emotions signifying a revival of hope and a reawakening sense of selfhood.

Levi acknowledged that experiencing the process of degradation and of recovery firsthand revealed terrible truths about humanity. Although the Germans were on the verge of defeat, and although civilization was revived, it was clear to him that mankind had a very dark side. Under such conditions, the depths to which prisoners must descend in order to survive can be understood, though not condoned. Thus, whoever waits for his neighbor to die so as to take his bread is not guilty. As a victim of circumstance, the one who waits has descended to an appallingly primitive level. What defines our humanity, according to Levi, is how we relate to and feel about others.

The Russians finally arrived on January 27, to find the Ka-Be inmates hard at work cleaning the latrine, preparing meals, and leaving the disposal of the dead to the end of the day. The distressing irony of Levi's story is that, during German captivity, only one of the men in the infirmary died, but, once in a Russian hospital at Auschwitz, five of the survivors died weeks later. The remaining survivors returned to the world, having overcome German deprivations. One can justifiably say that their illnesses saved them from the common fate.

In a conversation with Levi, Philip Roth remarks how he was impressed by the extent to which "thinking" contributed to survival in Ka-Be (180). Levi had approached his ordeal with "a practical, humane scientific-mind," and this frame of mind was instrumental in his survival. Roth differentiates this attitude from "brute biological strength or incredible luck." Levi's ability to withstand the rigors of the camp was rooted in his "professional character." Roth further describes him as "the man of precision, the controller of experiments who seeks the principle of order, confronted with the evil inversion of everything he values" (180). Levi responded to this encomium with the simple statement that he and companions were "willing to work ... for a just and human goal." Certainly, fortuitous events contributed to their survival (e.g., sulfa drugs, being sick at the time of deportation, the departure of the SS, and the availability of key items). And emotional discipline was of equal importance to the constructive efforts.

Levi did not retreat into himself, for morbid solipsism meant physical death. Instead, like Thucydides, he removed himself intellectually from the squalor and disease around him, recorded his experiences, and maintained his humanity throughout, all the while desiring to understand the aberrant reality around him. Throughout his experience, he apprehended the experience with the "curiosity of a naturalist who finds himself transplanted into an environment that is monstrous but new, monstrously new" (180). By insulating himself in the guise of an anthropologist, an explorer in a *terra incognita*, he was able to maintain his sanity and to utilize his intellectual gifts (180).

The primary difference between the survival stories of John McElroy and of Primo Levi is that the latter was able to reconstruct a viable society. Unlike the residents on Molokai whose well-being was in the hands of a competent government and medical establishment, the inmates of Levi's safe house owed their survival to analytical intelligence and to the predilection for teamwork. Because McElroy, London, and Levi stand at one intellectual remove from the diseased worlds of captivity, they were each able to describe the effects of diseases, the cost of human suffering, and the means of survival.

11. THE LANGUAGE OF REASON

Plague Extrapolations in Modern Fiction

The idea informing modern plague fiction, such as Sinclair Lewis's *Arrowsmith* (1924), Albert Camus' *The Plague* (1947), and Gwyneth Cravens' and John Marr's *The Black Death* (1977), is that the management of epidemic disease is a synergistic undertaking, the success of which depends on the joint effort of medical professionals, of civil authorities, and of an informed public. In this chapter, I will comment on the theme of collaboration in the fiction and compare each work to the scientific and historical facts. Writers who accurately represent biomedical facts are able to explore vicariously the devastating power of epidemic disease and humanity's struggle against it.

Sinclair Lewis's *Arrowsmith*

The central biomedical event in *Arrowsmith* is the discovery of bacteriophage, a virus that destroys bacteria. The bacteriologist Felix d'Hérelle, in 1917, invented the neologism *bacteriophage*, a Greek compound meaning, *eater of bacteria* (*Random House* 100). In reality, the phage virus does *not* eat bacteria. One form of the virus, for example, infects bacteria parasitically and, in the course of its own rapid reproduction, destroys the microbe it has penetrated. Composed of a protein head, an inner core of nucleic acid, and a hollow protein tail, the phage is specific to the bacteria it penetrates and usually affects one or a few related species (Stent [1963], 1–22; [1965], 73–87). Rather than to devour the bacterium, it attaches itself to its cell wall by its tail, a protein structure with long fibers; the fibers fix the virus to a specific receptor site on the bacterial cell wall, and the tail sheath, contracting like a syringe, injects the virus' nucleic acid through the cell wall into the cell membrane; the protein coat, meanwhile, remains outside the bacterium. The injected genetic material, however, takes over the chemical activity of the cell, producing viral enzymes and phage nucleic acid. In this manner, the original phage reproduces itself within, and at the expense of, the bacterial host. The newly-generated viral proteins and nucleic-acid molecules inside the host eventually assemble into as many as one hundred new phages. The effects of phage on visible, bacterial colonies appear as clear spots or *plaque*. Under a conventional microscope, ruptured and dying bacteria can be seen; and, under the electron microscope (developed by Hillier, Prebus, and Zworykin in 1932), the molecular activities of the phage are observable.

The scientists who were the first to see the dead cells rightly thought that the mysterious agent had medical uses. The challenge, at the outset, was to determine what the agent was, how it worked, and how its power could be harnessed. Typically, the cognitive history of early phage research began with the observation of an anomaly, from which scientists precipitously inferred that an invisible agent ate bacteria.

I would like to outline the historical background of early phage research as a standard against which to contrast Sinclair Lewis's imaginative treatment of the subject in *Arrowsmith*. In 1896 the British bacteriologist, Ernest Hanbury Hankin (1865–1939), while experimenting with the cholera-infected water of the Ganges and Jumna Rivers in India, noticed an anomaly. When he added a sample of river water to a culture dish of cholera vibrio, something in the water dissolved the bacteria. This was paradoxical since the river water, polluted with human waste, was known to have been contaminated with cholera. What accounted for this bactericidal activity in the water? Hankin tried but failed to isolate the mysterious agent, thought responsible for this effect, by passing river water through a fine porcelain filter that was designed to trap large micro-organisms. Despite his failure to isolate the agent, he continued to infer that its activity, naturally at work in the rivers, interrupted the growth of cholera ("Bacteriophage Therapy," *Biotech Journal*; Hankin 511).

The British microbiologist, Frederick William Twort (1877–1950), encountered a similar anomaly while searching for viruses. From 1912 to 1915, while at the Brown Institute (a research center for veterinary medicine), he attempted to culture viruses using laboratory techniques that were designed for bacteria (97–102). In cultivations of agar, egg, serum, dung, grass, hay, straw, and pond water, he found nothing unusual. The addition of chemicals or extracts from seeds and fungi did nothing. And though he covered the material with water, incubated it at 30 degrees C., filtered the solution, and inoculated it on different media, no "ultra-microscopic" organisms manifested themselves.

Realizing that these organisms could not be seen through a conventional microscope, Twort had to find a way of confirming their presence;

to this end, he experimented with tissue samples and exudate containing the organisms that cause vaccinia and canine distemper. Even though the pathogens that caused these diseases were ultramicroscopic, and even though they had not yet been isolated, their presence was confirmed by their effects on animals. The inoculum, which was derived from blood and tissue, contained the viruses; it could be extracted from animals infected with these diseases, and it could then be used for immunization and for experimentation.

For Twort, knowing the effect of the disease was not enough: he wanted to see what the invisible organisms looked like. So he tried, but failed again, to isolate them from the exudate. At this juncture, and with nothing to show for his work, he noticed something unusual in cultures of glycerinated calf vaccinia: amidst the field of visible bacterial colonies (the medium containing the vaccinia virus), there appeared "watery-looking areas" (98), which also appeared in inoculated agar tubes that had been incubating for 24 hours and at 37 degrees C. (98.6 F). The micrococci cultures exhibiting the glassy areas could not be subcultured and, in time, became completely "glassy and transparent" (98). Visible if stained reddish with Giemsa, the colonies were reduced to "minute granules."

Twort tried to replicate the anomaly under controlled conditions in order to understand its nature and function. Further experimentation was indicated. To make plated cultures, he inoculated water containing the agent into a series of test tubes filled with bacteria so that the inoculum floated over the surface of the medium. This done, he left the colonies of the first dilution alone. They, too, began to turn transparent, and the flourishing micrococci were, once again, reduced to "fine granules" (99). The dissolutive activity or *lysis* began at the outer edge of the colonies. Twort demonstrated that, if a pure culture of white or of yellow micrococcus extracted from the vaccinia culture dish came into contact with a minute sample of the glassy area in the bacterial colonies, the pure culture would also become transparent and glassy, and this condition rapidly spread over the entire growth. Sometimes, all of the micrococci were killed, leaving only granulated debris.

Twort discovered that the dissolutive process was more rapid and thorough with vigorous young cultures than with old ones, and that there was little or no activity on dead cultures, or on young cultures that had been killed by heat (at 60 degrees C.). When saline water was diluted to one part per million, the transparent material passed through the finest porcelain filters easily yet remained potent enough to destroy the micrococci. In fact, one drop of the filtrate deposited over an agar tube had dramatic bactericidal effects. If the micrococcus were inoculated down the test tube in a streak, the organism would grow, but transparent points would soon appear on the streaks and rapidly extend over the whole growth. In some cases, the bactericidal effect was so pronounced as to turn the micrococcus glassy on contact. The "condition or disease of the micrococcus," Twort affirms, can be transferred successfully to fresh bacterial cultures and for an indefinite number of generations.

If the agent were filtered from the exudate, it retained its lytic potency for over six months, was unattenuated even if emulsified and heated to 5 degrees C. for one hour, but was destroyed at 60 degrees C. A similar agent isolated from boils dissolved *staphylococcus aureas* and *staphylococcus albus*, but, interestingly enough, it did not have a similar effect on micrococcus.

Twort pondered the nature of phage: either it was a minute bacterium, an amoeba, a protoplasmic form, or an enzyme (100). Additionally, he suspected that the agent was part of, or issued from, the micrococcus. If that were true, the transparency could be a stage in the bacteria's natural development: the micrococcus might therefore have been catalyzed "to pass into the lytic stage" (100). Or perhaps the bacteria secreted a self-destructive enzyme? Since the agent could not be cultured independently of the micrococci, Twort could not test any of these hypotheses. Financial concerns prevented him from investigating bacteriophage definitively (101).

The bacteriologist, Felix d'Hérelle, brought Twort's work to fruition. Unlike Twort, d'Hérelle early in his research was interested not in viruses but in the use of bacteria in agriculture and for pest control. In his 1917 paper, "Bacteriophage," he recalls that, while investigating a locust plague in Yucatán, Mexico in 1910, he collected specimens of dead locusts to ascertain why they had suddenly died in large numbers (excerpts in Stent [1963], 1–22). He learned that sick locusts had blackish diarrhea that was caused by the bacteria coccobacillus, which could be harvested in pure state from the insect secretions. D'Hérelle cultured the locust disease in order to derive a specific insecticide from it. Theoretically, one could dust plants with powdered coccobacillus cultures to infect the feeding insects. From 1910 to 1914, he used his bacterial insecticide profitably in the Yucatán, in Argentina, in Colombia, in Cyprus, in Algeria, in Tunisia, and in Turkey (Summers [1999], 30, 33).

Like Hankin and Twort, d'Hérelle noticed a similar anomaly: plaque, two to three millimeters in diameter, developed in the midst of the coccobacilli. When he took samples of these spots for microscopic examination, he saw nothing. Whatever had formed the transparencies had passed through porcelain filters and was, therefore, smaller than bacteria.

In 1915, the anomaly inspired a hypothesis, and the opportunity to test it arose fortuitously (excerpts in Stent [1963], 1–22). The director of the Pasteur Institute, Dr. Emile Roux, famous for his discovery of the diphtheria toxin, requested that d'Hérelle investigate a dysentery epidemic afflicting a cavalry squadron. D'Hérelle filtered emulsions of the soldiers' feces, allowed the filtrates to act on cultures of dysentery bacilli, and then spread the solution out, after incubating it on nutritive agar petri dishes. As anticipated, the bacteria displayed transparencies. D'Hérelle applied this knowledge to dysentery cases in the Pasteur Institute, paying special attention to one particular case in order to calculate exactly when the dissolutive activity began. On the first day, he isolated *Shigella* dysentery bacilli from the bloody stools of patients. When he cultured the specimens and then added filtrate from the feces of the same patient, the results were negative, as they would be on the second and third days. On the fourth day, he again made an emulsion from the bloody stools and filtered it through a Chamberland filter so that only particles smaller than bacteria would pass through. He then added a drop of the filtrate to the dysentery culture that he had isolated on the first day. After spreading a drop of this mixture on agar, he incubated the broth culture tube and the agar plate at 37 degrees C. (98.6 F.). On the following morning, he was astonished to find that the infected broth was clear: all the bacterial colonies had vanished. The agar dish was also without *Shigella* growth. He assumed, at once, that "an invisible microbe," a filterable virus parasitic on bacteria, had been responsible for the plaque. The experiment suggested that a similar process had taken place in the sick man's body. Believing that the patient may also have experienced a cure, d'Hérelle rushed to the hospital to find that his belief had been confirmed.

D'Hérelle published his findings in the 1917 paper, "On an invisible microbe that is antagonistic to the dysentery bacillus" (157–59). Using the technique described in the abovementioned case, he tested secretions taken from dysentery convalescents. From their feces, he isolated microbes antagonistic to *Shigella* bacilli. D'Hérelle seeded tubes of broth, each with four to five drops of feces; he incubated the tube for 18 hours at 37 degrees C.; and he filtered the contents through a Chamberland candle filter. His initial observation was reinforced: "When a small quantity of an active filtrate is added to a broth culture of [*Shigella*] bacillus ... the culture is inhibited and the death of the bacillus through complete lysis occurs" (157–58). The identical phenomenon occurred if the antagonistic emulsion were taken from this dish and introduced directly into *Shigella* cultures. Since the first isolated strain was transferred fifty times, the antagonistic agent, he was convinced, had to be a living germ and not an enzyme. So intense was the activity of the antagonist that a single diluted drop of lysed culture (the new culture containing only one-millionth of a part of original lysate), if added to an agar slant and incubated, riddled a layer of dysentery bacilli with sterile plaque one millimeter in diameter. Undoubtedly, the spots circumscribed living, antagonistic colonies.

D'Hérelle ruled out a chemical agent because chemicals cannot concentrate activity in small areas. According to his calculations, a lysed culture of *Shigella* contained five to six *billion* filterable germs per cubic centimeter, one three-billionth of a cubic centimeter of a lysate containing a single germ, and this minute quantity, if added to *Shigella*, fully inhibited it (italics added). In five to six days, a minute quantity of antagonistic material was enough to sterilize ten cubic centimeters of the bacillus. Yet the antagonist could neither be cultivated in media devoid of the dysentery bacilli, nor did it affect heat-killed bacteria. Because it could be cultured in a suspension of saline-washed cells, d'Hérelle concluded that it was a parasite, and he labeled it an *obligate*, a term that had been invented, in 1870, by the German botanist, Heinrich Anton De Bary (1831–1888). The anti-*Shigella* obligate or bacteriophage was not only innocuous to laboratory animals, but it also conferred immunity: lysated cultures of *Shigella*, rich in obligate, immunized rabbits against doses of the same bacillus that killed control animals in five days. Obviously, the cultures had potential as both a bactericidal agent and as a vaccine.

In "On the Role of the Filterable Bacteriophage in Bacillary Dysentery" (1918), d'Hérelle advocated the clinical use of bacteriophage (excerpts in Stent [1963], 1–22). Early results against typhus, cholera, and plague were encouraging, but twenty years of research failed to establish phage as a pharmacological tool. William C. Summers remarks that "early trials of bacteriophage therapy for infectious diseases were confounded ... because the biological nature of bacteriophage was poorly understood" ([2001]: 5451; see also, Summers [1999], 51, 54, 56, 64, 109, 111–112, 117). Recently, scholars have attributed d'Hérelle's failure both to haste and altruism: he transferred phages from the laboratory to the hospital and community setting without including placebo groups of patients, perhaps because he was "reluctant to deprive anyone of therapy he believed could save his or her life" (Sulakvelidze 649–59).

Sinclair Lewis's (1885–1951) protagonist, Dr. Martin Arrowsmith, is portrayed as a contemporary of d'Hérelle and as an independent discoverer of bacteriophage, from which he, like his historical counterpart, attempts to manufacture anti-plague vaccine. While isolating a strain of staphylococcus, drawn from a patient's gluteal carbuncle, Arrowsmith learns that the lesion healed spontaneously and with "unusual rapidity" (307). To find out how this happened, he places the pus in broth medium, incubates the suspension, and finds, eight hours later, that the colony has grown; then he places the flask in the incubator (307). Some time later, and much to his surprise, he notices that the flask no longer contains any living bacteria. Suspecting a procedural error, he prepares a slide from the clear broth. To his astonishment, under the microscope he spies shadows, the thin outlines of dead organisms, "minute skeletons on an infinitesimal battlefield" (308), and concludes either that something external to the bacteria killed them or that the colony destroyed itself.

Arrowsmith claims to have searched, unsuccessfully, the American, English, French, and German literature on the subject (309). Unable to find a research precedent, he questions his method and assumptions: perhaps no living staphylococcus was in the pus extracted from the patient? To answer this question, he makes a glass-slide smear of the original pus, staining it with gentian-violet. One drop of the specimen appears, microscopically, as "grape-like clusters ... purple dots against the blank plane" (309). To his trained eye, this was unmistakably a rich colony of staphylococcus (310). Once certain that the original culture was staphylococcus, he lists all possible causes of the bacteria's spontaneous destruction (310). Like d'Hérelle, Arrowsmith considers possible causes: (1) an alkali in an improperly cleaned flask; (2) an unidentified property of the broth solution; (3) an unknown bacterial antagonist in the pus; or (4) a self-destructive agent issuing from the bacteria.

In order to test each possibility, Arrowsmith painstakingly sterilizes new flasks, clears them of antiseptics, plugs them with cotton, filters lysate into the flasks through a sterile porcelain filter, and then adds the lysate to his regular staphylococcus strains. In a group of differentially-conditioned flasks, all seeded with staphylococcus, he tests the four possibilities outlined above in order to determine the nature of the antagonistic agent. Each flask is incubated at body temperature. Despite his nervousness, impatience, and exhaustion, he proceeds systematically, recording each step of his experiment (311). On the following morning, he contacts the hospital to request more pus from the original patient only to hear that the carbuncle had entirely healed. Lewis definitely had d'Hérelle's work in mind, specifically the gradual and inexplicable recovery of the soldier afflicted with *Shigella dysenteriae*.

At 10 A.M., Arrowsmith finds that flasks containing broth from the original solution are clear of germs (312). With these positive results, he returns to the library to locate precedents but, again, finds none. At 6 P.M. the flasks containing the original broth remain devoid of bacteria. Those seeded with the original pus, at first, show abundant growth which disappears under the "slowly developing attack of the unknown assassin" (313). Not knowing what the agent is, he calls it the X Principle, inferring that it arrested the growth of several strains of staphylococcus.

Before Arrowsmith can ascertain if the agent can dissolve infectious bacteria other than staphylococcus (314), he must determine its nature: is it a germ, a chemical, or an enzyme? Two ancillary questions are: (1) whether the agent is transmitted from test tube to test tube or whether it reappears in the interim between transfers; and (2) whether it grows by cell division. He suspects that a "sub-germ" (Twort's adjective was "ultramicroscopic") infects the carbuncular bacteria (314), and he conjectures that the X Principle reproduces itself indefinitely or at least as far as the tenth test-tube transference.

When Arrowsmith discovers that the agent is unattenuated against staphylococcus, even after ten transferences, he seeks advice from Dr. Gottlieb, his senior colleague. Characteristically thorough, Gottlieb poses a series of questions regarding temperature variation, the effect of the growth medium in use, the X Principle's effects on dead bacteria, and its capacity to replicate itself (315). Resuming work, Arrowsmith encounters a secondary anomaly: pus retrieved from boils on the arm, on the leg, or on the back is insensitive to the X Principle (316). Gottlieb thinks that the X Principle coming from the carbuncle is probably specific to gluteal boils which contain bacteria from the intestinal tract. Gottlieb's simple deduction puts his young associate on the right track. Extending his investigation to the intestinal group of organisms, he learns that the X Principle in the test tubes does indeed work against common intestinal flora.

At this point in Arrowsmith's intellectual journey, he commits an unbelievable breach in protocol by volunteering the X Principle for clinical use in a Manhattan hospital. Dr. Gottlieb chastises him for using the untested agent clinically *before* definitively analyzing the relationship between it and staphylococcus (316). The use of the agent in the hospital subverts the ongoing research, but this is half of the problem. Once the word gets out, the Institute's director, Dr. Tubbs, unjustifiably proclaims that the Institute has a bactericidal agent. Despite Arrowsmith's incomplete findings, the director hails the X Principle as another Salvarsan (a chemical therapy for syphillis, relapsing fever, and tropical diseases like yaws) and precipitously declares it to be a miracle cure for staphylococcus, typhoid, and dysentery. He boasts of how he and Arrowsmith shall become "the dictators of science" (322).

Instead of rushing into print, Arrowsmith procrastinates. During this interval, history and fiction intersect one another. Lewis writes of how d'Hérelle beat Arrowsmith to the punch by publishing his findings on the bacteriophage, presumably in the famous 1917 paper, "An invisible microbe that is antagonistic to the dysentery bacillus." In reality, Lewis's character was far from a codiscoverer of phage, a point upon which I will expand upon briefly.

Lewis either failed to research the subject thoroughly, or he deliberately abridged the research history of phage. It is difficult to believe that Gottlieb, even though a bacteriologist, would be unfamiliar with groundbreaking research on ultramicroscopic organisms. Since Jenner's day, viruses were being used in immunization, although practitioners had no idea what they were and how they worked. Of Latinate origin, the word *virus* literally means "slimy liquid, poison, offensive odor or taste" (*OED* XIX: 243; "virus"). From the late seventeenth to the beginning of the twentieth century, the word was synonymous with venom from poisonous animals, and, later in that period, was thought of as being a "morbid principle" or poison *produced* by a disease, especially "one capable of being introduced into other persons or animals by inoculation or otherwise and of developing the same disease in them" (*OED* XIX: 243; "virus"). What we now know to be an infectious, ultramicroscopic agent that reproduces in living cells (*Random House* 1471) had been confused historically with toxins, such as those produced by tetanus and diphtheria, and was identified solely by its capacity for transmission via inoculation.

In early virological texts, though the term *virus* is used loosely and often muddled in translation, it was also defined as a toxin and not as a parasitic micro-organism. In 1898, Friedrich Löffler and Paul Frosch, while working on foot-and-mouth disease, confirmed Dmitri I. Ivanovski's 1892 discovery of filterable viruses (Oldstone 96). Yet, for Löffler and Frosch, whatever caused foot-and-mouth disease was "a germ-free toxic substance" [150], and the word *virus* does not appear in the Brock translation of their groundbreaking paper (149–53). The word *virus* does appear in Martinus W. Beijerinck's pioneering 1899 paper, A *Contagium vivum fluidum* as the cause of the mosaic disease of tobacco leaves." In addition to the archaic phrase *Contagium vivum fluidum* ("living germ that is soluble" [153]), which describes the cause of tobacco mosaic disease, is the word *virus* which appears liberally in the Brock translation (e.g., "The amount of virus which is sufficient to infect a large number of leaves is quite small" [15]); however, if Beijerinck had used the ambiguous German word *Gift* ("poison, toxin, virus, venom" [*Cassell's New German Dictionary* 199]) for the infectious agent, then it is possible that he, too, was thinking of an unstable chemical compound rather than of a living organism.

Etymological concerns notwithstanding, the fictional world of Arrowsmith exists in the context of early virological research, and this is what makes it so evocative. In response to Gottlieb's disclosure that "Someone else has ... [discovered phage]," Arrowsmith incredulously replies, "They have not! I've searched all the literature, and except for Twort, not one person has ever hinted at anticipating—[the discovery and use of phage]" (327). Clearly,

Arrowsmith (and Lewis) missed Hankin's 1896 paper, published by the prestigious Pasteur Institute, and did not appreciate Twort's detailed account of 1915, which appeared in the equally prestigious journal, the *Lancet*. Since Lewis chose to interpolate the life and work of Arrowsmith into the historical envelope of phage research, he was obligated to represent the theoretical background of the story comprehensively. Had he done so, the significance of Arrowsmith's discovery would have been cast in a less grandiose light. It would also have become clear that Lewis' protagonist had merely stumbled across a twenty-year-old finding.

The most significant stage of the discovery for Arrowsmith, as it was for his historical counterpart, d'Hérelle, was to find out if the X Principle could be used clinically, especially under epidemic conditions. Given the technological void and the desperate need for new medicines, what choice was there but to strike out in a "new direction" (to paraphrase Robert Koch)? Even though Arrowsmith's finding amounts to a footnote, Dr. Tubbs realizes that the race was on: d'Hérelle et al. could be outdistanced if the Institute sponsored the clinical trials of phage in an epidemic of typhoid or plague (330).

Arrowsmith's clinical trial of phage will take place in the midst of the third plague pandemic (c. 1850s–1959) on the Caribbean island of St. Hubert. Lewis' use of St. Hubert is medically and biographically significant in that St. Hubert is the patron saint of rabies victims and the site of an abbey in northern France which Felix d'Hérelle had visited in adolescence (Summers [1999], 1, 2, 187n.). In the interest of historical verisimilitude, Lewis positioned St. Hubert on the epidemiological map of the third pandemic.

Lewis writes that the outbreak in St. Hubert originated in Yunnan China, was carried through human migration across the Himalayas into an American missionary compound, arrived at Bombay via shipping, killed off wharf rats and a guard during an epizootic, and was transported amidst a cargo of wheat to Marseilles, France (340–41). From there, the plague steamer sailed to Montevideo and berthed next to the freighter *S.S. Pendown Castle*, bound for St. Hubert. The disease wended inexorably from ship to ship in the bloodstreams of rats. During the voyage to St. Hubert, a Goanese boy and a mess-room steward died of "influenza" — a misdiagnosis suggesting the pneumonic form of the disease. Of greater significance is the fact that rats died on deck. Yet none of these events raised an alarm, which is difficult to understand since the fictional time-frame of the novel is 1917, when much was known about the etiology of plague.

Even when the disease is fully manifested, the Surgeon General of the Island, Dr. Inchcape Jones, obstinately denies its existence. Dr. Stokes, his colleague, proves that plague is active, establishing this diagnosis in the laboratory (by isolating *Y. pestis* from dead rat fleas), and from clinical symptoms consistent with the disease (depression, anorexia, fevers, aches, vertigo, and buboes) (344). Factionalism among medical and civil authorities allows the plague to gain headway. The idea of politicizing the epidemic is not original, but Lewis, in this regard, did his research well since he had in mind a similar set of circumstances in turn-of-the century San Francisco. The notorious Governor Henry T. Gage scandalously impeded the medical establishment there to protect businesses that presumably would have suffered had the plague epidemic been officially acknowledged (Kohn 293–94). Jones has much in common with Gage, for the former is overly concerned with political and economic repercussions if the health authority were to enact aggressive measures, such as burning bodies (364).

The debate permits the disease to progress. Fear spreads as the pestilence becomes firmly entrenched in areas where rundown habitations, overcrowding, and insanitation exacerbate the problem (368–69). Jones's emphasis shifts from socio-cultural to economic issues. For example, the isolation of patients would adversely affect the powerful merchants who control the House of Assembly (370). To safeguard their pecuniary interests, the merchants deny Jones the authority to manage the crisis, deciding instead to deal with it in conjunction with the Board of Health (370). The newspapers back the merchants, calling Jones a tyrant and vowing not to persuade the public to take precautions against rats and ground squirrels (370). The merchants obstruct the doctors in the interest of profit. Specifically, they reject the plan to fumigate warehouses with sulfur dioxide, an efficient way of killing rats and fleas, because the gas would damage fabrics and paint (371). Their lobbying forces the Board of Health to adopt a wait-and-see attitude, the worst possible reaction to a plague outbreak. Even if Jones had been authorized to carry on, he would have been at a disadvantage, since he lacked the trained personnel necessary to locate plague foci (371). In addition, racism plays a role in the story: Jones who is white does not trust the judgment of Drs. Stokes and Marchand who are black.

With mercenary logic, Sondelius brings the procrastinating Board of Health to its senses. Judging from his experience with plague in Mongolia and India, he points out that, if left unchecked, the disease could become endemic to the region and, in that event, would destroy its lucrative tourism industry, along with interrupting smuggling profits. In light of this compelling information, authorities begin using hydrocyanic gas in warehouses over the merchants' protests (371–73).

Arrowsmith can not fight the plague aggressively and maintain scientific standards at the same time. Conducting clinical trials in the midst of a medical disaster, he discovers, is a daunting task. The first problem is that ground-squirrels can easily pick up infected rat fleas and transport them to Port Carib (374). With its stinking cottages and palm-thatched huts made of cow-dung plaster, and with roosters and goats everywhere, Port Carib is a perfect habitat for rat and flea infestation. The immunization experiment raises a second concern: the protocol requires Arrowsmith to treat only one-half of the infected population while using the other half as a control (375), a problem similar to one that vexed d'Hérelle.

Arrowsmith hopes that common sense will prevail, so he presents his plan to a Special Board of the government. Though the plan is sound, Dr. Sondelius opposes it because he believes that experiments are for the laboratory and not for the field (376). On ostensibly humanitarian grounds, he argues for the wholesale use of the agent. Arrowsmith retorts that it would be best to save at least half of the stricken population and, in the process, "to test for all time the value of phage" (377); those in the control group who do not receive the phage, he points out, would receive other regimens. His arguments, however, are futile: the Board ignorantly believes that he possesses a miracle cure (the most serious effect of the Institute's false advertising campaign), one that he plans to withhold for discreditable reasons. Consequently, everyone denounces Arrowsmith unjustly. Sondelius calls him a fanatic (377); Ira Hinkley, the missionary, who would die of the disease four days later, calls him a liar and a fool (377); and Inchcape Jones demands that Martin administer phage to everyone who needs it.

Sondelius' argument sways Arrowsmith. When the morbidity rate in Port Carib reaches an alarming 33 percent, the latter begins to administer the phage to the village (379). But, as the epidemic begins to slacken there, Arrowsmith considers the possibility of conducting the trial at the alternative site of St. Swithin's (379). Sondelius, meanwhile, orders the burning of Port Carib because of ground-squirrel infestation. Upon his return to Blackwater, he, too, succumbs to plague, his dying wish being that Martin treat his people (380–81).

After Jones commits suicide, Stokes is appointed Surgeon General. More amenable to Arrowsmith's work, Stokes appoints him as medical officer in St. Swithin's Parish (383). Conditions in St. Swithin's identify it as a possible secondary test site. Arrowsmith promptly divides the population into two equal parts, injecting one with plague phage and leaving the other without; and he begins to notice improvement (386). As expected, the plague strikes the untreated population more severely than it does the treated group. The sufferings of the control group distress Arrowsmith to the point that he strikes a balance between ethics and protocol: he dispenses the phage to half of the untreated victims, in effect, treating three-quarters of the people (386–87).

The secondary experiment, so promising at its inception, is brought to an abrupt end. An unforeseen tragedy interrupts Arrowsmith's experiment. A maid at his residence knocks a plague test tube over, spilling its lethal contents onto one of his wife Leora's cigarettes (390–91). Her death breaks Arrowsmith's resolve: "he raged, 'Oh, damn experimentation!' and ... he gave the phage to everyone who asked" (392). Though he aborts the trials, Drs. Stokes and Twyford carry on with the experiments and record their findings (392). However, Lewis is ambiguous over the efficacy of the vaccine. Since the epidemic ceases six months after Arrowsmith's arrival (395), there is no definitive proof that the phage vaccine, derived from plague sera, made the difference. The profiteers trumpet his success, nevertheless, and assert that the vaccine worked. But Martin knows the truth, admitting to Gottlieb "that he did not have complete proof of the value of the phage" (397). He finds comfort in the acknowledgment that planning clinical trials in a laboratory and carrying them out in the midst of suffering and death are starkly different activities. Those lacking plague experience, he avers, simply cannot appreciate how difficult it is to remain calm and to follow the rules (400). He is content to salvage what he can from the experience in St. Swithin's.

A number of factors subvert Arrowsmith's anti-plague work. The first is his anxious tendency of jumping to conclusions and of by-passing experimental criteria; throughout the novel, emotions interfere with scientific procedure. Second, the McGurk Institute puts profit before sound biomedical practice by publicizing the phage as a wonder drug. The publicity, in turn, undercuts clinical trials on the island of St. Hubert as authorities balk against the use of control groups, a comparative means of assessing morbidity and mortality rates in an untreated segment of the population. And finally, personal tragedy overwhelms Arrowsmith at a point of impending success at St. Swithin's, the alternative site for clinical trials. An imaginative work set against the background of the third plague pandemic, *Arrowsmith* reveals all that can go wrong during an epidemiological crisis.

Albert Camus, *The Plague*

According to reliable historical records, the Algerian city of Oran, setting of Albert Camus' *The Plague*, had never experienced an outbreak of plague — that is, until the summer of 2003. According to a BBC report of July 10, 2003, medical teams from the WHO, along with other international agencies, traveled to Oran to investigate an outbreak of bubonic plague, which began in June 2003 ("Algeria," BBC). Eleven cases (eight of the bubonic and two of the septicemic form) were identified. When laboratory

studies determined the source of the disease, Algerian and French authorities enforced sanitary controls to prevent contaminated rats and insects
from arriving on ships. Thus, a synergistic response was able to stop the
disease.

Although the epidemiological content of *The Plague* does not correspond to an actual event, it is possible that other outbreaks may have
inspired Camus. In the 1940s, for example, while Camus was living in the
region, two preventable epidemics broke out concurrently, one in Oran and
the other in northern Algerian areas (Kohn 5–6). From 1943 to 1946, a
relapsing-fever epidemic arose. This acute, lice-borne disease killed 2000
of the 32,000 people afflicted with it. Relapsing fever, caused by the spiro-
chete bacterium, *Borrelia recurrentis*, induces high fever lasting two to nine
days. In the northern department of Oran, at the time an overseas province
of France, the infection spread widely because of malnutrition, lice infestation, and a shortage of soap. The epidemic peaked in July 1945. A typhus
epidemic, also due to lice, lasted from 1942 to 1944. This outbreak which
was more serious than the Oranais event killed almost 13,000 of the 52,000
who were infected. Because of cold weather in February 1942, people in the
northern departments of the cities of Algiers, of Oran, and of Constantine
wore contaminated attire and bathed infrequently; consequently, typhus
was contracted through bites and from lice feces. The mortality rate among
white Europeans was the highest of all ethnic groups. On the basis of this
information, it is likely that *The Plague* owed much to Camus' experiences
with these outbreaks.

Bernard Rieux, M.D., the chronicler of the novel, claims to have maintained a tone of impartiality throughout. In a way, this standpoint is reminiscent of Thucydides,' whose account of the Athenian plague greatly
influenced Camus. Rieux's perspective is very intriguing. Ideally situated
to provide a "true account of all he saw and heard," he stands at one remove
from the medical and psychological impact of the plague (271).

The prevailing conditions in Oran are similar to those Arrowsmith
faced and are analogous to the real experiences of Yersin and of Kitasato.
Rieux records what he experiences, avoids suppositions, and stoically weath-
ers the crisis. Arrowsmith and Rieux, however, face the plague in radically
different ways. On the one hand, Arrowsmith is optimistic that biomedi-
cine can arrest the immediate outbreak and erase the disease altogether
from human history. But the greed, short-sightedness, and bigotry of his
colleagues frustrate his inspired efforts. Other factors contributing to the
failure of the phage experiment are the McGurk Institute's poor planning,
its false advertising campaign, and its inadequate material support for
Arrowsmith who must, unbelievably, house live bacilli at his personal res-

idence. At the outset, Arrowsmith is disadvantaged, very much like Yersin whose laboratory was ramshackle, and whose equipment was inadequate. These conditions allow the disease to gain a foothold in Lewis's novel and force medical and civil authorities to call for the universal application of phage.

Rieux weighs evidence carefully, suspects plague, but foregoes diagnosis until probability or crisis warrants it (12, 28). When he encounters patients with enlarged inguinal lymph nodes and with fever, and when two die in a 48 to 72 hour time-frame, his suspicions intensify, although he avoids a diagnosis; the involvement of inguinal or groin lymphatics is especially suspicious since fleas commonly bite and infect the lower extremities. Inferring that a serious disease process is at work, he contacts his colleagues to inquire about similar cases and learns that they, too, have encountered patients similarly afflicted, almost all of whom died. Eventually, however, probability moves Rieux to action: ratfall, the classic symptoms, and the high fatality rate, prompt him to advise Dr. Richard, chair of the local medical association, to put new cases into isolation wards as a precaution — against *what*, he does not say. When Richard questions the grounds for supposing that there is danger of contagion, Rieux responds that there are no definite grounds, but the alarming symptoms call for this precaution (32).

Inexorably, isolated symptoms coalesce into a syndrome. Vomiting, high fevers, delirium, darkened patches under the skin, and engorged, excruciating lymph nodes that either burst or have to be suppurated confirm Rieux's suspicions, but he does not articulate a diagnosis publicly. Instead, he checks plague vaccine inventories, only to find Oran's pharmacological supplies at a low level. When it becomes evident that this "strange malady" is indeed an epidemic, Rieux's senior colleague, Dr. Castel, a veteran of the 1920s plague outbreaks in China and in Paris (no historical referent found), enunciates Rieux's suspicion: "Everything points to its being plague" (33).

Rieux's historical survey of the plague, which follows at this point in the narrative, suggests that he is far from optimistic about the situation. The cumulative death toll, a hundred million fatalities in thirty outbreaks, is incomprehensible. No sensationalist, he is doubtful about the veracity of Procopius' claim that ten thousand people died in one day in Constantinople, and he has no opinion on the estimate that, in Canton China in the 1870s, forty thousand rats died. Acknowledging that these exempla do not shed light on the Oranais' disease, he reaffirms the need for "serious precautions" to prevent the unidentified outbreak from worsening (36). He recalls morbid scenes, for example, the charnel houses of Athens that Thucydides describes, the convicts of Marseilles who piled up rotting plague corpses, the plague episode in Lucretius' writings, and cartloads of the dead in London (38). In human experience, according to Rieux's survey, the plague has been a surreptitious, irrepressible, and ubiquitous force (38).

Thirteen centuries of human experience with plague, Rieux implies, has furnished no practical insight into how to manage the immediate crisis. He realizes that, in order to gain some degree of control over the impending crisis, one has to narrow one's scope to the present moment, for a strategy of containment depends upon "observed facts." Case histories have to be compared with textbook descriptions of the disease. The Oranais' symptoms (stupor, prostration, buboes, thirst, delirium, enlarged organs, irregular pulse, and high mortality) match the description of plague in Rieux's medical handbook; incidentally, they are consistent with the CDC's description of symptoms, notably "fever, chills, headache, and extreme exhaustion" and an incubation period ranging from two to six days for the bubonic form of the disease. When the lungs are affected, the patient may experience high fever, chills, cough, and breathing difficulties ("Plague," CDC).

Despite Dr. Castel's pronouncement, Rieux calls for precautions commensurate with a confirmed diagnosis, a decision he bases on probability. Even from this standpoint, Rieux fails to convince the medical authorities to act and is drawn into a time-consuming debate over public-health strategy (44–7). Some doctors reject the possibility of plague outright, while others hesitate to take prophylactic measures. Castel backpedals, making a public-health program contingent upon the definitive diagnosis of plague. Intent upon avoiding public alarm, Dr. Richard suggests that it may just be a special type of fever that is causing the lymphatic swelling. There is something to be said for this view in that the symptoms of the louse-borne infections can resemble bubonic plague. On the basis of his Asian experiences, Castel flip-flops and calls for drastic steps.

The position of Rieux and Castel gains support when preliminary laboratory findings arrive. Analysis of excised pus drawn from Rieux's patients confirms that it is indeed plague, although this specific strain possesses "certain modifications," not corresponding to classic *Yersinia pestis* (45). The anomaly encourages the skeptics. Dr. Richard questions the propriety of raising a public alarm on the basis of a single laboratory report; instead, he would rather await the results of further testing. Rieux's attitude changes radically at this point since his colleagues are becoming dangerously complacent. He argues compellingly against inaction: in three days' time, the microbe can quadruple the volume of the spleen, swell mesenteric ganglia to the size of oranges, and reduce these structures to the consistency of gruel. Worse yet, if left unchecked, the infection may kill off half of Oran in two months. The only logical course of action remaining for them is to prevent this from happening. The precise identification of the microbe is a secondary concern (45–6).

Rieux's appeal to common sense and his dire warning do not dissuade Richard from the specious argument that the disease is not likely to be contagious since relatives living in the same home reputedly have not been affected. Richard apparently does not realize that contagion with the *bubonic* form of the disease is usually sporadic since infected fleas transmit the microbe directly into the human body, usually biting lower extremities. Rieux corrects Richard when he says that contagion is never absolutely predictable. Nonetheless, the latter rejects Rieux's call for prophylactic measures, contending that publicity risks panic. On the basis of the clinical, epidemiological, and serological data, Rieux reiterates that precautionary measures are justified. The stakes are simply too high, inasmuch as delay risks the lives of tens of thousands (46). Richard does not understand that plague infections increase exponentially, and that the more treatable form of the malady can give rise to the untreatable, pneumonic form which is communicated from person to person. Yet he stubbornly resists Rieux's argument. The government and medical establishment, fortunately, enact precautionary measures (47).

Judging from the plague's historical record, Rieux is justifiably pessimistic about the chances of defeating the disease. The only hope, he drearily reflects, is that it will subside naturally (56). Nevertheless, the doctor approaches public health aggressively. Though the historical record is discouraging, he believes that a reasonable anti-plague strategy can be devised, based on all that is known about the illness, and in view of the medical resources at their disposal; hence, he tells Castel that concrete measures rather than words are needed to set up "a real barrier" against the plague (57). With Dr. Richard sidetracked on the irrelevant question of who commands authority during the crisis, Rieux predicts that the epidemic will worsen. The prophecy is self-fulfilling: within three days, both hospital wards are full, apparently with bubonic cases. Rieux abandons the debate to excise buboes (a palliative measure), while awaiting the arrival of the prophylactic serum.

The Prefect instructs Rieux to draw up a report to the central administration of the colony that will include statistics and a diagnosis. New regulations are to be initiated. Under Rieux's direction, all cases of fever must be declared; isolation of the sick will be compulsory and enforced; residences where plague is active are to be disinfected; households where plague exists are to be quarantined; and burials are to be controlled by local authorities. Rieux's thinking corresponds to today's actual recommendations. Reducing the possibility of flea bites, of contact with infective tissues and exudates, and of exposure to pneumonia patients, for example, are primary concerns in the management of plague (Chin 383–86). Epidemiologists recommend educating the public in enzootic areas, such as the southwestern United States, on how the disease is transmitted from animals carrying infected fleas. In addition, sanitary programs to reduce rodent populations and to destroy fleas and then rats, especially in cargo ships, on docks, and in warehouses, and instructions on the use of appropriate gloves when handling wildlife are essential. Moreover, cases are to be reported to the local health authority, patients are to be isolated, and clothing and baggage are to be confiscated. Soiled articles of clothing must be disinfected, and bodily secretions must be destroyed. Because bodies and carcasses carry communicable infection, they must be handled under strict, aseptic conditions. Quarantine is indicated for those residing in infected households or who have had face-to-face contact with pneumonic plague victims. The original or index case and whoever that patient has contacted must be identified and examined. In a full-blown epidemic (what Camus creates in Oran), health-care workers are to investigate all suspected plague deaths and, where indicated, conduct serological and clinical examinations. Facilities for diagnosis and treatment are to be established. Public hysteria is to be controlled through the dissemination of information in news media. Intensive flea control is to be instituted in expanding circles, widening from disease foci. Rodents and other animal carriers are to be destroyed after the insects are killed. Finally, workers are to be informed that social upheaval, crowding, and unhygienic conditions exacerbate the problem (Chin 383–86).

It is unclear whether Rieux et al. have antibiotics at their disposal. Since anti-plague vaccine is the only medical treatment available in the novel, the plan is to immunize those *not yet infected* and to isolate patients with active disease in order to reduce the possibility of contagion (italics added). At this crucial juncture in the narrative, insecticides and scrupulous sanitation are to be employed to control fleas. But the vaccine supplies are woefully inadequate, and the emergency stocks are depleted. Because it takes time to prepare a new supply, the Prefect has no choice but to close the town (58). In 1947, the year of *The Plague*'s publication, antibiotics were available, but Camus is not specific about their use in the story. In *1948*, however, streptomycin (produced by a mold in soil and discovered in 1942 by Selman Waksman) became, and has remained, the antibiotic choice for all forms of the disease, with intravenous chloramphenicol as adjunctive therapy; tetracycline is used orally in mild cases, with doxycycline as a possible alternative (McGovern and Friedlander 497; italics added). In all cases, antibiotic treatment has to be started within eighteen hours of the onset of symptoms; otherwise, a 60 percent fatality rate is to be expected for bubonic plague, and 100 percent for both the septicemic and pneumonic forms of the disease (McGovern and Friedlander 497). An additional point is that insecticide has to be used widely and *prior* to the use of rodenticide. Fleas have to be killed before the rats; if the reverse is done, the parasites immediately seek other mammalian hosts. The use of cyanide gas (as in *Arrowsmith*), simultaneously destroying rats and fleas, is recommended. Overall, Camus has nothing specific to say either about antibiotics or vaccine.

The development of plague vaccine antedates that of plague antibiotics. The first vaccine, consisting of killed whole cells, was developed by a Russian physician, Waldemar M. W. Haffkine, who worked in India during the 1896 outbreak there (Hays 198–99). Christopher Wills explains that, although Haffkine successfully vaccinated thousands of Indians, nineteen people in a remote village died from what was later determined to have been contaminated medicine; according to Wills, a local health-care worker was to blame for this incident. The damage, however, was done, and the tragedy virtually destroyed Haffkine's credibility and career (98–9). Karl F. Meyer, in 1942, developed the vaccine used today (McGovern and Friedlander 498). The serum that Rieux would have ordered from France is likely to have been this kind. It is important to note that the vaccine prevents or destroys bubonic plague but has no effect on the pneumonic form (498). Camus is not clear on whether Rieux alludes to the Haffkine, to the Yersin, or to the Meyer vaccine. Nor can we be certain that Camus understood that the vaccines were ineffective against pneumonic plague.

Quarantines, Camus was aware, have been used throughout history to interrupt the progress of plague. No one escapes the quarantine in Camus' Oran. One character, Rambert, castigates Rieux for upholding the law and for refusing to allow him to leave. He decries Rieux for using "the language of reason" rather than of the heart, and of living in a world of abstractions. Rambert seriously misjudges his friend. On the contrary, Rieux acknowledges subscribing to "the language of the facts as everybody could see them"; yet, in so doing, he has taken the ethical high ground: to violate the quarantine is to permit the plague to spread (79–80). Despite the mounting difficulties, Rieux applies himself to clinical practice, injecting serum, lancing nodes, rechecking statistics on morbidity and mortality, mapping locations of disease, and consulting with patients (81). Rather than to retreat into hopelessness, he resists the plague on his own terms, one patient at a time. He realizes that his general practice has been expanded into an epidemiological dimension (82).

Other events spell disaster. The Paris serum, apparently derived from a strain different from Oran's, is even less effective than the depleted supply at hand (as it turns out, an indigenous vaccine would have worked best). Moreover, it is impossible to administer prophylactic inoculations widely: they are earmarked for households in which the disease is already present. Another problem is that lymph nodes harden, which means that they can not be suppurated to relieve patients. Finally, the situation takes an ominous turn: two cases of pneumonic plague are diagnosed, raising the possibility of inhalational contagion.

Although Rieux describes his situation as "fumbling in the dark" (116), he continues to fight the plague systematically (116). Father Paneloux's idea of Creation as God's design and theodicy contrasts sharply with Rieux's idea of nature as being amoral and of man as a creature. Since "The order of the world," Rieux reflects, "is shaped by death," any victories achieved against the plague, though they are to be pursued, remain transient ones. The plague cannot be eradicated from the Earth, but man must resist it when it appears. When Rieux remarks that the plague is a "never-ending defeat" (118), he is not being a pessimist; instead, he is drawing an axiom from history and from his daily experience with victims. The imperative is to save the greatest number of people, even if Oran is inexorably reduced to the likeness of a fourteenth-century European city (122)

Rieux attributes the subsidence of the epidemic to prophylactic vaccinations (212), though it lingers long enough to kill Tarrou. Rieux's wife, sequestered in a sanatorium, also dies at that time, though not of plague (260, 263). The physician-epidemiologist remains to bear witness to the plague of Oran, and he presents the chronicle as a memorial to "what had to be done" (278). The struggle, Rieux states, has been against pathogens hidden in the fabric of human civilization. In this statement, however, Camus misconstrues the etiology of plague. *Y. pestis* is endemic to certain regions on Earth, and human beings are relatively safe during the enzootic phase of the cycle because the pathogen is endemic to rodent populations in specific regions. The *X. cheopsis* flea, a rodent parasite primarily, carries an abundance of *Y. pestis* in its abdomen and disgorges the microbes into rats through bite-wounds. In this cycle, therefore, man is a host of opportunity. In an epizootic state, a rodent population is destroyed by *Y. pestis*. When the host population (rats, squirrels, or prairie dogs) is decimated, fleas *which do not feed on a host carcasses* then seek new mammalian bloodsources, human beings included (McGovern and Friedlander 487–88; italics added).

Camus misrepresents the biological facts further when he states that the plague bacillus lies dormant in "furniture, linen chests, bedrooms, cellars, trunks, bookshelves," waiting for an opportunity to be the bane and enlightenment of man (278). This statement is blatantly erroneous: *Y. pestis* can survive on inanimate objects briefly, but only if coughed out or if secreted. In its aerosolized state, the pathogen degrades rapidly and dies in the air and sunlight (we recall the experiments of Kitasato). There is some truth, however, in the statement that germ-engorged fleas can survive in linen and bales of hay, which is one way they can be transported without the rat as its carrier.

Gwyneth Cravens and John Marr, M.D., *The Black Death*

The thought of bubonic plague erupting in a major urban environment sounds like the plot of a B movie. But the possibility is a real one. On November 6, 2002, the Department of Health and Mental Hygiene of the City of New York diagnosed bubonic plague in a middle-age couple from New Mexico who were traveling in New York City (Health Alert # 36). They reside in Santa Fe County, New Mexico, a region "known to be an enzootic focus for plague" (#36). It was believed that they contracted the disease after being bitten by the fleas of a woodrat which had been found in their backyard in July 2002; both the carcass and the fleas it carried tested positive for plague. After arriving in New York City on November 1, 2002, they became ill, and they were hospitalized on November 5. Examinations revealed fever and swollen inguinal lymph nodes ("buboes"). Sophisticated laboratory tests (the polymerase chain reaction test, direct fluorescent antibody testing, and others) confirmed the diagnosis. Both patients were treated and recovered. Since neither patient showed signs of plague pneumonia, it was not necessary for authorities to track their contacts down; laboratory staff who handled specimens followed Biosafety Level 2 precautions. The New York Health Department points out that the plague, endemic to Arizona, California, Colorado, and New Mexico, exists naturally in ground squirrels, in prairie dogs, and in other wild rodents. The report concludes with the statement that "there has not been a case of plague in New York City in at least 100 years." John S. Marr, M.D. and Gwyneth Cravens, coauthors of the thriller *The Black Death* (1977), plausibly extrapolate a plague epidemic in New York City, from an index case to a catastrophic extreme.

Although aggressive public-health measures against an outbreak of bubonic plague are seriously impeded at the outset of *The Black Death*, the medical establishment, in cooperation with the public and with local (not Federal) authorities, manages to save a portion of New York City's population. The lineage of the plague outbreak in the novel is traced to the third pandemic, specifically to the plague of San Francisco that spread to the southwest, and especially to New Mexico, where it became endemic.

David Hart, M.D., of the Bureau of Preventable Diseases, is assigned to keep track of outbreaks and epidemics (32). He once idealistically believed that "nature could be turned around": that medical science, in other words, was more than a match for any disease. After the death of his wife, however, he became disillusioned with medicine. In this regard, his outlook has much in common with that of Rieux: Hart's practical goal as an epidemiologist is to contain disease, to work as well as one can, and to use every available resource to isolate the disease-causing organisms and to medicate victims. Despite this energetic approach, he realizes that often a contagious disease will run its course, despite the best scientific effort. Acknowledging the limitations of the discipline, he views medicine as a craft, and he seeks both to hone his skills and to optimize the chances of success.

With a healthy respect for the power of nature, Dr. Hart meets his greatest challenge: an outbreak of *Y. pestis* in New York City, in the period from September 2 to 12. The epidemiological crisis in the fiction begins with a single case, unlike that which was reported in Health Alert # 36 of 2002, which involved two people. The biggest difference between the two scenarios is that the index case in the fiction develops the highly contagious and untreatable pneumonic plague *before* being identified. By that time, the disease had already been communicated to others who did not have access to adequate medical care.

The index case in *The Black Death* is a young woman who picked up the disease from a ground squirrel that she had handled during her travels in the southwestern United States, possibly in New Mexico where plague is endemic among rodents. The man and his wife contracted the disease the very same way. The fictional character has flea bites on her extremities, but emergency-room physicians fail to recognize them as such and mistake them for needle marks. When Dr. Hart views blood cultures, sputum, and other bodily substances of the patient, he appears to recognize the bacteria: its red stain (Gram-negativity) and oval structure identify it as a coccobacillus, and it has a bipolar shape (41–2). All of the clinical and microscopic evidence suggests plague, although Hart (like Rieux) does not jump to conclusions. Only the definitive fluorescent antibody test on the sputum will dispel any doubt about the disease. However, this important phase in the investigation must wait since New York City, in the1977 fiction, is unequipped to run the test; thus, a critical delay is unavoidable (42). In the 2002 Health Alert, on the other hand, the New York City DOHMH's Public Health Laboratory, on the evening of November 6 (twenty-four hours after the patients were admitted), ran the fluorescent antibody test, along with other tests, in conjunction with the CDC.

Like Simond, Hart is a clinical detective. He finds what looks like finger-nail scratches and insect bites on the woman's extremities which had been confused with needle tracks. The sputum culture is sent to the CDC for the final proof (44–5); meanwhile, the resident nurse-epidemiologist is summoned, and efforts are initiated to identify the girl and to trace all of her contacts which must be done in the case of pneumonic plague (46). Hart mulls over the dire situation unfolding before him: twenty-four hours have passed since the girl's death. By this time, any contacts she had had would be in danger. But what could be done? Hart encounters a dilemma similar to what Arrowsmith and Rieux faced. If he contacts the media before the antibody-test results, he can cause a panic (hospitals would be overwhelmed with people who mistakenly thought they had the disease) (48). He decides to question the emergency-room physicians who treated the girl the day before, only to discover, quite ominously, that they both called in sick. His request for immediate autopsy results from the Medical Examiner devolves into a bureaucratic debate (49). His nurse assistant, however, manages to track down vital information: she estimates a total of eighty-two contacts, seventy-seven of whom are known (50). Jane Doe's backpack and outdoor clothing indicate that she was in a wilderness area when she was bitten by a flea. The autopsy indicates possible insect bites, suppurating lymph nodes or buboes in the armpits and groin, typical of the plague, and, worst of all, plague-infected lungs (81). Without immediate and effective measures in place, the disease is likely to spread exponentially — "in a breath, a touch, a sneeze, a handshake, a curse" (57). Medical intervention, Hart knows, can work but only if there is no delay: in the early stages of the disease, the antibiotics tetracycline and streptomycin work. But budget cuts and the lack of trained personnel in New York City mean that the capacity to fight a major epidemic, to strike when the outbreak is manageable, is no longer possible (58); moreover, everyone in the Health Department has gone home on September 5, so Hart finds it difficult to mobilize staff at this crucial moment (62).

Dr. Hart has no choice but to take the initiative. He sets up a station in the emergency room to dispense antibiotics and, with the help of Dr. Vincent Calabrese, Commissioner of Health, begins to put an organized procedure into effect (69). They check morgues and emergency rooms for people showing up with plague-like symptoms and realize that unlimited resources and the cooperation of the City government are essential if the plague is to be stopped (76–7). On September 5, *Y. pestis* is definitively diagnosed as the florescent antibody test results come in (89). Hart concludes that the index case, Sarah Dobbs, had bubonic *and* pneumonic plague.

Hart and Calabrese decide to go public with the news because a leak would create rumors and precipitate panic (115). Before the announcement on September 7, they plan to have set up facilities throughout the city in district health centers. Meanwhile, the CDC begins checking nationwide for reports of rodent die-offs, for that information could pinpoint the origin of the outbreak and help other States prepare themselves (118). Intent on stopping the plague's progress in its secondary and tertiary stages, Hart and Calabrese determine that Dobbs had been infectious for at least forty-eight hours before her death (i.e., the period from September 2 to 4), and that anyone she infected would, in turn, be infectious from twenty-four to thirty-two hours afterwards (118). On September 7, police reports come to their attention of two suspicious cases, both dead on arrival at the hospital. A pimp and a prostitute each presented with plague-like symptoms. Hart could not have known that, when Dobbs arrived at the Port Authority Bus Terminal on September 2, she was accosted by a pimp who tried to recruit her, and she sneezed in his face (1). By September 7, it is confirmed that Sarah Dobbs contracted the plague from infected fleas she had picked up from a ground squirrel while vacationing at Point Lobos, a fictitious location somewhere in the American southwest (there is a *Puerto Lobos* in Argentina). The contagion wards at Hart's hospital, meanwhile, have reached capacity (169). But that day, Dr. Hart encourages the Mayor that the epidemic can be stopped within a few days if help and cooperation are forthcoming; otherwise, he cautions, people will die in a mass panic. By September 12, 1,208 exposures have been documented (191). At this point in the narrative, the reader anticipates the heroic triumph of modern medicine over the plague: Dr. Hart's indefatigable company will no doubt overcome political, social, and logistical obstacles to conquer the disease. But the authors choose a different tack. Instead of demonstrating the courage and resourcefulness of Hart's group, they show how the most complex, technologically-advanced society on Earth can be overwhelmed by an ancient, ineradicable disease.

From the beginning of the campaign, Hart's efforts are precarious. Confused priorities and administrative stupidity hamper him at every turn. Eventually, the disease becomes unstoppable when Dr. Hart, whose small group had been resisting it single-handedly, contracts plague himself; but he survives, thanks to the immediate use of antibiotics. The third-person narrator conveys Dr. Hart's thoughts and his slide into febrile disorientation:

> Talk to Strohman, reopen Sydenham Hospital, a couple of others. Use stretchers on the floors.... And the dead — the morgues must be filling up. Cremation. Make a note, a not, a knot, an ought, the lights, the lights, too bright, his mind was sliding sideways, the headlights bled over

his eyes ... he was right, he was right, his father would not listen, he was right, he would write, in the bright, write in the bright book of life ... [195].

Hart's thinking fragments into meaningless associations, and his mental state reflects the disintegration of the urban environment around him. As the infection continues to spread, the city deteriorates. Panic ensues, and the mass exodus of urban dwellers threatens to spread the disease into the outer boroughs and suburbs, and suburban dwellers prepare to leave their homes (202). According to the CDC in the fiction, by September 8, six days after Dobbs had stepped off her bus at the Port Authority Bus Terminal, 312 people have died of the pneumonic plague, and four to ten times that number are estimated as being infected, including Dr. Hart.

Hart is incapacitated for three days. To describe his situation in detail, the authors look within his body and trace the influx of the organism, how Hart's immune system responds, how antibiotics interrupt microbial reproduction, and how the germ momentarily rejuvenates as the antibiotic level in the bloodstream declines (212–13). We are taken into Hart's febrile nightmare and experience his disordered thoughts, the melding of Viet Nam memories and eschatological images from the Bible. Injections of streptomycin ensure Hart's recovery (226–27), but he awakens after three days (on Sunday, September 10) to find the hospital abandoned and littered with corpses. The government is dysfunctional, law has broken down, and mobs roam the streets. Two possibilities for the city's rapid decline are as follows: that the public-health system, inadequate to begin with, collapsed without Hart's rallying leadership and that his team could not sustain the effort without him; or that the plague spread relentlessly, despite the efforts of public-health workers. I am inclined to accept the second possibility: Hart's indisposition is likely to have coincided with the plague's gaining of momentum, as it spread rapidly through the community and ignited a medical, social, psychological, and civil crisis.

On the day of Hart's recovery, he finds survivors and the remnants of his team. The work of organization begins in Central Park as the Health Department staff supervises the digging of latrines, the burial of the dead in slit trenches away from fresh water sources, the wide-scale use of insecticide to kill fleas, the setting up of makeshift hospitals in tents where gasoline generators, taken from abandoned hospitals, are used to provide electricity. Sodium hypochlorite is used in the drinking water, food is rationed, and the survivors of every walk of life pitch in to help (303). When it is discovered that the Federal government plans to gas the city to wipe out suspected carriers of the plague, Hart's team conducts a mass exodus of thousands through City Tunnel Number Three, which is twenty feet in diameter and five to six hundred feet below the surface. It extends through Central Park and nine miles into Queens and has elevator and tunnel shafts at 78th Street and at 102nd and Columbus (333–34). Equipped with individual injectors of atropine (an antidote to the nerve gas), the exiles make their way to safety. To prevent any carriers from spreading the disease into Queens, they set up a health station at the Ridgewood Reservoir, the exit point. There, they treat all who emerge (340).

The novel concludes on the somber note that, although Hart heroically mobilizes his team to save lives and to contain the epidemic, and although the introduction of nerve gas via helicopter eliminates rodent vectors in Manhattan, the plague can never be eradicated entirely. It appears to burn itself out, irrespective of human efforts. Thus, the speaker concludes that there is no reason why the organism stopped with its last victim and went no farther, even before the nerve gas was dispensed (353–54). The authors personify the plague at this point: "If it had chosen to continue, nothing could have halted it in its course. It vanished as suddenly as it had come. And nothing could prevent its return" (354).

The message of these imaginative works is that epidemic diseases such as plague can appear unexpectedly, progress relentlessly, and defy health measures. But from the human experience with plague have come valuable insights. The response against deadly, infectious diseases, as exemplified by the Legionellosis outbreak in 1977, and by the plague-infected travelers in New York City in 2002, must be carefully planned and be a interdisciplinary endeavor. In contrast to the ideal situation, Arrowsmith's efforts are ill-advised, poorly coordinated, understaffed, underequipped and fore-doomed. Even though Rieux practices medicine judiciously, advocating reasonable precautions prior to definitive diagnosis and aggressive ones thereafter, ignorant and conflicted colleagues, along with the lack of medical resources, allow the epidemic to gain momentum.

The fiction I have selected here has great value as a learning tool because writers can imaginatively explore what can go wrong on every level of human activity during an epidemic crisis. For this reason, students of epidemiology can profit greatly from hypothetical scenarios, as long as the facts are credibly represented.

12. A Just and Proper Tale
Figurative Language and Epidemiological Discourse

The pre-conceptual interpretation of epidemics and the use of figurative devices, such as personification (the convention endowing pestilence with human characteristics and sensibilities), reflect the ancients' inability to make sense of infectious disease. Outbreaks struck without warning, slew with brutal efficiency, demolished families, societies, even nations, and then simply receded. The cause(s) of these disasters defied all reason: pestilence was ubiquitous, it was invisible, it disfigured, it killed, and it could not be stopped. Since pre-scientific communities were understandably terrified and helpless in pestilential times, their tendency to blame (or to invoke) supernatural power and to envisage epidemics in anthropomorphic terms was commonplace, as we have seen in both imaginative and historical writings.

Scholars have long been interested in the way language is used in scientific writing. Michael A. Arbib and Mary B. Hesse, for example, in *The Construction of Reality*, state that "scientific revolutions" are essentially "metaphoric revolutions" (156). In *Rhetorical Figures in Science*, Jeanne Fahnestock examines the influence of figurative language on scientific argumentation from antiquity to the present and argues that figures of speech have played a constructive role in scientific discourse, contributing to our understanding of how language and reasoning interrelate with one another. With the exception of Koch's postulates, however, Fahnestock devotes limited attention to the use of figurative language in modern biomedical science (162–65). I hope to demonstrate in this chapter that figurative language should be used sparingly, if at all, in modern epidemiological texts because it can be misleading.

Susan Sontag wrote two influential books on the relationship between disease and language, and I would like to give some attention to her commentary on HIV/AIDS, primarily because she believes that metaphor (defined in the Aristotelian sense as "the transfer of a word belonging to something else" [*Poetics*, 1457b]) can misrepresent biomedical reality (93). We know that the writers of antiquity freely used figurative language to describe the epidemic experience. Even though they could not understand the experience, they still had to put their suffering into concrete terms. Writers in the tradition of Thucydides, however, eschewed subjective interpretations and figurative language, preferring instead to record the palpable effects of epidemics on the health of individuals and on society. The question at issue here is whether or not figurative language has a place in modern biomedical discourse.

Sontag's analysis suggests that, if one is to analyze scientific discourse accurately, one must have a balanced understanding of language *and* of the science it purports to represent. Selecting three passages from popular essays (none of them is bibliographically cited), she tries to show that the inaccurate use of figurative language obfuscates the reader's understanding of the molecular processes leading to HIV infection (104–112).

Sontag begins by criticizing the militaristic language of the first passage (105): the HIV virus is described as a minuscule "invader"; the macrophage (a phagocytic blood cell and component of the immune system) as a "scout" alerting the system when it finds "the diminutive foreigner"; and the warning "mobilize[s] an array of cells," which produce antibodies "to deal with the threat." The AIDS virus, meanwhile, pursues its objective "single-mindedly" and, in the process, "ignores" certain blood cells, "evades the rapidly advancing defenders," and "homes in on" a T cell, which is called "the master coordinator of the immune system" (105).

Although criticism of the first passage is warranted, Sontag fails to explain *why* the military analogy does not correspond to the microscopic events happening in the body. Instead, she utters a platitude about "the language of political paranoia, with its characteristic distrust of a pluralistic world" (106). In my view, the passage is suspect not for its militaristic imagery and language, *per se*, but because its author *personifies* the virus (a parasite) and the human cell it infects (a host). The language, in other words, is biologically inaccurate: HIV does not *evade* certain cells (i.e., to avoid by deceit or cleverness) and *home in on* others (i.e., to target consciously). Nor does it move through the bloodstream, *single-mindedly* intent upon finding a vulnerable cell. The point is that HIV knows nothing; it has no political aim. Genetic material housed in a membranous coat, it is driven by complex biochemical impulses. Its innate drive is to sustain and replicate itself. Heinz L. Fraenkel-Conrat's definition of *life* as the "highly organized interplay of enzymes and genetic material, of energy and blueprints" (205; "Synthetic Mutants" 191–205) efficiently describes the life-force and motives of the HIV particle. To experts like Dr. Joshua Lederberg, several of whose essays we will look at in this chapter, HIV is a primitive parasite: paradoxically, its biochemical affinity for T cells is disadvantageous to itself, since its life-cycle weakens its host who succumbs to opportunistic infections, and since it does not have the capacity to protect the host from microbes that threaten their common environment. By causing its host's demise, the virus and its burgeoning colony paradoxically destroy the very environment that could have sustained it had an evolutionary balance been attained between the needs of the parasite and the integrity of the host. That, essentially, is Lederberg's point. In this light, Sontag's popular and political readings of molecular biology are tangential at best.

Sontag's reading of the second passage (from an uncited 1986 *Time* magazine article on AIDS) exemplifies the idea that effective criticism of scientific discourse requires one to have a reasonable understanding of the subject matter. To point out the deficiencies in Sontag's interpretation, I will section the passage she critiques, interpolate the critic's comments, and then, for comparison, paraphrase an authoritative description of how HIV organizes and penetrates a cell.

The second passage begins as follows: "On the surface of [a] cell, [HIV] finds a receptor into which one of its envelope proteins fits perfectly, like a key into a lock. Docking with the cell, the virus penetrates the cell membrane and is stripped of its protective shell in the process"(106). Sontag objects on the grounds that the language belongs to the lexicon of "high-tech warfare," evokes video-game imagery, is in keeping with "the fantasies of our leaders" (i.e., with the Reagan Administration's Star Wars missile-defense plan), and is reminiscent of science-fiction literature (106–07). The image of an HIV particle "docking" with a host cell (which suggests two space vehicles) or of fusing like a key in a lock does not seem to strike Sontag as being biologically imprecise: rather, she is more concerned with the political and popular associations of these figures. I maintain that the only sure way to test the viability of figurative tropes such as these is to determine the degree to which they communicate the scientific truth undistortively to the average reader. The political subtext to which Sontag repeatedly refers is biologically irrelevant.

I have chosen an article published by the National Institutes of Health ("HIV, How [It] Causes AIDS") as the standard against which to test the excerpt, along with Sontag's reading of it. To begin with, HIV cannot *find* anything because *to find* presupposes cognition, the having of an object in mind. More appropriately, HIV *is drawn to* a receptor that accommodates the virus' connective protein. The outer membrane of an HIV particle, its envelope, consists of fatty molecules (lipids), derived from the membrane of a previously infected human cell, within which it had gestated and from which it had originally emerged; in addition, the virus particles retain gestational substances from dead host cells. From the surface of HIV protrudes protein spikes—prong-like projections, each consisting of a cap and an anchored stem (on average, seventy-two such structures per particle). The replication cycle commences when the HIV particle is drawn to a potential host because of the latter's surface molecule, called CD4+; a potential host, the T cell (e.g., T 4) is a component of the immune system that normally kills parasitic cells like HIV. HIV, however, has a biochemical affinity for, and compatibility with, the T cell. On the surface of the T cell, two CD4+ receptors bind together with molecules on the HIV spike-caps. At this junction, the virus particle and the large cell fuse (hence, the lock-in-key simile and the docking metaphor), and the virus penetrates the cell.

The lock-in-key and docking figures, which are intended to convey the complex activities of proteins and of viral particles, are efficient enough to give the reader a general idea of what happens on the molecular level. The interested reader will usually ask questions: *what* causes the parasitic virus to move to T cells? And *how* exactly does the biochemistry work to enact this fusion? The reader can then consult more sophisticated sources to answer these questions. Our concern here is whether or not the simile and metaphor obscure or misrepresent the general idea that the virus attaches to, and penetrates, the host cell. I believe that, for the general reader, the lock-in-key and docking figures are acceptable, while Sontag's comments on popular culture and on Republican politics are irrelevant.

Sontag strongly objects to another passage from the second text:

> the naked AIDS virus converts its RNA into ... DNA, the master molecule of life. The molecule then penetrates the cell nucleus, inserts itself into a chromosome and takes over part of the cellular machinery, directing it to produce more AIDS viruses. Eventually, overcome by its alien product, the cell swells and dies, releasing a flood of new viruses to attack other cells ... [106].

For Sontag, the portrayal of HIV as alien invader (as found in "science-fiction narratives") is unacceptable. In her view, the excerpt misrepresents the replicative process; however, she misreads the passage entirely. Her claim that the "body's own cells *become* the invader" (a science-fiction motif) is blatantly incorrect. What actually happens is that HIV, a retrovirus (and a parasite), encodes its genetic material into the host's DNA, and with the help of certain enzymes, the virus copies itself by using the host's genetic processes. In effect, the virus has become situated in a gestational environment, one in which a new generation of HIV particles comes into being. The host cells, though they carry the HIV virus, *are not transformed* into them.

The choice of words in the above-quoted *Time* magazine excerpt, with the exception of *naked* (which pertains to humanity and could be replaced by a word like *denuded*), corresponds closely to the NIH description. According to the official document, when HIV enters the cytoplasm of the host cell, it loses its protective membrane. From that point on, the author of the excerpt, like the NIH writer, correctly describes the process by which HIV replicates itself within a cell. According to the NIH article, the replicative process has five stages: (1) an HIV enzyme (reverse transcriptase) converts viral RNA into DNA, once the virus is inside the host; (2) the newly-formed HIV-DNA, which is not yet infectious, moves into the nucleus of the cell and is spliced into the DNA of the host; (3) once its genetic material is fixed in the host's chromosomes, HIV begins replicating itself by transcribing new RNA copies (using the host's own enzymes!), and the copied RNA (called *messenger-* or mRNA) becomes the genetic material of a new generation; (4) *translation* follows *transcription*: the genetic language of HIV encoded in the newly-produced mRNA is transported to the host's cytoplasm; and (5) the molecular parts of the new HIV particles—proteins and genomic RNA— collect inside the cellular membrane; the viral envelope which will house the new HIV virus particles also forms within the host's membrane. When the immature viruses bud off from the cell, they are individually enveloped in membrane containing both cellular and HIV protein. Another HIV protein, protease, then cuts large HIV proteins into smaller ones that go into the new viral particles. The replicated particles emerge in large numbers and spread into the bloodstream, vacating the dead host cell.

Whereas I agree with Sontag that militaristic language distorts the biological content of the first excerpt, her objections to the second and third excerpts as being misrepresentative are wholly unfounded. In reality, the *Time* magazine description of HIV's organization and replication is factually accurate, devoid of popular and of political overtones, and the language, with a single-word exception, is appropriate to the readership. The most important point to observe is that, in the second and third excerpts, figurative language is used sparingly, and the author conveys the biological process of HIV replication perspicuously.

As we take a step back from Sontag's book (about 1500 years back), the question arises: why would an author use figurative language to describe the epidemic experience, if conventions such as these obscure biological realities? To appreciate where figurative language is helpful (or an only choice) in biomedical writing, let us, once again, consider the Byzantine historian Procopius' eyewitness description of a plague which broke out in

A.D. 543 (known also as the plague of Justinian) (Marks and Beatty 44–8). To this classical prototype, I will compare modern works.

According to Procopius, the plague broke out among the Egyptians in Pelusium and spread in a northeasterly direction to Palestine, eventually encompassing "the whole world" — that is, the world as demarcated by the borders of the Eastern Roman Empire (Bk. II.xxii: p. 453). Procopius suggests that the Byzantine plague moved by "fixed arrangement" (p. 454), remaining in each country for a "specified time." This implies that the pestilence planned its movement from region to region. In order to discern a pattern of dissemination, one would have to study such things as demography, ecology, public health, and so on. Procopius' strategy, however, was much different. He ascribes the geographical pattern not to the possibility that human beings carried infected fleas in their travels, but to the deliberations of the invasive entity itself as it presumably drifted over vast expanses of land and sea in the form of a poisonous cloud.

When the historian notes that the plague-entity also followed a predictable route along coastlines, this raises the possibility (for us) that its dissemination had more to do with overland and maritime trade routes than with the calculated drift of a miasmatic cloud. That it diffused itself widely as if the plague-entity was careful not to miss "some corner of the earth" (p. 455) could mean that there were multiple infection sites and that this virulent disease was quickly disseminated. And to say, as he does, that it stalked human beings in every abode (cave, mountain, and island) implies that the disease was especially contagious wherever human beings congregated, and that human behavior and living conditions were somehow implicated in the cycle of contagion.

Another phenomenon intriguing the Byzantine historian was that disease recurrence was characterized by a kind of malicious thoroughness: the plague reafflicts severely those whom it had barely touched in its initial sweep (p. 455); conversely, and as if seeking parity, it attacks lightly those severely stricken during its initial visitation. Procopius perceives significant anomalies; his interpretation of them, however, goes nowhere since anomalies are comprehended in the context of sixth-century thinking.

To humanize the destructive force into an entity is not out of the ordinary. Thus, the pestilence is perceived as having a human quota, never vacating an area altogether until that region had "given up its just and proper tale of the dead" (p. 455). To the modern reader, this observation suggests that the Byzantines were familiar with the disease from earlier experiences, that they kept mortality records, and, in comparing these statistics, determined that the death rate in A.D. 543 was basically equivalent to those of earlier outbreaks. So, beneath the pre-conceptual surface, an inquiring eyewitness uses anecdotal and folkloric knowledge to find patterns, to disclose anomalies, and ultimately to make sense of the event, relative to his experience and knowledge.

Whereas the epidemic persona that Procopius creates is formulaic and a practical way of envisioning the outbreak, on a deeper level it reflects the activities of the scientific investigator trying to deduce the cause of the disaster from its frightening, uncontrollable effects. In Procopius's history, the metaphoric representation of plague dominates the foreground, yet, as the historian makes clear, the medical establishment of the times was also busy gathering crucial information about its effects on patients (as we have seen in an earlier chapter). The work of observation and of inquiry would eventually clear away the pre-conceptual surface. In the final analysis, the personification of the plague is historically appropriate to Procopius' milieu.

In many ways, the personification of micro-organisms and of disease is incongruent with the spirit of the modern scientific commentary. Ferdinand Cohn's influential essay, *Bacteria: The Smallest of Living Organisms*, is a case in point. F. J. Cohn (1828–1898), German botanist, bacteriologist, and pioneer in the field, demonstrated that bacteria do not generate spontaneously and that some can actually arise from spores, a theory he proved, in 1876, using *Bacillus subtilis*, a species that he discovered (Brock 55). In his *Studies on Bacteria* (1875), his most significant contribution to the field, he articulated a fourfold bacterial taxonomy.

Cohn certainly understood that bacteria are microscopic, unicellular organisms, which (at the time) were believed to be either plant-like or to belong to a distinct heterogeneous phylum. His work paved the way for the work of later taxonomists and to the contemporary formulation that bacteria belong to a distinct taxonomic kingdom altogether, the Prokaryotae, to which blue-green algae also belong. If Cohn had been able to see one hundred years into the future, it is likely he would have agreed with the zoologist, Ernst Mayr, who in 1982, called the Prokaryotes "the most challenging frontier of descriptive systematics" (140). From his vantage point in the late 1870s, Cohn had before him an equally challenging frontier. He had no doubt that he was studying living organisms, manipulating them in the laboratory, and classifying them systematically. There is no question as to Cohn's pioneering efforts in, and contribution to, the history of microbiology. Unexpectedly, however, in the midst of his watershed paper on bacteria, he personifies the epidemic, and the results are counterproductive.

Cohn writes of how insights into "the secret life energies of bacteria" have shown that these organisms "rule with demoniacal power" over the life and death of man. In a sense, this statement has some validity: micro-organisms certainly control or dominate human existence. It is essential, however, to keep in mind that the vast majority of bacterial flora is either harmless or beneficial to man. Andrew Spielman, a specialist in tropical diseases and in entomology, writes that "Microbes are everywhere. They make up about a twentieth of our weight, filling our intestines, covering our skin, and lining our mouth and nasal passages.... A suitable microbial mix is essential to our well being. If certain of these microbes that have colonized us are destroyed, as by excessive antibiotic use, our microbial balance may be upset, which can result in [illness]" (19). If one accepts Spielman's estimates, it is difficult to resist calculating how many pounds of bacteria make up or share one's body mass (the idea inclines one to bathe in sodium hypochlorite). This idle thought illustrates the widely-held misconception that "the word 'bacteria' automatically means disease" (Koob and Boggs 32). Certainly, if the two thousand existing species of bacteria were eliminated from the Earth, there would be no bacterial diseases. But under such conditions, organisms such as fungi, held in balance by bacteria, would proliferate to dangerous levels and threaten health. For man, starvation would be the most catastrophic effect of global bactericide since bacteria are essential to digestion. Because bacteria and blue-green algae convert atmospheric nitrogen for plant and animal utilization, their absence would cause crops to fail and lead to famine (32). Moreover, since bacteria and fungi are essential to decomposition, dead organisms would accumulate, leaving the planet "a heap of corpses, and the human race ... part of the pile" (32).

Although a pioneer in bacterial taxonomy, in 1872 Cohn invokes the image of bacteria as a malevolent, undifferentiated mass-organism and employs the pre-conceptual phrase, "demoniacal power," to describe the kingdom's relationship to man. Furthermore, to call pestilence the "scourge of God" is to suggest to the unlearned that epidemic disease is a means of divine chastisement and its wielder a punitive, extranatural entity. One wonders if Cohn was thinking of Procopius when he alludes to the epidemic in the indefinite third-person singular pronoun as an *It* that, with unrelenting "progress," wanders from city to city and from land to land. This characterization suggests that *It* is a desultory predator.

Unfortunately, Cohn overextends the epidemic metaphor: the outbreak becomes a cunning, inscrutable being. Diminishing in intensity in one place "as if exhausted" and seeming to disappear, the epidemic then employs a feint: "in order to carry on its work," it arises unexpectedly in a new location, its brief subsidence disguising an intended point of attack. The entire epidemic pattern — i.e., dissemination, intensification, and diminution — comprises a fanciful strategy; for Cohn, the epidemic is at "work" in a systematic fashion and with an implicit goal: the destruction of its human victims.

Even if this portrayal is not taken so literally, it undoubtedly promulgates the stereotypical impression that epidemics, certainly dreadful in their physical, emotional, and social effects, are inexplicable and unnatural. It is one thing to call the epidemic a phenomenon, the understanding of which lies *within* the range of scientific inquiry, and quite another to describe it pre-conceptually as a "scourge," a nonhuman entity, ubiquitous in its movements, unpredictable in its behavior, and invariably lethal to man. As a "scourge," epidemic disease not only inflicts devastation, but it is also the living embodiment of affliction, punishing humanity to satisfy some outstanding transgression. Cohn's use of figurative language, then, is definitely at cross-purposes with his scientific pursuits. On the one hand, he depicts bacteria as an undifferentiated predatory mass, yet, on the other hand, he labors to classify bacteria into genera and species by painstakingly documenting their distinctive physical features. I cannot begin to guess why Cohn revived pre-conceptual language and sentiment in a pioneering work intended to enlighten readers and to dispel common misconceptions.

A similar inconsistency exists in Hans Zinsser's well-known, 1934 history of typhus, *Rats, Lice, and History*. His employment of personification contradicts his intention of writing a natural history of the disease. Hunting microbes is described whimsically as a sport for enthusiasts, and the microbes themselves are portrayed as "ferocious little fellow creatures"; and these *fellows* "lurk in the dark corners and stalk us" in the bodies of rats, mice, domestic animals, and insects, awaiting the opportunity to "waylay" us (14). The reader who may have rudimentary knowledge of the subject is burdened with the misperception that all microbes are ferocious, uniformly hostile to man, and capable of ambush; consequently, Zinsser obfuscates the parasite-host relationship and how human behavior, such as crowding and insanitation, contributes to typhus epidemics.

According to the chapter headings, the natural history of typhus is comparable to a heroic biography, outlineable in five developmental stages: (1) birth, childhood, and adolescence; (2) earliest exploits; (3) young vigor; (4) contemporary life; and (5) prospects of future education and discipline. Obviously, the metaphors of ferocity and of heroism are incongruent with one another: the ubiquitous predator is somehow praiseworthy and robust, and the European typhus epidemics of World War I (1914 to 1918) constitute a *"triumphant"* (italics added) period in its natural history (300), which means that it has been a successful adversary of mankind.

After World War I, however, the *hero* inevitably becomes a fugitive, one whom medical science relentlessly pursues. Vicious when cornered, the fugitive turns upon its pursuer, and (using Zinsser's metaphor) stops him in his tracks. This is likely an allusion to the tragic death of Howard Taylor

Ricketts (1871–1910), the American pathologist who, as noted earlier, discovered a group of micro-organisms, later called *Rickettsia* (named in his honor), which includes Rocky Mountain Spotted Fever and typhus. In his pursuit of Spotted Fever, he successfully proved, in 1906, that human beings contract the disease from a particular species of tick. In 1908, he isolated the causative organism in the bloodstream of infected animals and in the bodies and eggs of ticks. While in Mexico, he demonstrated that lice gave typhus to human beings, but there, in 1910, he caught the disease and died from it (hence, the microbe stopped its pursuer). Since then, Zinssner continues, others have tracked typhus down "to all corners of the world," determining where "his tribe is established," and its "hiding places" within animal and insect vectors (300).

Although the fugitive remained a dangerous adversary in the post-War years, much had been learned since then about the cycle of contagion or, as Zinsser puts it, "His method of attack." Once the "method" is fully comprehended, scientists will be able to forge weapons to "repulse him." Eventually, as its freedom of action is progressively curtailed, typhus will be confined, "like other savage creatures," to "the zoological gardens of controlled diseases." Once again, typhus is portrayed as a surreptitious agent: it is an entity with a plan and not a parasitic organism. From the author's standpoint in the 1930s, it is to be eradicated from the natural world and its remnants preserved as living curiosities.

Zinsser's use of personification should not suggest that he seriously entertained pre-conceptual beliefs. The rhetorical eccentricities he exhibits — i.e., ironic anthropomorphism and persiflage (satirical banter on a serious topic) — give the book great appeal, but the imagery also reinforces the mistaken notion that all micro-organisms cause disease. The injudicious style, tone, and rhetoric, in effect, conflict with the gravity of the subject: the history of a disease that, by the end of World War II, had caused sixty-six recorded epidemics world-wide.

Surprisingly, Laurie Garrett, author of the informative book, *The Coming Plague*, employs personification. Warfare, she writes, is constant on the microscopic level. In fact, the microbial world is "a frantic, angry place, a colorless, high-speed pushing and shoving match" (619). To call microbial behavior frenzied and belligerent is to personify, and her language choices move perilously close to anthropomorphism: thus, microbes work together to combat a shared enemy by "swapping" genes (*to swap* is to barter or trade one thing for another) in order to counter an antibiotic; or they secrete a chemical inside a useful host to allow the parasite to be comfortable (she refers to protein coats that prevent blood cells from responding to pathogens). Symbiosis and the exchange of genes enhance the survival of a micro-organism under attack by the body's defenses. But no accord (in the denotative sense of the word) is reached between organisms; there is no cooperation or mutual defense pact between microbes. Moreover, by gene swapping, are we to understand that organisms interchange genes mechanically on *a quid pro quo* basis? Garrett attenuates her description further when she calls microbes "sophisticated" if they can "outwit or manipulate" the human immune system. The adjective "sophisticated" works well if it denotes a complex or intricate system and a biological process— although *to outwit* or to manipulate denotes superior ingenuity or conscious adaptability. Personification, in this case, propagates the obsolete notion that, in relation to man, infectious organisms are self-conscious, competitive, and antagonistic. Certainly, neither Cohn, nor Zinsser, nor Garrett thinks that pathogens are intelligent creatures. To the uncritical reader, on the other hand, their use of language may suggest otherwise.

The most obvious reason for using figurative language is to make microbiological phenomena apprehensible to the general reader. My point has been that a careful balance must always be maintained in this discourse between the edifying use of language and the factual integrity of the science. The writer must always be aware of the effects his or her language will have on the reader.

With the advent of molecular biology, new metaphors would be used to characterize micro-organisms, not as predators, but as coinhabitants of the biosphere. In basic texts, writers routinely use analogies to convey these invisible realities. But, in this endeavor, a delicate balance has still to be maintained. Robert DeSalle's essay, "Natural History of Infectious Disease," for example, promulgates the idea that human beings and microbes coexist with one another ecologically, but the author uses contradictory metaphors to convey how mankind relates to micro-organisms: one is the seesaw (symbolizing ecological balance) and the other, borrowed from Cold War terminology, is the arms (or armaments) race.

In De Salle's construct, the seesaw is the ecosystem, with mankind and microbes sitting on opposite sides of the plank. The plank will not balance unless the principals are of equal weight, that is, unless they are adapted to one another. If one principal is heavier than the other, the seesaw becomes imbalanced, and a series of adaptations are called for to adjust it. In a stable ecosystem, the seesaw is balanced, despite momentary fluctuations that can be naturally counterbalanced. But when an excessive fluctuation occurs— due to flood, war, or microbial mutation — the balance can be so radically altered as to threaten one or both of the principals and affect the entire ecosystem. Disequilibrium of this magnitude, therefore, requires "more substantial repositioning by both on the ecological seesaw" (2).

What does this mean in evolutionary terms? Unlike microbes that genetically adapt to changing conditions through rapid reproduction, human adjustments (De Salle explains) are artificial, taking the form of biochemical or of technological interventions, for example, the creation of new medicines, of pesticides, and of sanitary techniques to control and to prevent the spread of disease. De Salle also points to human culture — to politics, as well as to economic, social, and behavioral responses to disease — as a significant realm of human-microbial interaction. In this complex relationship, man is at a disadvantage, for microbes adapt on a molecular level rapidly, making "new evolutionary adjustments that human populations must cope with" (2–3). For this reason, according to DeSalle, evolutionary biologists have described the microbial-human interaction as an *arms race* having three possible scenarios: (1) mutually-beneficial coexistence (as, for instance, between man and intestinal *E. coli* bacteria); (2) hostile stalemate (as in the case of Ebola virus which kills too efficiently to be propagated); and (3) the protracted struggle (as in the case of human beings and the bacilli that cause tuberculosis). Because the metaphor of the arms race revives the image of the predatory germ and contradicts De Salle's fulcrum image, it requires closer scrutiny.

The question to be answered here is whether the historical concept of an arms race accurately represents the human-microbe interaction. Bradford Lee defines an arms race as "a rapid, competitive increase in the quantity or quality of instruments of military or naval power by rival states in peacetime." The arms race is a way of maintaining the balance of terror. During the Cold War, "Neither antagonist would knowingly invite suicidal destruction by unloosing nuclear weapons ... the side that first did so would soon learn that a counterattack would prove equally lethal" (May 535).

The relationship between man and microbe is also a matter of survival. But the analogy between pathogen-host and adversarial superpowers is imprecise. First and foremost, the microbe is not a conscious antagonist of man, although the reverse is true. Whereas mankind is just now realizing how misconceptions about infectious disease have contributed to human vulnerability, the germs are not conscious participants in the struggle. To imply as much is to restore the arcane notion of disease-causing microbes as rapacious invaders. Today, scientists have come to recognize that human activities, such as deforestation, the overdevelopment of natural areas, pesticide or antibiotic overuse, and personal behavior are, in large part, to blame for outbreaks of contagious disease. As I see it, the analogy between an arms race and the human-microbe nexus translates this way: man suppresses or eradicates disease-causing germs, while the germs become resistant to these innovations through natural selection. The arms-race analogy may have worked better had De Salle been talking about parity between two aggressive microbes.

The Cold War analogy unjustifiably personifies micro-organisms and over-emphasizes the predatory idea. To its credit, the analogy draws attention to how biotechnology has tried to keep pace with natural selection on a micro-organic level. In this sense, the survival of both principals, microbe and man, depends upon efficient adjustments (armaments): on the one hand, in the DNA makeup of the microbe and, on the other, in scientific experimentation, the latter (an artificial innovation) adjusting to the former (a random, unconscious process).

The implicit paradox of the arms races of the twentieth century (from 1904 to the Cold War) is that the dynamic struggle between opponents created an increasingly dangerous world and the high probability of unanticipated conflict. Whether this paradox obtains in the history of the human-microbe interaction is an interesting proposition. Would there ever come a day when the pharmaceutical industry will find itself unable to outdistance an especially adaptive germ? It takes time to manufacture and test a new generation of antibiotic or of anti-viral drugs; it takes hours for bacteria or viruses to produce a new generation of offspring. De Salle's thought-provoking analogies illustrate how challenging it is to achieve a logical balance between tenor (the meaning of a metaphor) and vehicle (its embodiment).

Two essays by Dr. Joshua Lederberg, molecular geneticist and 1958 Nobel laureate, show that an effective revision may require the deletion of figurative language altogether. In a redaction of the Address from the International Conference on Emerging Infectious Diseases, delivered in Atlanta, Georgia, on March 8, 1998, (re-entitled, "Infectious Disease an Example of Evolution" [revised in 1999]), Lederberg invites his audience to look at the relationship between man and pathogens as "an evolutionary drama." The word *drama* invokes the idea of conflict between protagonist and antagonist, and Lederberg begins on familiar ground. On the one hand, he writes, is man; on the other, "are the bugs." The connection between them is one of predator and prey: "They are looking for food; we are their meat in one sense or another. How do we compete with them?"

Lederberg describes the struggle between man and microbe. The "bugs" have enormous evolutionary advantages over their prey because they reproduce rapidly, outnumber us, and, by virtue of their ability to propagate themselves, have a greater tendency to acquire "advantageous adaptations." In addition, they have the potential to make toxins, to defend themselves against antibiotics, and to alter their proteins so as to elude the immune system. Lederberg then poses the question: why is man still around? The answer is that, despite common misconceptions, "our microbial adversaries have a shared interest in our survival." By destroying the human environment that nourishes them, infectious agents die off unless communicated to another host: "Almost any pathogen comes to a dead-end when we die; it first has to communicate itself to another host in order to survive." According to this argument, the worst outbreaks in history — the Black Death of the fourteenth century (which killed twenty-five million) and the influenza pandemic of 1918 (which killed forty to sixty million) — were *curtailed* by extreme lethality.

Lederberg identifies an evolutionary trend in the pathogen-host relationship, through which "the host species acquires factors for resistance and the parasite species becomes less virulent to the host species" (14). This trend permits the host to survive longer after infection has disappeared; as a result, "the time the parasite can survive in the host" is extended (14). As Lederberg explains it, if a pathogen allows its host to live, it also allows itself to propagate further, and this increases its chances of spreading to a new host (14–15). HIV, for example, can infect the body for a long time, during which many cycles of coadaptation occur "between the evolving population of HIV viruses and the body's population of antibodies to these viruses." The coadaptive cycles eventually break down, however, when HIV mutates beyond the body's defensive capabilities and as the immune system is progressively weakened. If the host-parasite balance is upset under these conditions, then the host will die, not from HIV, but from the opportunistic infections that overcome the weakened immune system (15).

Lederberg distinguishes between the predatory microbe that restricts its own survival and evolutionary development, on the one hand, and the germs that have benignly adapted to human hosts, on the other. In making this distinction, however, he unjustifiably humanizes the microbial "parasite." Thus, it is said to face a "dilemma" (a difficult problem). As if the germ had the capacity to decide which course of action to take, Lederberg explains its two choices: (1) the pathogen can spread rapidly but kill its host in the process (rapid dissemination has its advantages only if the germ were easily transmitted to a new host); and (2) a microbe that "adopts the strategy of proliferating slowly" is vulnerable to the host's inherent defenses, hence the dilemma. Through rapid adaptation, the micro-organism can develop new "tactics," such as evolving a protein coat to prevent the body's immune system from recognizing it as a "'foreign invader.'" That Lederberg emphasizes the phrase *foreign invader[s]* with quotation marks makes it apparent that he is deliberately using metaphor to communicate a complex, molecular phenomenon in easily understood terms (italics added). But his employment of figurative language is admissible only to a degree.

The image of the hegemonic germ is not the issue: it is certainly a living invader of the body, inasmuch as it enters the host and causes injury (though it does not act deliberately). Personifying the microbe as a problem-solver (a "dilemma") and its genetic adaptation as a deliberate solution (a "strategy"), however, harkens back to the language of pre-conceptuality. The military language — e.g., adopting tactics (i.e., genetic adaptations) to serve a strategic end (i.e., survival) — is less problematic in that microbes have "the enormous capacity for genetic plasticity" (14), a central point in Lederberg's address. Although the author most certainly does not subscribe to the idea that micro-organisms have higher intelligence, the use of personification to describe how pathogens respond to hosts reinforces archaic ideas of how infectious diseases act. I am reminded of Ernst Mayr's words: "Since we have no way of determining which of the animals (and plants) have intentions or consciousness, the use of these terms adds nothing to the analysis; indeed, it only obfuscates it" (51).

It is instructive to compare the 1998 *Address* to Lederberg's treatment of the same thesis in his essay, *Infectious History* (2000). Once again, the author's point is that the pathogen-host relationship is best understood in evolutionary, coadaptive terms rather than in the conventional misrepresentation of predator and prey. In the 2000 essay, however, personification is conspicuously absent. His exposition takes the form of a historical survey of medical microbiology from 1880 to the present and of its place in biological studies.

The paramount issue, according to Lederberg, is what the natural history of disease can tell us about biology and evolution. The fundamental premise upon which inquiries of this kind depends is that man cohabitates with animals, plants, and microbes. From this premise, one can then try to comprehend how ecological and evolutionary instabilities arise. It is an incontrovertible truth that altering the physical and biological environment affects our relation with microbes. The alterations can be demographic, hygienic, or even therapeutic, as in the overdispensing of antibiotics. The population explosion in the twentieth century (a 73 percent increase in world population, 1900 to 2000) is an example: it has been directly responsible for crowding, for the destruction of forests, for suburbanization, and for similar trends which have brought people into close contact with viruses, and with vector-borne diseases to which they are vulnerable. International commerce and long-distance travel bring infected people to remote places and spread communicable diseases quickly. A genetic dimension to this phenomenon is that the mixture of peoples and cultures will redistribute their inherited predispositions, their immunities, and pathogens that may otherwise have remained dormant in the country of origin. Defense against the rapid global transmission of pathogens, Lederberg maintains, must begin with an intellectual reorientation, with a revolution in how we think about disease-causing microbes.

The reorientation Lederberg espouses has its roots in the past. Germs, he emphasizes, are alive and evolve. It is a fact that evolutionary processes change microbial genotypes as well as their hosts. Our knowledge of hereditary adaptation to infectious disease is not new. We even have an insight into a genetic alteration that provides some protection against HIV/AIDS. But human evolution cannot compete with the evolution of microbes, the genetic composition of which can change more rapidly than that of man. The human immune system, though robust, has changed very little in two hundred million years. Whereas germs which overcome antagonists will preserve and replicate successful genes that are part of their immediate heritage, our immunological adaptations cannot be passed on to our progeny. "If our collective immune systems fail to keep pace with microbial innovations in the altered contexts we have created," Lederberg concludes, "we will have to rely more on our wits" (8).

Well-adapted microbes, Lederberg reiterates, are best served if they *do not kill* the host whose system sustains them (italics added). To domesticate or to coexist with the host is the ideal situation: symbiosis is the balance. Lederberg therefore proposes that we accept our biological status as hosts, the microbes' as parasites, and the best relationship between the two as coexistence. From this perspective, he envisages the microbial and human genome as a unified system — one that, to my mind, is a kind of chimera; but, in Lederberg's mind, it constitutes a life-sustaining amalgam of heterogeneous life forms. At present, the relationship between man-the-host and the microbial parasite is a life-or-death struggle. Responses on either side can be excessive, as mutant pathogens can kill a host and itself in the process, while a host may suffer from autoimmunological side-effects caused by an infection. So how can man approach a balance?

Lederberg contends that, if we are to understand human-microbial symbiosis as a way of rendering pathogens innocuous, research is necessary. The problem is that, since germs and man have evolved at very different rates, the microbe alone has the capacity for genetic adaptation. The first step in the manipulation of microbes, therefore, would be to invent appropriate experimental models of infection. This is necessary since the worst zoonoses (i.e., animal diseases that spread to man) are maladapted to their hosts, since parasite and host have only just recently come into contact with one another through genetic, sociological, or environmental changes. In effect, mankind and certain germs lack a coevolutionary history, a heritage of adaptive adjustments. For Lederberg, a successful parasite will evoke an immune response that will do two things simultaneously: kill off competitive microbes yet allow the invader to live. From this perspective, HIV is a primitive, maladapted virus because it destroys its own host and because it cannot prevent opportunitistic infections from overwhelming the host that it inhabits.

Lederberg's 2000 revision, an exemplary biomedical essay, expands the scope of the 1998 Address. It improves upon the earlier essay because the idea of coadaptation is surveyed within its intellectual contexts, and, most important of all, because figurative language (i.e., the predator-prey metaphor and the personification of microbial activity) is virtually eliminated. Even when skillfully managed, figurative language in epidemiological discourse promulgates misconceptions about mankind's relationship with microbes.

We have seen, thus far, that biomedical discourse is a demanding craft, one in which the integrity of scientific facts is preeminent. I would like to direct our attention from a survey of metaphoric passages to the rhetorical incarnations of smallpox, which run the gamut from precise denotation to personification. On one end of the spectrum is the authoritative, biomedical report. The CDC, the WHO, and the writers of handbooks and of specialized studies provide the public with a wealth of general of information about the etiology, history, and treatment of the disease. The CDC's *Smallpox Overview*, for example, includes a general history of the disease, as well as information about its origin, its mode of transmission, and its clinical stages. Its content is efficiently presented and worth summarizing because, like the NIH article on AIDS, it is a linguistic standard by which to judge other modes of smallpox discourse.

According to the *Overview*, scientists now know that smallpox can spread through coughing, just like the common cold. The virus enters the body through the lungs, invades the bloodstream and organs, and spreads to the skin where it causes a distinctive rash, progressing from spots to scabs. During an incubation period of from seven to seventeen or from twelve to fourteen days, a person is not contagious and has no symptoms. Initial symptoms, appearing in the prodromal phase, last from two to four days. In this period, fever, malaise, head and body aches, and sometimes vomiting occur. Fevers range from 101 to 104 degree F.; patients can be contagious at this time. When the early rash emerges, red spots appear on the tongue and in the mouth, and the patient is contagious; the spots develop into sores which break open, spreading the virus. The early rash which lasts for four days erupts on the skin, spreading from the face to the arms, legs, hands, and feet. With the appearance of the rash, the fever begins to fall. The blisters fill with thick fluid and have a characteristic, central depression. Until scabs form over the blisters, fever can rise again. The bumps eventually become hardened pustules, crust off, and scab in the next phase which lasts about five days. By the end of the second week after the rash emerges, most of the sores will have scabbed over. They resolve over the next week, leaving pitted scars. From prodrome to resolution, the patient is contagious, but the danger of contagion disappears once the scabs fall off (the scabs themselves are a source of infection). During this ordeal, some patients develop secondary bacterial infections, internal bleeding, and even blindness.

Two clinical forms of the disease have been identified: variola major, the worst and most common form, brings on an extensive rash and high fever. It has four subtypes: the ordinary form, accounting for 90 percent of cases; the modified form, which is mild and occurs in previously vaccinated patients; the flat form; and the severe, hemorrhagic form. Smallpox kills nearly 30 percent of those it infects (statistics vary); flat and hemorrhagic smallpox are fatal; the rate of survival for those stricken with variola minor, the second and mildest form of the disease, is 99 percent.

I have paraphrased the CDC Report to underscore its emphases on descriptive language, on clinical facts such as symptoms, and on phases and subtypes of the disease. All of this information is skillfully interwoven in the text and designed to communicate the facts from historical, medical, and epidemiological perspectives. The CDC Report and documents of its kind are incisively written. Historical, clinical, and epidemiological perspectives are included, providing the reader with an outline and basis for further study. In such a tightly-knit text, personification is an extrinsic element.

Several writers who survey the history of smallpox use personification as a way of describing man's relationship with the disease. Laurie Garrett, for example, personifies the disease as a *fugitive* (italics added). In her survey of smallpox's eradication in the Third World, the virus is pursued and eradicated in remote, natural strongholds. The pioneers of eradication, scientists and physicians such as Donald Henderson, Daniel Tarantola, and David Heymann, braved inhospitable environments, religious and tribal resistance, civil wars, global power politics, bureaucratic obduracy, shortages of medicine, famines, wars, and their own doubts and fears, to eradicate the disease in many places in Africa and Asia (Garrett 40–7). The highlights of the campaign include Henderson's announcement, in November 1975, that a three-year old Bangladeshi girl, Rahima Banu, had been cured. Hers was "the last case of wild variola major in human history" (45). The world's last cases of variola minor were found among Somali Moslems. February 1977, was a critical juncture in the campaign (45). In November, thousands of infected Somalis were expected to pilgrimage to Mecca where they would have intermingled with some two-million fellow Moslems from all over the world, and this event would have spread this strain of the disease and would have defeated the campaign (46). With a ten-month window, the international team focused its efforts on the region of Ogaden, Somalia (46). Under the direction of Dr. Isao Arita, they tracked down the last case of variola minor in Merka, Somalia: Ali Maow Maalin would be the last person to be cured, and smallpox was conquered (46).

To portray smallpox as a fugitive, as Laurie Garrett does, is to say that it is on the run from authorities. The metaphor unintentionally creates confusion. The virus was being pursued in remote corners of the Third World, not because it was trying to evade its pursuers, but because it was endemic to these regions and had to be expunged through the immunization of residents. The real fugitives who had to be pursued were infected individuals who resisted treatment. Had the human carriers not been tracked down, the virus would have remained alive in the ecosystem in the bodies of its carriers. The personification of the virus misleadingly shifts the emphasis away from the human populations at risk (and the elusive human vectors) to the virus itself, which is portrayed as a conscious entity.

A second example of smallpox personification portrays the virus as an incarcerated killer. Once smallpox was contained and eradicated in the wild through immunization, living remnants of the virus were kept for study and as a natural resource for vaccine. The aftermath of one of the most important events in biomedical history is summed up in Jonathan Tucker's chapter, "Monster on Death Row." Tucker personifies the remaining stocks of smallpox as mass murderers in maximum-security facilities, one of which is in Atlanta. The incarcerated specimens are being held in padlocked freezers at the CDC. Four hundred and fifty samples of the virus in frozen suspended animation sit like condemned prisoners in solitary confinement, awaiting execution "for the torture and death of millions of people" (1). A second set of samples is secured in a vault at a Russian laboratory in Siberia. To this day, the world debates whether to extend this stay of execution or to destroy the last remaining samples. The debate over the disposition of these samples is complex, as scientists have been weighing the dangers of accidental release against the requirements of research and of vaccine development (Tucker 166–169).

Tucker's mass murderer is a darker variant of the fugitive, and he seems to be saying that smallpox has a place in a notorious line of mass murderers from Vlad the Impaler to Pol Pot. Neither national boundaries nor time have confined the ravages of smallpox, and this quality magnifies its image as a mass murderer. The analogy makes some sense if we consider why authorities are keeping the virus on ice: so that its genetic material remains accessible for vaccine experimentation and as a resource for study should a weaponized form of the virus be manufactured by terrorists or hostile nations (some believe that strains of the virus are unaccounted for). Why keep a real mass murderer imprisoned for life? One reason is to understand his or her motives and psyche, perhaps. In the final analysis, endowing a virus with human characteristics has dramatic appeal, but it is fundamentally misleading.

The fugitive and mass murderer becomes a *chimera/chimaera* in the hands of biowarfare experts. To depict weaponized smallpox as a heterogeneous animal is not as far-fetched, figuratively, as one might think, and I would like to explain why. The term comes from the feminine form of the Greek word *chimaros* which means *goat* (*OED* II: 348; "chimera"). A chimera is a mythological, fire-breathing monster, having a lion's head, a goat's body, and a serpent's tail, or it is any monster having disparate parts. In biology, the word has two meanings: "an organism composed of two or more genetically distinct tissues, as an organism that is partly male and partly female, or an artificially produced individual having tissues of several species" (*Random House* 234). To the ancient Greeks, chimera was the fire-breathing aggregate of lion (head), of goat (body), and of serpent (tail). A variant found in Hesiod's *Theogony* is of a "swift-footed" beast with the heads of a lion, of a goat, and of a serpent (pp. 12–13); in the genealogy of the Greek gods, it is the inbred offspring of the Hydra of Lerna and her canine brother, Orthos. Ovid's creature which prowls the hills of Lycia with "lungs of fire" has a lion's breast and head and a dragon's tail (*Metamorphoses*, IX: lines 645–46, p. 119).

The microbiological chimera, also a monster, is the product of paranoia and of technological inventiveness. I am referring, specifically, to the clandestine operations of the Soviet virologist, Sergei Netyosov, who is reported to have been working on a genetic experiment, begun in 1985, that combined microbes and toxins (Alibek 259–60; Tucker 158–61). His aim was to create what he aptly termed a chimera virus. The specific project was to insert the genetic material of Venezuelan Equine Encephalitis (VEE), the cause of a severe brain disease, into cowpox. Publicly, Netyosov and his colleagues claimed that their work was connected to the development of vaccines. Recombinant genetic research using microbes was begun with the aim of alleviating human suffering and of understanding why certain strains of viruses cause disease while others do not.

The scientific lineage of the chimera concept is both intriguing and ironic in that the genetic monster created by the Soviets gestated in, and sprang from, a legitimate area of research. Bacteriologists discovered the phenomenon of genetic recombination accidentally in the 1920s. Gerald

Messadié points out, in the article "Genetic Recombination," that studies of the pneumococcus bacteria revealed that several types of this microbe existed and could be identified in terms of the biochemical composition of the capsule which was secreted as a way of protecting the bacteria from the host's immune system (79–81). Classification of bacterial biotypes led to ways of producing medicines to overcome their natural barriers and to kill germs.

In the process of experimentation, scientists noticed an anomaly: the ability to produce this capsule was lost in certain colonies of pneumococci, cultured in the laboratory (80). Dr. Fred Griffith of the British Ministry of Health discovered that germs with a rough capsule (called R) did not sicken mice, whereas those with a smooth capsule (called S) killed them. After killing the S bacteria with heat, he incubated it with R. One would logically expect that the commingling of a dead microbe and of a benign one would produce something innocuous. But when he inoculated the hybrid microbe into mice, several of them died from bacterial infection. Although Griffith and his colleagues did not understand what had happened on a molecular level, the effects were undeniable: R and S had interacted genetically; unpredictably, a virulent organism arose from the genetic crossing of benign R and dead S strains. In the 1930s, scientists inferred that the dead S bacteria were still able to communicate a lethal genetic element to the live R. In 1944 the American scientists, Avery, McLeod, and McCarty, proved that viable DNA from S had indeed been communicated to R, and they suspected that this process could occur with other bacteria as well.

Precisely how the transference happened remained a mystery until 1955 when a Japanese woman with bacillary dysentery, caused by the *Shigella* bacilli, did not respond to antibiotic treatment (80). At the time, the possibility of an antibiotic-resistant strain of *Shigella* alarmed the medical community. In 1960, *Shigella* resistance was tracked down to its interaction with ordinary intestinal bacteria. Resistant genetic material, it turned out, came from an ordinary germ residing in the intestinal tract; the resistant *Shigella* germ then communicated this factor to its colony. The vehicle for transmission, which Dr. Joshua Lederberg discovered in 1952, was a tiny piece of genetic material he called a *plasmid*; he subsequently learned that the plasmid was itself enveloped in a chromosomal fragment (called *episome*). In 1965, the episome and the plasmid were conclusively connected to one another (81). Thus, it became evident that genetic recombination made certain germs resistant to antibiotics, and that this process took place when plasmids were transferred from one cell to another, thus endowing bacteria with the capacity to secrete enzymes responsible for antibiotic resistance.

Technology brought this work full term. With the discovery of biochemical properties intrinsic to cell life, such as restriction enzymes (like protease which cuts up HIV-RNA during replication), scientists learned how to section a piece of DNA precisely and to perform genetic grafting: that is, to insert a DNA sequence having a particular property worthy of study (e.g., one regulating the synthesis of certain substances) into a host cell (81). The cell with the transferred DNA within it will manufacture important therapeutic substances. In short, simple bacteria such as *E. coli* can be engineered into pharmaceutical factories and used to battle refractory diseases.

The biomedical tradition in which Dr. Netyosov had been trained was devoted to the *prevention* of disease. Netyosov and company, however, had other ideas. When they inserted VEE into vaccinia virus, they found that cowpox could actually *manufacture* VEE cells. They pondered a forbidden possibility: if VEE can be rendered compatible with cowpox, it might also be combined with smallpox. Why would anyone think of tampering genetically with variola to make it *more* dangerous than it is in its natural state, especially after the extraordinary work of Tarantola, of Henderson, and of others to eradicate it in the wild? Research into the use of smallpox as a biological weapon, it turns out, had been the stated goal of the Soviet program, and accidental releases of the germ in 1971 demonstrated how recklessly they handled these dangerous agents (Alibek 259–60). The truth behind the Soviet program was partially revealed by the 1992 disclosures of Ken Alibek. A specialist in epidemiology, infectious disease, and microbiology, and the former director of the Soviet bioweapons project (called *Biopreparat*) from 1988 to 1992, Alibek who defected to the United States in 1992 revealed Netyosov's purpose: to explore the military use of smallpox; in so doing, the latter wanted to find a way of *defeating* vaccines and of rendering naturally-occurring smallpox strains *more* lethal than they already were (i.e., fatal in more than 30 percent of natural cases); indeed, this had been the goal of Soviet research from 1981 to 1985.

Netyosov's teams tried to clone and insert Ebola genes into cowpox, and they also used cowpox as the vehicle of morphine-like brain peptides, of conotoxin genes (a lethal nerve agent derived from a marine snail), and of fragments of myelin basic protein (which induces allergic reactions causing brain damage) (Alibek 261–62). According to Alibek, Netyosov's cowpox chimera was the prototype of an even greater monstrosity: Ebola-smallpox, a real fire-breathing, leonine beast. Alibek believed that Vector, the main Soviet installation, had not yet tested the stability of such an aerosolized chimera and its effects on primates. Recalling the Hesiodic beast and the hydra-headed creatures of *The Revelation of St. John*, chapter 13, Netyosov's chimera features three heads (one for each pathogen) and had been manufactured to target the brain and nervous system of its victims.

As a zoomorphic composite, is the chimera an appropriate symbol for weaponized smallpox? Unlike the fugitive or the mass murderer, the analogy between the mythological chimera and the virological weapon is a logical one. In the lexicon of biology, chimera has been used to describe artificial combinations of disparate tissues and organisms. This is precisely what the Soviet project entailed: the creation of a *sui generis* agent composed of incongruent elements, one of which was smallpox. By definition, Netyosov's monster is a chimera. In the final analysis, the zoomorphic depiction of smallpox succeeds because it does not ascribe self-consciousness to the organism.

13. A Tangible Something
The Yellow Fever Construct

An efficient approach to understanding the process of discovery is to read the then-contemporary discourse concerning a specific campaign and to determine the means through which knowledge was obtained. Periodic documents will show that the defeat of an epidemic disease often proceeds with reticular rather than with unilinear motion. Though scientific inquiry is a temporal process and its course unpredictable, a kind of cognitive momentum can keep the process of discovery on track, as we have seen in the systematic problem-solving of the germ theorists. In this chapter, I have selected papers, memoirs, letters, and a drama that tell the story of the Havana yellow fever epidemic of 1899–1900. The yellow fever construct, consisting of periodic texts, documents the inexorable process through which great scientists and their associates identified the source of the disease and devised a method for prevention.

Carlos Finlay: Inference to Hypothesis

The Havana Yellow Fever Epidemic of 1899–1900 was a severe outbreak among United States troops occupying Havana after the Cuban War of Independence (1895–98) and the Spanish-American War (1898) (Kohn 137; Snodgrass 244; Oldstone 58–66). The medical establishment, at the time, was unaware that the mosquito spread the disease from person to person. Instead, they thought that dirt and decay were responsible for keeping yellow fever endemic to Cuba. They were surprised to find out that, even though Havana had been cleaned up in the summer of 1900, the epidemic was undiminished (1400 cases were reported). To find out what was behind the pestilence, the United States dispatched Walter Reed, M.D., to Cuba as head of an Army board of enquiry, which had been established by Carlos Juan Finlay, M.D., a Cuban physician. In 1881, Finlay theorized that the *Stegomyia fasciata* mosquito (now known as *Aëdes Aegypti*) transmitted the virus. Often dismissed by contemporaries as being highly conjectural, Finlay's pioneering work is the focus of this section.

On August 11, 1881, Dr. Finlay delivered a watershed address to the Royal Academy of Sciences of Havana, "The Mosquito Hypothetically Considered as an Agent in the Transmission of Yellow Fever Poison." In this paper, he rejects any theory attributing the origin or propagation of yellow fever either to atmospheric, miasmatic, or meteorological influences, and he dismisses theories implicating sanitation and hygiene. Calling these explanations "primitive beliefs," he proposes to submit for peer review "a new series of experimental studies" in entomology and histology, to be undertaken "with the view of ascertaining the mode by which the yellow fever poison may be propagated." Finlay infers that there exists "a tangible something"—an organism that has to be communicated from the sick to the healthy. The focus of his study is "the medium or agent by which the pathogenic material of yellow fever is carried from the bodies of the infected to be implanted in the bodies of the non-infected." In other words, he was looking for what we know to be a carrier or vector.

When Finlay found anomalies in long-standing topographical and meteorological theories about yellow fever, he pursued the mosquito-vector hypothesis in earnest. He questioned several of the anomalies: how can one attribute the disease to miasmatic conditions if it traverses oceans, if it occurs in cities distant from one another, and if it appears where meteorological conditions vary considerably from one another? And why is it that yellow fever tends not to spread beyond limited epidemic zones, he asks, "even if the meteorology and topography of nearby localities are quite similar to one another"? He concludes that "an agent of transmission" *other* than atmosphere or topography exists to explain these "anomalies" (italics added).

Because yellow fever causes vascular lesions and physico-chemical alterations of the blood, Finlay rightly suspected that contagion was due to insects penetrating "into the interior of the blood vessels," to "suck up the blood together with any infecting particles contained therein, and carry the same from the diseased to the healthy." Comprising two inferential steps, this "hypothesis" warranted experimentation.

Finlay ingeniously speculated that the mosquito contracted a virus when ingesting diseased blood and, in the process, injected the virus-contaminated blood into a healthy person. Five experimental attempts at inoculation with a single bite yielded positive results: one case of "benign yellow fever," two cases of "aborted yellow fever," and "two light ephemeral fevers, without definite character." The mildness and indefinition of these positive reactions, Finlay realized, were due to the fact that live volunteers were each subjected to a single bite. On the basis of preliminary experiments, Finlay "infer[s] that a single [bite] from the mosquito is insufficient to reproduce the graver forms of yellow fever," but that his "final judgment in regard to the efficacy of mosquito inoculations must be postponed until we are corroborated by experimental evidence in absolutely decisive conditions, i.e. outside of the epidemic yellow fever regions." He realizes that these "suspicions and conceptions" must wait for "the decisive evidence furnished by direct experimentation." The story of this decisive trial follows.

John J. Moran and the Reed Commission: Etiology and Experimentation

The etiological phase of the investigation is told by a participant. John J. Moran (1876–1950), clerk at the Headquarters of General Fitzhugh Lee in western Cuba, was one of fifteen volunteers to take part in human experimentation on yellow fever from November 30, 1900 to January 31, 1901. Moran's autobiographical writings give us a unique inside-look at the yellow fever trials. Of the fifteen volunteers, eight were bitten by infected mosquitoes in quarantined locales, seven were inoculated with the blood sera of yellow fever patients, and three were housed for nearly three weeks in an infected-bedding house. The purpose of the experiments was to establish that the mosquito carried the disease. Human experimentation was the only available way, at that time, to prove this definitively since the agent, specific to primates, could not be isolated in the laboratory. The concomitant purpose was to test the contact theory of transmission. As I noted above, many professionals at that time believed that yellow fever was communicated through the air or through excreta. George M. Sternberg, M.D. (1838–1915), the Surgeon General of the United States, entertained this view in 1894. In a letter of January 19, 1894, to Walter Reed, M.D. (1851–1902), Sternberg advocated the idea that yellow fever patients exuded "something" from their bodies that under favorable "local" and "meteorological" conditions multiplied outside of the body and created an epidemic. Like typhoid fever or cholera, this "something" was likely "a living germ," present in the excreta of sick individuals. The microbe, it was believed, multiplied rapidly in the excreta and permeated the ground in ditches and latrines. Sternberg reasoned, therefore, that precautions similar to those taken against cholera and typhoid had to be taken against yellow fever; therefore, infected immigrants had to be isolated from the general population and their soiled clothing destroyed.

The individual efforts of Reed's colleagues to prove the mosquito theory, though admirable, were methodologically flawed (see "Yellow Fever and the Reed Commission"). The need for a collaborative effort and for foolproof controls is underscored by the futility of Drs. James Carroll (1854–1907) and Jesse William Lazear (1866–1900). Both subjected themselves to infected insects but did so outside of secure test conditions; consequently, even if they had contracted the illness, mosquitoes could not have been definitively identified to be the cause. Reed even chastised Carroll for not remaining in quarantine for ten days before being bitten because the objection could legitimately be raised of his having been infected before, not during, the experiment (see "Letter of Walter Reed to James Carroll" [September 24, 1900]). The experiment was further jeopardized because Carroll traveled to another locale *after* being bitten which raised the legitimate possibility of infection taking place subsequent to the experiment and not necessarily as a result of mosquito bites received under controlled conditions.

In the construction of two mosquito-proof buildings, Reed had devised a way of testing all three theories of transmission (i.e., the atmospheric, the contact, and the insect-vector theory, respectively). Three procedures were planned: (1) uninfected volunteers were to be bitten by infected mosquitoes in a protected environment; (2) uninfected volunteers were to be injected with the blood sera of infected human patients; and (3) uninfected volunteers were to be exposed to yellow fever secretions.

John J. Moran's story is told in a letter of February 15, 1900 and in a 1949 memoir. A version of the story also appears in Paul de Kruif's *Microbe Hunters* (1926), and Sidney Coe Howard's *Yellow Jack: A History* (1933) is a dramatic rendition of the story (which became the basis of a major motion picture). We will begin with Moran's succinct, retrospective autobiography in a letter of February 15, 1907. After his honorable discharge from the United States Army on July 3, 1900, Moran was appointed as clerk to General Lee in Western Cuba. At about this time, Robert Post Ames, M.D., an Army surgeon, approached him with a proposition: Moran would receive $500 if he were to participate in a yellow fever experiment in which he would be bitten by infected insects. Ames encouraged Moran to take part by emphasizing how the money would help defray the cost of a medical education, which Moran hoped to pursue at a later date. Moran volunteered on the next day but refused any remuneration. It is not clear from the letter as to why he made this unusual decision.

Two weeks after entering camp, Moran was bitten by infected mosquitoes that were in a test tube. He was held for observation to allow the virus to incubate; however, the first exposure was negative, and Moran admits to having become bored during this process. About six weeks later, he was placed in the mosquito house, a muslin-lined shack with three doors. Reed, Carroll and others observed him from outside through a screened window. On the first morning, seven infected mosquitoes bit Moran; five or six, in the afternoon. On Christmas day, at 11 A.M., Moran developed a temperature of 101 degrees F.; by noon, it was 102 degrees F. In the afternoon, after being diagnosed, he was sent to the yellow fever ward. He describes having diffuse bodily pain. But he recovered and was discharged fourteen days later. To make certain that he indeed had had yellow fever, they injected him with the blood serum of an infected man. If he had contracted the disease from mosquitoes and had recovered, then he was theoretically immune to yellow fever, whether from mosquito bites or from tainted blood serum. Reed was correct: Moran was indeed immune to injected blood products that were tainted with virus.

Paul de Kruif's version of the story corroborates Moran's. De Kruif writes that Moran and his friend Private Kissenger (1877–1946) approached Reed personally and offered to volunteer "for the cause of humanity and in the interest of science" (314). They surprised Reed by refusing to be compensated (de Kruif mistakenly cites the sum as between $200 and $300). Both were placed in "preparatory quarantine" to certify that they carried no disease before the experiment commenced. On December 5, five infected mosquitoes were let loose in the house (de Kruif does not mention the negative results of bites administered from test tube mosquitoes). Kissenger, who developed the disease in five days, exhibited classic symptoms. Fortunately, he recovered.

Moran was placed in the house at 12 o'clock on December 21, 1900, and was set upon by fifteen infected mosquitoes that had been set loose in the room five minutes before he had entered. These insects had previously fed on the blood of yellow fever patients at Las Animas Hospital, Havana. Within thirty minutes, he was bitten seven times. He then left the shack for a time, returning at 4:30 P.M. for further exposure. As a control, two healthy volunteers were housed in the same building but in a separate room that had a mosquito-proof screen. Their isolation was intended to prove that sharing the same air had no effect on yellow fever transmission. The disease, Reed's Commission thought, was blood-borne. On December 25, Moran became severely ill with yellow fever, but he withstood the disease.

Through these experiments, Reed proved Finlay's theory: infected mosquitoes transmit the pathogen through the blood. Warren G. Jernegan, Levi E. Folk, and James L. Hanberry, all of the Hospital Corps, emerged from the infected-bedding house with no signs of infection. This aspect of the experiment was successful as well: it proved that secretions could not communicate the disease. Reed was relentlessly thorough, and it paid off. For example, Jernegan is said to have submitted himself to a triad of exposure: he was twice bitten by mosquitoes, exposed to bedding, and then inoculated with serum. The results were negative for the first and second experiment, but the serum brought on a severe attack of the disease from which he recovered.

John Moran's "Memoirs of a Human Guinea Pig" (1949), written at the age of eighty-three, expands upon the 1907 letter. In this extensive account, Moran explains that, in 1899, efforts had been made to isolate the yellow fever microbe, supposedly present in the blood of patients, by passing sera through a filter. Since it was a virus (a fact unknown to scientists at that time), and since it was small enough to pass through the filter, the agent could not be isolated. In consultation with Finlay, Reed expressed his desire to test the mosquito theory. Finlay was elated to hear this, so he gave Reed a supply of mosquito eggs of the species *Stegomyia* (now known as *Aëdes Aegypti*). Reed hatched the eggs, nursed the larvae, placed them in test tubes, fed them, identified each by number, and used them as vectors that would be fed the blood of yellow fever patients. Throughout, Reed and his coworkers kept accurate records on each insect.

One October afternoon, Moran recalls, Dr. Ames approached him about the experiment. Reed's "missionary and scout" for prospective volunteers, Ames knew about Moran's need to save tuition money, so he offered him $500 to participate, adding that this would be "a fitting start for a young man bent on studying medicine." Moran recollects that, "Neither of [them] gave very much thought to a possible death lurking in the background." Nevertheless, Moran decided to join.

Reed left Washington, D.C., for Cuba after Dr. Lazear had died of yellow fever, on September 28, 1900. Lazear contracted the disease, either through voluntary or accidental exposure, while infecting mosquitoes (i.e. while allowing them to feed on the blood of yellow fever patients) in the ward of Las Animas Hospital. Moran broke the news of Lazear's death and of the impending experiment to his roommate, Private John R. Kissenger of the Hospital Corps. Lazear's death did not dissuade Moran; rather, the situation emboldened him to forego pay and to volunteer for the sake of medical science. To this seeming impetuosity, Kissenger replied that Moran was a fool and that such an act would be misconstrued by some as grandstanding. Not lacking in moral courage, Kissenger, too, decided to join his friend and to forego pay as well. Hearing this, Moran pointed out that their situations were different: he (Moran) wanted to study medicine, so volunteering would be in line with his life's work, but Kissenger had no such ambition. The two friends discussed the issue for the better part of the night, ultimately deciding that it would be "a joint venture." This account, as we shall see, is quite different from Howard's portrayal of it in *Yellow Jack*. In the play, O'Hara (Moran) entertains delusions of grandeur and persuades a rather shallow roommate to volunteer for glory. No mention is made of Kissenger's objection or of their candid discussion throughout the night.

The volunteers surprise Dr. Reed with their decision, Moran adding that they were doing this for "medical science and humanity." Reed was jubilant. The two volunteers then chose the mosquito over the infected-bedding test. Major Reed wanted no fatalities to occur, so the volunteers underwent rigorous physical examinations to make sure that they were up to the ordeal. The plan to use human guinea pigs was quietly undertaken. Publicity was avoided to preclude the hue and cry of anti-vivisectionist groups. Although Moran believed wholeheartedly that the sacrifice of a half-dozen lives to save millions was justified, they anticipated criticism of their plan on ethical grounds. Encouraged by the enthusiasm of Moran and Kissenger, Ames was able to sign up a dozen more participants at the Hospital Corps Detachment. Two sets of experiments were to be undertaken concurrently at Camp Lazear.

On November 20, 1900, Camp Lazear was ready. It had a barbed-wire fence around the perimeter and a military guard for the dual purpose of keeping intruders outside and the participants inside. The experiment itself took place in two twenty-by-fourteen-foot buildings, Number 1 being adapted for the infected clothing test and Number 2 for the infected mosquito test. The first trio, Dr. Cooke, Mr. Folk, and Mr. Jernegan, slept twenty nights in Building No. 1, "on sheets, pillow slips and convalescent suits used and worn by severe and fatal cases of yellow fever, some of which were saturated with 'black vomit.'" When it was over, they emerged in good health.

Moran states that Reed had prepared him for a fool-proof experiment using fifteen mosquitoes, since earlier exposures were negative. This test brought on the infection. In an April 1901 Address to the Medical and Chirurgical Faculty of the State of Maryland, Reed speaks admiringly of "a plucky Ohio boy" named John Moran who,

> clad only in his night shirt, and fresh from a bath, entered the room containing the mosquitoes, where he lay down for a period of thirty minutes.... Within two minutes from Moran's entrance, he was being bitten about the face and hands by the insects that had promptly settled down upon him. Seven in all bit him at this visit. At 4.30 P.M., the same day, he again entered and remained twenty minutes, during which time five others bit him. The following day at 4.30 P.M., he again entered and remained fifteen minutes, during which time three insects bit him, making the number fifteen that had fed at these three visits.... On Christmas morning at 11 A.M., this brave lad was stricken with yellow fever, and had a sharp attack, which he bore without a murmur ["Yellow Fever," 484].

While the experiment continued, and even after Kissenger was successfully inoculated via the mosquito route, the doctors of The United States Public Health and Marine Hospital Service on duty in Havana, and backed by Surgeon General Walter Wyman, M.D., discredited Major Reed's work, even to the point of trying to halt the experiment (484). They obdurately clung to the belief that yellow fever, certainly a contagious disease, was not contracted through mosquito bites. Nevertheless, General Wood, the Military Governor of Cuba and a captain in the Medical Corps of the Army, supported Reed with money and equipment. Moran confides that the attacks against the mosquito-theory proponents were acrimonious.

Major Reed ended his mission in Cuba on or about February 15, 1901 ("Yellow Fever," 479–84). He came to a number of significant conclusions: (1) if a mosquito is to be infected with yellow fever by biting a human being, the transmission of the virus from human blood to insect could only take place within three or four days *after* the onset of symptoms in the patient; (2) the infected mosquito being prepared for use in experiments had to be kept twelve to fourteen days in isolation so that the virus could incubate to a communicable stage within the insect; (3) after that period of time, the insect was a danger to non-immune people and remained so for up to 80 days under favorable conditions; and (4) the carrier insect usually fed at night and was a domestic species. Moran, who called his illness on December 25 a Christmas gift, deduced that his first exposures were negative because he had been bitten in the incubation period and not later when the vector was dangerous.

Finlay had initiated the conquest of yellow fever when he focused on anomalies in historical literature that did not correspond to the miasmatic theory. These anomalies led him to surmise that insects transmitted the agent and were part of a contagious cycle. When he studied both mosquito physiology and human pathology, he concluded that insects were adapted to transmitting contaminated blood from sick to healthy persons and that the skin was initially affected when bitten. These distinct inferences generated a hypothesis, a premise to be subjected to experimental trials. Finlay successfully transmitted yellow fever from sick to healthy patients via the mosquito in an experiment conducted from late June to early September 1880. His limited success became the groundwork of definitive trials undertaken in 1898. The process beginning with inference ended with praxis, as William Crawford Gorgas, M.D., undertook a successful program of mosquito prevention in Havana, and it is to his work that we shall turn.

William Crawford Gorgas: Prevention

Early knowledge about yellow fever causation was about to be put into practice in the tropics. In the winter of 1901, the hypothesis that the mosquito is the intermediate vector of the disease had been established, and the Walter Reed Commission announced this discovery to the American Public Health Commission. When Reed and Carroll induced the disease in non-immune volunteers using the filtered sera of yellow fever patients, they demonstrated conclusively that the agent was a filterable virus. This was the first time that a filterable virus had been implicated as the cause of a specific disease in human beings. Their experimentation also proved that the virus was inviable on inanimate objects or in human secretions and could not be transmitted in the air; its mode of transmission, therefore, was unlike cholera, typhoid fever, or smallpox. This was a significant conclusion, for now it was realized that a comprehensive sanitation plan, though effective for the control of other serious diseases, was useless against yellow fever, unless it was aimed at controlling the breeding grounds of mosquitoes. With this new information, the Commission directed a campaign that oiled and screened over drainage ditches in the city, and they covered clean water supplies, especially during the warm months, since insects thrived in climates over 72 degrees F. (Garrett 67). By the summer of 1902, yellow fever had been virtually eliminated from Havana. In 1904 Dr. Gorgas would be sent to Panama to fight mosquito-borne diseases, and his efforts greatly contributed to the completion of the Panama Canal. Gorgas' paper is the preventive phase of the construct.

In the April 15, 1908 report, "Method of the Spread of Yellow Fever," which Gorgas read before the Medical Association of the Panama Canal Zone, he recounts his experiences in both Havana and Panama. In this report, Gorgas reiterates Finlay's belief that the bite of the female *Stegomyia* mosquito transmitted yellow fever from an infected to an uninfected person. The disease had been endemic in Havana for one hundred and thirty years and would have continued so since a large number of the 250,000 people who lived there were not immune; in addition, as many as 20,000 non-immune people arrived every year, and the birth-rate was around 6000 per year; so, at the minimum, 10 percent of the population was vulnerable to the disease. The mosquito campaign began in February 1901 and was effectively concluded in September 1901. The eight-month campaign owed its success, Gorgas explains, to a rigorous threefold strategy to prevent *Stegomyias* from breeding (which meant that water sources had to be treated to kill larvae), to destroy infected female mosquitoes, and to prevent uninfected mosquitoes from biting infected humans (ironically, Gorgas had to protect the mosquitoes from the patients).

Gorgas's team subdivided the city into districts, each to be overseen by an inspector whose workers saw to it that breeding places were destroyed; to this end, they proscribed standing water. In order to destroy infected mosquitoes, they visited every house in which the fever was reported and fumigated it, along with contiguous dwellings. Those who already had the disease were quarantined in screened hospital wards so that uninfected mosquitoes would not contract the virus from them and, through bites, pass it along to healthy people.

Recounting how he planned the same strategy in Panama in 1904, Gorgas was surprised to learn that the Panamanian epidemic was difficult to manage. It seems that the Havana campaign had the benefit of "a most excellent machine" which had been ready for deployment when Gorgas arrived there; however, in Panama, the machine had to be built from the ground up, delaying the effort considerably. Gorgas does not explain the nature or purpose of the machine, but one can reasonably surmise that it was a fumigation device or one that sprayed oil on water to kill larvae.

One impressive aspect of Gorgas' plan is its quantitative emphasis. He calculated, for example, that the disease could be controlled if the number of mosquitoes per square yard were reduced to what he called "the yellow fever point," that is, ten infected mosquitoes per square yard. No matter how many non-immune or infected persons were present, if the number of insects was less than the threshold previously mentioned, "yellow fever cannot spread." In Panama, in 1905, yellow fever did not spread and eventually disappeared because the mosquito population had fallen below the threshold. It was obvious that the number of mosquitoes had to be reduced drastically. Gorgas acknowledged that it was impossible to eliminate the *Stegomyia* completely, although fumigation of homes offered protection. Attacking the mosquito at vulnerable stages in its life-cycle, especially during the aquatic stage, remained the most promising approach.

As Gorgas plainly demonstrates, disease prevention is a direct outgrowth of scientific investigation and historical study. The correlation between breeding grounds and concentrations of disease-carrying insects, Gorgas knew, was convincingly illustrated by the great yellow fever epidemics in Philadelphia, New York, Boston, and Quebec. Ships transported *Stegomyia* from the tropics, the mosquitoes bred in open water sources, and the epidemic followed. The problem disappeared once a piped water supply was introduced, thus interrupting the life-cycle of the carrier.

Sidney Coe Howard: Dramatic Extrapolation

In chapter eleven, I argued that, if an imaginative epidemic is to have edifying value and credibility, it needs to be grounded in biological reality. An extrapolation through which the reader may vicariously experience the biomedical drama should, therefore, faithfully represent the facts. In Sidney Coe Howard's well-known recreation of the story, however, we find that the personality of John Moran is misrepresented.

In the prospectus to the play, Howard expresses interest in describing the experiment step by step in order to get its "personal side." He communicates this intention in a December 17, 1931, letter to Colonel Albert E.

Truby, whom he had contacted for information. Writing to Moran himself, Howard reiterates how much he valued "the little details and anecdotes that make a story human," and that are often never written down. However, Howard admits to his uneasiness about writing a "historical play or picture" about "living characters." The problem, for the playwright, was to balance the facts with aesthetic imperatives. Writing once again to Moran, on January 12, 1932, Howard speaks about coming "as near as possible to what actually happened and to what the real characters were actually like," a strategy preferable to making up "both characters and incidents for [himself] out of whole cloth." He tells Moran that other participants in the trial, namely Mr. Truby and Mr. Kissenger, had helped him in his pursuit of factual accuracy.

Once the play had been published, however, Howard confessed that he had not recreated the historical facts as he had received them. To achieve a measure of dramatic coherence, he had to restructure the events. Thus, he made up "a story about soldiers ... which would run along with the experiment and keep both elements going together until they finally meet at the moment of volunteering." Howard's dilemma, in effect, was to create a world for the volunteers, which entailed fashioning believable characters from a meager amount of information. In order not to represent Moran, Kissenger, Folk, and Jernegan as "doing anything [they] never did," he decided to make fictional counterparts for each man. The names were changed, therefore, to provide room for dramatic license. In the Preface to the 1933 edition of *Yellow Jack: A History*, Howard writes that, "since the play is in part concerned with the deeds of four American soldiers, whose heroism should not go unrecorded," he used new names: O'Hara (for Moran), Brinkerhof (for Kissenger), McClelland (for Jernegan), and Bush (for Folk). Because he did this reputedly to celebrate rather than merely to represent their "heroic conduct," he did not expect any of them to object to these pseudonyms.

But was Howard true to his stated purpose of representing the "heroic conduct" of the participants? The dramatic portrayal of William H. Dean, a volunteer, raises serious questions about Howard's aim. Dean, known to the Commission by the initials X.Y., was bitten by infected mosquitoes on September 6, 1900. De Kruif writes that the Commissioners exposed him to four mosquitoes (311). John H. Andrus, a fellow volunteer, mentions in his memoir that Dean was bitten by the very same mosquito that had infected Carroll, as well as by three other insects, all resulting in a mild attack. The point of contention is Howard's version of how Dean was recruited into the program. In the play, the Commissioners not only coerce Dean into submitting to exposure, but do so without having apprised him of the life-threatening dangers. Dean's character is portrayed as naïve and even slow-witted. Dr. Lazear orders Dean to roll up his sleeve, but the private naturally recoils: "No, no, I don't think I'd care to do that doctor. Just something about it don't strike me" (100). Instead of respecting Dean's decision, Finlay downplays the danger ("You're bitten by mosquitoes every day!"). Dr. Lazear, an officer, then orders the private to comply: "Come on, now, Mr. Dean! Roll up your sleeve!" Dean reluctantly follows orders. Finlay interjects that Lazear is, in fact, "offering him a great honor." Obviously, Dean was being duped (he utters the line: "I don't get this!").

Howard's depiction of Drs. Finlay and Lazear as having coerced an enlisted man to volunteer for a dangerous experiment did not go unnoticed. Walter De Blois Briggs, writing to Howard, on July 23, 1934, expressed his concern about the scene, requesting that Howard not include it in a movie since it was untrue. Based on the testimony of another Commissioner, Aristides Agramonte, who was an eyewitness to the Dean interview, Briggs contends that, "Dean was not forced into the experiment against his will and I am certain, out of all fairness to Dr. Lazear's memory and to his family now living, you will be unwilling to allow any implication to stand, should the play appear in the moving pictures, that there was anything unethical in this glorious experiment for the benefit of humanity." The dramatic rendition raises ethical questions, since it reduces Dean from heroic volunteer to dim-witted victim and Drs. Finlay and Lazear from dedicated professionals to unethical administrators.

While not degrading the persona of O'Hara/Moran, Howard distorts him into a two-dimensional heroic figure. O'Hara's opinion on yellow fever and on similar afflictions is that they are "questions of fate." Biomedical science, he asserts, offers the only hope for finding a cure (28), so therefore he is willing to sacrifice himself for the cause. In this vein, he tells Bush and McClelland that, should he die from yellow fever, he would gladly offer his remains "to the service of science and not waste them buried whole beneath grass or marble!" (31). Announcing that a special kind of nobility is needed in the struggle against yellow fever (32–3), he fearlessly enters the mosquito house and speaks of his "vision of service," as well as of his "passionate conviction" about the medical profession (54). On another level, O'Hara feels that he is participating in an esoteric undertaking, the comprehension of which belongs to a scientific elect, of which he is a member (69). As a participant, he has no regrets about "dying for science," for sacrifice is glorious (116). And though the monetary reward is tempting, he has to remain true to his idealism and to reject compensation (128). Overall, the dramatic persona seems oblivious to, if not ignorant of, the real risks involved (129).

Brinkerhof/Kissenger, a fellow participant, comes down with yellow fever on schedule while O'Hara remains uninfected, despite having been bitten repeatedly. To encourage his friend, O'Hara quotes a well-known passage from *Julius Caesar*:

> Cowards die many times before their deaths;
> The valiant never taste death but once.
> Of all the wonders that I yet have heard,
> It seems most strange to me that men should fear,
> Seeing that death, a necessary end,
> Will come when it will come.

[II.2:32–7]

Howard's choice of this passage is confounding. The idea that valor or stoic fatalism can rationalize away a serious illness is thought-provoking in the abstract but a rather strange sentiment to express to someone in Brinkerhof's condition. Moreover, O'Hara's stilted and euphoric exclamations render him an unrealistic figure, whose advice on medical matters is untrustworthy and naïve. There is no mention of the dangers— e.g., of high fever, renal failure, and black vomit — all of which O'Hara had witnessed, time and time again, in the Ward where he worked.

The Caesarian allusion is also misleading. If we assess Caesar's motives in context, we see that he is self-deluded and oblivious, not only to the dangers surrounding him, but also to the premonitory warnings of those who wish to preserve his life. For O'Hara to evoke Caesar, then, is highly ironic: it suggests that Moran was stumbling into a life-threatening situation, comforted by his grandiose ideals. Caesar was blind to the political machinations of his enemies, and he dismissed portents. On the night before the conspiracy is to be carried out, prophets disclose ominous, apocalyptic omens (II.2: 13–26); his wife Calpurnia has an ill-omened dream about his statue bleeding profusely while Romans bathe in his blood; and although she convinces him to stay home, her advice is overridden by Decius Brutus, a chief conspirator who reinterprets the portents and dreams in favorable terms so that he can lead Caesar to the Capitol and to his death (II.2:83–90). Finally, in Act III, Caesar ignores the last-ditch warning of the soothsayer, Artemidorus, who bears irrefutable evidence of the plot (III.1:1–8). If we read the Shakespearean scenes in conjunction with O'Hara's opinion, then it seems that the latter has done a grave disservice to Brinkerhof/Kissenger who, swayed by O'Hara's delusions, now had only his robust constitution to count on. In the case of Dean and O'Hara, the spirit of volunteerism is tainted, even though the latter makes a grand gesture at the end of the play.

Since O'Hara, a non-immune patient, does not develop yellow fever as Brinkerhof had, the experimental results are compromised. Realizing this, the former takes the initiative and allows carrier mosquitoes to bite him again. This brings on the fever and seems to prove that mosquitoes are the vectors. But on this point Howard is gravely mistaken. Since O'Hara's re-exposure occurs *outside* of controlled conditions, Reed's chief critics in the context of the play could certainly have challenged its validity. In fact, as in the cases of Lazear and Carroll who ignored the possibility of prior or of subsequent exposure to sources other than insects, O'Hara voids experimental conditions and his effulgent gesture is useless. Nonetheless, O'Hara exults in his achievement as he is carried away: "Now science and humanity become one in the person of Johnny O'Hara! And no shadow of gain for him but his own satisfaction, and only the hell and vanity of that!" (149).

The literary and philosophical aspects of the play detract considerably from its realism and from the facts surrounding Walter Reed's experiment. The actual story, in my view, is sufficiently dramatic without the Shakespearian allusions. Unlike the plague novels, Howard's drama is not true to the background of the story. Nor does the play enlighten the reader as to the contributions and struggles of actual participants. The extrapolative or imaginative aspect of the yellow fever construct is therefore anti-climactic.

The WHO Fact Sheet

I would like to review a document reflecting what is now known about yellow fever in order to give the reader some idea as to how far we have come from the days of Walter Reed. An incisive text, the WHO "Fact Sheet" reflects the comprehensive understanding we now have of yellow fever. It treats viral taxonomy, symptomology, morbidity/mortality, etiology, and entomology/ecology, all in easily understood language.

According to the "Fact Sheet," the virus has four genetic types, two that are endemic to Africa and two to South America (100). After one is bitten by an infected mosquito, the disease incubates in the body for a period of three to six days. Some infections produce no symptoms at all. However, when symptoms occur, the patient usually goes through an acute phase of discomfort (fever, muscle aches, backache, headache, shivers, nausea, and vomiting). After three or four days of this, 85 percent of the patients recover. Fifteen percent, however, experience the toxic phase, suffering fever, jaundice, bleeding from orifices, and kidney dysfunction; patients in this state produce the characteristic black vomit. Within 10 to 14 days, 50 percent of the toxic-phase patients die, with only 7–8 percent recovering without significant organ damage. Encouragingly, some 92–93 percent of those coming down with yellow fever will recover.

A blood test or serology assay is one of several ways of identifying the disease. This test detects antibodies that are the body's immune response to the invading virus. The virus which affects man and monkeys has two pathways of transmission: in horizontal transmission, a biting mosquito (the vector) carries the virus from one animal to another; in vertical transmission, mosquitoes pass the virus to offspring via infected eggs; the eggs then function as protective spores in the sense that they are resistant to drying and, lying dormant through dry conditions, hatch in the rainy season. The mosquito then is the reservoir of the disease. In South America, the *Aëdes* and *Haemogogus* species are the indigenous vectors. These mosquitoes can be domestic (breeding near houses), or wild (breeding in jungles), or semi-domestic (breeding in both areas). Three transmission cycles have been identified for the disease. Sylvatic or jungle yellow fever strikes monkeys which contract the virus from bites. Intermediate yellow fever occurs in humid or semi-humid plains in Africa and can affect many villages. In this cycle, semi-domestic insects infect both monkeys and human beings. This kind of outbreak can lead to the more severe urban epidemic if domestic insects contract the virus and feed on unvaccinated, non-immune people. The *Aëdes aegypti* species, which is domestic in habitat, is a known carrier.

14. THE DYNAMIC OF FEAR
AND THE MECHANISMS
OF RESISTANCE

The emotion of fear, in all of its behavioral manifestations, links together epidemic events throughout history. Public fear in the midst of an epidemic catastrophe exhibits a developmental pattern that begins with alarm and that intensifies to panic and hysteria, a kind of collective fight-or-flight response. There is also the tendency that a level of emotional equilibrium will be reached, once the afflicted population has marshaled all resources at its disposal in the hope of resisting medical adversity. The intensity of fear, which is the focus of this chapter, is a barometer of the popular resolve: it indicates the degree to which a population has faced the disease and has discovered ways of countering it.

The yellow fever outbreak of Philadelphia, in 1793 and the Ebola epidemic of western Africa, beginning in 1976, exemplify the idea that fear is a universal and chartable aspect of the epidemic experience. Emotional reactions to the Philadelphia yellow fever epidemic of 1793 greatly intrigued the historian, J. H. Powell. In the definitive account, *Bring Out Your Dead*, he observes that an epidemic "is compounded not of disease alone, but of people's reaction to disease, how they recognize the pestilence, how they fear it or flee from it or fight it, how they are unnerved or gather resolution to conquer it" (26). During the calamity, the people of Philadelphia "acquired the habits of living with fear," and they began to snub acquaintances, not to shake hands, and to avoid contaminated houses (46). Exploring the dynamics of fear in a pivotal chapter entitled "Panic," Powell remarks how "Terror and numb dismay overwhelmed people," as Philadelphians gave in to "a coarsening fear" (90). With bodies littering the streets and with orphaned children wandering around, civil government broke down (91–3). Fear even led to persecution: African-Americans who volunteered to help white citizens were scapegoated and decried as disease carriers and as predators (95). Fear intensified into panic and hysteria (103).

Although fear "was in everyone's heart" (112), it reached a saturation point in September 1793 (112). On September 15, the worst day of all, the public attitude reputedly changed, and people developed "mechanisms of resistance," counteracting "the operation of fear" (112). After September 15, Philadelphians were then able to view the outbreak more objectively, as "a fact to be confronted, and overcome." Despite the steady increase in the death rate, "the citizens were about to find resources within themselves to develop a program of control and achievement" (112).

The emotional pattern in Powell's account (from fear, to panic, to resistance) emerges in Laurie Garrett's narration of the 1976 Ebola outbreaks in western Africa. With the eruption of Ebola in a remote Zairean village called Yambuku, health-care workers and residents, over a very brief period of time, experienced steadily-intensifying fear that reached the level of panic. The sudden appearance of hemorrhagic fever overwhelmed the staff of the local missionary hospital, and the fear it induced spread outwardly, having a palpable effect. "Panic spread," writes Garrett, "as village elders spoke of an illness, unlike anything ever seen before, that made people bleed to death" (103). The disease threatened to trigger "a mass exodus of terrified, infected villagers." When nuns became infected, fear among the staff became "contagious" (105), and when the mission's priest succumbed to the disease, the beleaguered group was "virtually paralyzed by anxiety" (107). As if fear were an infectious disorder, it reached all the way to Belgium, when blood samples that had been sent to a laboratory for analysis arrived damaged and in "a soup of melted ice" (111). In England, a scientists named Geoffrey Platt, while transferring Ebola virus from one animal to another, accidentally jabbed himself with Ebola-infected blood and contracted the disease one week later. When his colleagues at Yambuku learned of the accident, "collective fear" arose to the point that it impaired their research efforts. And when Peace Corps volunteer Del Conn caught the virus on November 26 while working at Yambuku, a radio message was as follows: "You can't imagine the fear here" (139–40). All but one CDC expert declined the Zairean assignment "out of fear" (142). The epidemic subsided naturally in November 1976. Its spread was successfully precluded by sealing off the region, but the original source of contagion was not determined (Snodgrass 325).

By the 1990s, much had been learned about the hemorrhagic virus that had caused such acute suffering. Scientific discovery gradually stemmed the emotional contagion: it was learned that the virus was contracted through the consumption of tainted primate meat, and that outbreaks could be controlled through isolation and with a well-provisioned, medical response. The benefits of this knowledge can be seen from 1996 to 2001. Of the one half-dozen Ebola outbreaks in this period, the original source of contamination for most was shown, definitively, to be the consumption of tainted primate meat. Abstention from this food source, therefore, was an obvious remedy. Although the source of a recurrence in N'zara, Sudan, in early August 1979, was not found (Snodgrass 327), the April 1995 outbreak in Kikwit, Zaire, was traced to a man who prepared infected monkey meat; five mission workers contracted the virus and died, along with the index case.

The effects of fear, though predictable, had to be included in the epidemiological strategy against Ebola. While the WHO was mobilizing to contain the outbreak, terrified natives ran away and spread the disease, with hundreds dying as a direct result (340). Though it was known that primate meat could harbor the virus, and though warnings to that effect were posted, people at Mayibout, Gabon, ate chimpanzee meat anyway, became ill, and died of Ebola. The virus continued to spread. On July 13, 1996, it hit Booué, Gabon, killing nineteen of twenty-seven victims, and traveled southeast to Johannesburg, South Africa, killing a nurse. Its dissemination was contained by a concerted international response and by the timely arrival of supplies and experts (343). In September 2000, it reappeared in northern Ugandan villages, killing half of its four hundred and twenty-eight victims. Once again, strict regional isolation limited its dissemination (355). On December 11, 2001, it flared up in a Gabonese village, prompting an international response (360). And on June 13, 2002, at Oloba in northwestern Congo, five people who ate contaminated monkey meat died of Ebola, creating panic in Central Africa. Once again, the government banned primate meat consumption, but the natives objected because it was a staple of their diet (364).

In terms of the dynamics of fear, Ebola's history from 1976 to 2001 parallels the yellow fever outbreak of August to November 1793 in Philadelphia. In both cases, the paralytic effects of fear gave way to panicked flight. In both cases, disaster was averted when the pathogen was viewed as an objective phenomenon, the effects of which could be assayed to determine its cause and to formulate a method of prevention. Whereas the embattled civic and medical agencies of eighteenth-century Philadelphia dug in their heels against the calamity, using every known resource, western virologists in the twentieth century identified the Ebola pathogen, were prepared to respond to each renewed flare-up, were at work training local agencies in its management, were informing the public (with varying success on compliance) about the source of infection, and used isolation to prevent the fear-stricken from carrying the disease beyond the affected region. As these examples show, the dynamic of fear in an epidemiological crisis is a universal reaction, transcending both time and place.

The threefold aim of this study has been to reveal the inherent unity of epidemiological thought in the West; to suggest that critical readings will show how scientists formulated strategies to overcome diseases; and to encourage students of medical history to appreciate the informative value, not only of the scientific essay, but also of histories and of imaginative works. I have tried to suggest several approaches to the appreciation of epidemiology in its socio-historical contexts. Compiling periodic texts of all kinds and . reading them critically is extremely useful. Comparing one construct to another will bring to light extraordinary similarities in the human response to contagious disease. To suggest how fruitful this approach can be, I have compared the 1793 Philadelphia yellow-fever outbreak to African Ebola epidemics in the late twentieth century, using a common pattern of fear to link the episodes to one another.

I have also tried to suggest why pre-scientific writers depended on figurative language to concretize their experiences and that the use of such figures in modern texts can unintentionally create misconceptions about science. For the creative writer who observes scientific verisimilitude, the history of epidemiology provides an unparalleled opportunity to explore medical crises vicariously and to test possibilities. But imaginative works can not be accepted at face value, since a genuinely critical assessment must take into account the degree to which the fiction conforms to, or deviates from, biomedical fact.

Works Cited

"Algeria hit by plague outbreak." *British Broadcasting Company News.* 10 July 2003. http://news.bbc.co.uk.

Alibek, Ken, with Stephen Handelman. *Biohazard: The Chilling True Story of the Largest Covert Biological Weapons Program in the World — Told from the Inside by the Man Who Ran It.* New York: Random House, 1999.

Andrus, John H. "The tale of a guinea pig" (1942), *Philip S. Hench Walter Reed Yellow Fever Collection.* http://etext.lib.virginia.edu.

The Anglo-Saxon Chronicle. Translated with an introduction by G. N. Garmonsway. New York: E, p. Dutton, 1977.

"Anthrax." Division of Bacterial and Mycotic Diseases. Centers for Disease Control. http://www.cdc.gov.

Arbib, Michael A., and Mary B. Hesse. *The Construction of Reality.* Cambridge Studies in Philosophy. New York and Cambridge: Cambridge University Press, 1986.

Aristotle. *Poetics.* Translation and analysis by Kenneth A. Telford. Chicago: Henry Regnery, 1961.

Augustine, Saint (Aurelius Augustinus). *Concerning the City of God Against the Pagans.* Translated by Henry Bettenson. Introduction by John O'Meara. New York: Penguin, 1984.

"*Bacillus anthracis.*" *Basic Laboratory Protocols for the Presumptive Identification.* www.bt.cdc.gov.

Barry, John M. *The Great Influenza: The Epic Story of the Deadliest Plague in History.* New York and London: Penguin, 2004.

Bede, Saint. *A History of the English Church and People.* Translated with an introduction by Leo Sherley-Price. Revised by R. E. Latham. (1955.) Harmondsworth, Middlesex, England: Penguin, 1960.

Beijerinck. M. W. "A *Contagium vivum fluidum* as the cause of the mosaic disease of tobacco leaves" (1899). In Brock, *Milestones in Microbiology,* pp. 153–59.

Bergin, Thomas G. *Boccaccio.* New York: Viking, 1981

_____."An introduction to Boccaccio." *The Decameron by Giovanni Boccaccio: A New Translation. Contemporary Reactions, Modern Criticism.* A Norton Critical Edition. Selected, translated, and edited by Mark Musa and Peter E. Bondarella. New York and London: W. W. Norton, 1977. pp. 151–171.

Beveridge, W. I. B. *The Art of Scientific Investigation.* (1950.) New York: W. W. Norton, 1957.

Boccaccio, Giovanni. *The Decameron.* Translated with an introduction by G. H. McWilliam. 2nd edition. New York and London: Penguin, 1995.

Bradford, William. *Of Plymouth Plantation.* Edited with an introduction by Harvey Wish. New York: Capricorn, 1962.

Branca, Vittore. *Boccaccio: The Man and His Works.* Translated by Richard Monges and Dennis J. McAuliffe. Foreword by Robert C. Clements. New York: New York University Press, 1976.

Breisach, Ernst. *Historiography: Ancient, Medieval and Modern.* Chicago and London: University of Chicago Press, 1983.

Brickman, Marla Jo. "Agents of infection." In De Salle, *Epidemic! The World of Infectious Disease*, pp. 43–49.

Briggs, Walter DeBlois. Letter to Sidney Coe Howard. July 23, 1934, p*hilip S. Hench Walter Reed Yellow Fever Collection*. http://etext.lib.virginia.edu.

Brock, Thomas D., translator and editor. *Milestones in Microbiology: 1546 to 1940*. 1961. Washington, D.C.: American Society for Microbiology, 1998.

Bruce, F. F. "Seeing." *The Interpreter's Dictionary of the Bible*. Volume 4, pp. 261–62.

Burdon, Kenneth L., and Robert P. Williams. *Microbiology*. 6th edition, 1932. New York: Macmillan, 1968.

Bury, John Bagnell. *A History of Greece to the Death of Alexander the Great*. New York: Modern Library, 1913.

Caird, George B. Introduction and Exegesis. "First and Second Books of Samuel." *The Interpreter's Bible*. Volume 11, pp. 853–1176.

Camus, Albert. *The Plague*. Translated by Stuart Gilbert. (1947.) New York: Modern Library, 1948.

Carlyon, Richard. *A Guide to the Gods: An Essential Guide to World Mythology*. New York: William Morrow, 1981.

Chin, James, editor. *Control of Communicable Diseases Manual*. 17th edition.Washington, D.C.: American Health Association, 2000.

Cohn, Ferdinand. *Bacteria: The Smallest of Living Organisms*. Translated by Charles S.Dolley. Introduction by Morris C. Leikind. (1872.) Baltimore: The Johns Hopkins University Press, 1939.

_____. "Studies on bacteria" (1875). Translated by Thomas D. Brock. In Brock, *Milestones in Microbiology*, pp. 210–15.

_____. "Studies on the biology of the bacilli" (1876). In Brock, *Milestones in Microbiology*, pp. 49–56.

Cohn, Norman. *The Pursuit of the Millennium*. (1957.) Revised edition. New York: Oxford University Press, 1977.

Conley, Nancy, et al., editors. *Fields of Writing: Readings Across the Disciplines*. 2nd edition. New York: St. Martin's, 1987.

Corney, R. W."Abiathar." *The Interpreter's Dictionary of the Bible*. Volume 1, A-D, pp. 6–7.

Cowley, Geoffrey. "The plan to fight smallpox." *Newsweek*, October 14, 2002, pp. 45–52.

Cravens, Gwyneth, and John S. Marr. *The Black Death*. New York: Ballantine, 1977.

Crosby, Alfred W. *America's Forgotten Pandemic: The Influenza of 1918*. (1976.) Cambridge and New York: Cambridge University Press, 2003.

Da Rocha-Lima, H. "On the etiology of typhus fever." In Hahon, *Selected Papers on the Pathogenic Rickettsiae*, pp. 74–78.

Davies, G. Henton. "Ark of the Covenant." *The Interpreter's Dictionary of the Bible*. Volume 1, A-D, pp. 222–26.

De Kruif, Paul. *Microbe Hunters*. Introduction by F. Gonzalez-Crussi. (1926.) San Diego, New York, and London: Harcourt, Brace, 1996.

De Salle, Robert. "Epidemics and pandemics." In De Salle, *Epidemic! The World of Infectious Disease*, pp. 153–56.

_____. "Natural history of infectious disease." In De Salle, *Epidemic! The World of Infectious Disease*, pp. 19–22.

_____, editor. *Epidemic! The World of Infectious Disease*. New York: The New Press, 1999.

De Salle, Robert, and Marla Jo Brickman. "Outbreaks." In De Salle, *Epidemic! The World of Infectious Disease*, pp. 113–16.

De Sanctis, Francesco. "Boccaccio and the human comedy." *The Decameron*. A Norton Critical Edition. New York: W.W. Norton, 1977, pp. 216–29.

D'Hérelle, Felix. "An invisible microbe that is antagonistic to the dysentery bacillus" (1917). In Brock, *Milestones in Microbiology*, pp. 157–59.

_____. "On the role of the filterable bacteriophage in bacillary dysentery" (1918). Excerpts in *Molecular Biology of Bacterial Viruses* by Gunther S. Stent. San Francisco and London: W. H. Freeman, 1963, pp. 1–22.

Dictionary of the Bible. Edited by James Hastings. Revised by Frederick C. Grant and H. H. Rowley. New York: Charles Scribner's Sons, 1963.

Dimsdale, Thomas. "An account of the inoculation of Catherine the Second [1729–1796], Empress of all the Russias." http://www.library.ucla.edu.

Diogenes Laertius. "Letter to Herodotus." *The Epicurus Reader. Selected Writings and Testimonia.* Translated and edited by Brad Inwood and L.P. Gerson. Introduction by D. S. Hutchinson. Indianapolis and Cambridge: Hackett, 1994, pp. 5–19.

Dombroski, Robert S. "Introduction." In *Critical Perspectives on The Decameron.* Edited by Robert S. Dombroski. London and Sydney: Hodder and Stoughton, 1976, pp. 1–13.

Dondero, T. J., Jr., et al. "An outbreak of Legionnaires' disease associated with a contaminated air-conditioning cooling tower." *New England Journal of Medicine* 307.7 (February 14, 1980): 365–70.

Driver, G. R. "Leprosy." *Dictionary of the Bible,* pp. 575–78.

Dubois, Marguerite-Marie, with the collaboration of Charles Cestre et al. *Modern French-English Dictionary.* Edited by William Maxwell Landers, Roger Shattuck, and Margaret G. Cobb, Paris: Librairie LaRousse, 1960.

Dubos, René. *Pasteur and Modern Science.* Garden City. NY: Anchor, 1960.

England, A. C., et al. "Sporadic *Legionellosis* in the United States: the first thousand cases." *Annals of Internal Medicine* 94.2 (February 1981): 64–70.

"Epidemic dysentery." *Cholera and Epidemic-prone Diarrheal Diseases.* World Health Organization. http://www.who.int/csr/disease/cholera/en.

Eusebius of Caesarea. *The History of the Church from Christ to Constantine.* Translated with an introduction by G. A. Williamson. Harmondsworth, Middlesex, England: Penguin, 1965.

Fahnestock, Jeanne. *Rhetorical Figures in Science.* New York: Oxford University Press, 1999.

Fetrow, Charles W., and Juan R. Avila. *The Complete Guide to Herbal Medicines.* New York and London: Pocket, 2000.

Fields, Barry S., et al. "*Legionella* and Legionnaires' disease: 25 years of investigation." *Clinical Microbiology Reviews* 15.3 (July 2002): 506–26.

Fleming, Alexander. "On the antibacterial action of cultures of a Penicillium, with special reference to their use in the isolation of *B. influenzae*" (1929). In Brock, *Milestones in Microbiology,* pp. 185–94.

Fox, Robin Lane. *Pagans and Christians.* New York: Alfred A. Knopf, 1987.

Fracastoro, Girolamo. "Contagion, contagious diseases and their treatment (1546)." Translated by Wilmer C. Wright. In Brock, *Milestones in Microbiology,* pp. 69–75.

_____. "The fever called *Lenticulae* or *Puncticulae*." In Hahon, *Selected Papers on the Pathogenic Rickettsiae,* pp. 1–3.

Fraenkel-Conrat, Heinz L."Synthetic mutants." In Stanley and Valens, *Viruses and the Nature of Life,* pp. 191–205.

Fraser, D. W., et al. "Legionnaires' disease: description of an epidemic pneumonia." *The New England Journal of Medicine* 297.22 (December 1, 1977): 1189–97.

_____, et al. "Sporadic *Legionellosis* in the United States: the first two thousand cases." *Annals of Internal Medicine* 94.2 (February 1981): 164–170.

Frazer, Sir James George. *The Golden Bough: A Study in Magic and Religion.* Volume 1. (Abridged edition, 1922.) New York: Macmillan, 1951.

"Gangrene." MayoClinic.com./invoke.cfm.

Garrett, Laurie. *The Coming Plague: Newly Emerging Diseases in a World Out of Balance.* New York and London: Penguin, 1994.

Gerhard, W. W. "On the typhus fever. Which occurred at Philadelphia in the spring and summer of 1836..." (1837). In Hahon, *Selected Papers on the Pathogenic Rickettsiae,* pp. 4–26.

Glyn, Ian, and Jenifer Glyn. *The Life and Death of Smallpox.* New York: Cambridge University Press, 2004.

Goebel, Lynne, and Henry Driscoll. "Scurvy." *Medicine: Instant Access to the Minds of Medicine.* http://www.emedicine.com.

Gold, V. R. "Beth-Shemesh." *Dictionary of the Bible,* p. 101.

_____, "Kiriath-jearim." *The Interpreter's Dictionary of the Bible.* Volume 3, K-Q, pp.37–8.

Gorgas, William Crawford. "Report: method of the spread of yellow fever" (April 15, 1908).

Philip S. Hench Walter Reed Yellow Fever Collection. http://etext.lib.virginia.edu.

Grant, Michael. *The Myths of the Greeks and Romans.* (Revised edition, 1962.) New York: Mentor, 1986.

Gray, J. "Beth-shemesh." *Dictionary of the Bible,* p. 101.

_____. "Dagon." *The Interpreter's Dictionary of the Bible.* Volume 1: A-D, p. 756.

_____. "Vanity." *The Interpreter's Dictionary of the Bible.* Volume 4, R-Z, pp. 746–47.

Greenfield, J. C. "Philistines." *The Interpreter's Dictionary of the Bible.* Volume 3, K-Q. pp. 791–95.

Greenfield, Stanley B. *A Critical History of Old English Literature.* 1965. New York: New York University Press, 1974.

Gregory of Tours. *The History of the Franks.* Translated with an introduction by Lewis Thorpe. New York and London: Penguin, 1974.

Hahon, Nicholas, editor. *Selected Papers on the Pathogenic Rickettsiae.* Cambridge: Harvard University Press, 1968.

Hankin, Ernest. "L'action bactericide des eaux de la Jumna et du Ganges sur le vibrion du cholera." *Annals of the Pasteur Institute* 10 (1896): 511.

"Hansen's disease (leprosy)." *Disease Information: Division of Bacterial and Mycotic Diseases.* Centers for Disease Control. http://www.cdc.gov.

Harrison, R. K. "Leprosy." *The Interpreter's Dictionary of the Bible.* Volume 3, K-Q, pp. 111–13.

_____. "Plague." *The Interpreter's Dictionary of the Bible.* Volume 3, K-Q, pp. 821–22.

Hays, J. N. *The Burdens of Disease: Epidemics and Human Response in Western History.* New Brunswick, NJ: Rutgers University Press, 2000.

"Head lice infestation (pediculosis)." Centers for Disease Control. http://www.cdc.gov.

Hellemans, Alexander, and Bryan Bunch. *The Timetables of Science: A Chronology of the Most Important People and Events in the History of Science.* (1988.) New York: Simon and Schuster, 1991.

Henle, Jacob. "Concerning miasmatic, contagious, and miasmatic-contagious diseases" (1840). In Brock, *Milestones in Microbiology,* pp. 76–9.

Herbert, A. S. "Abiathar." *Dictionary of the Bible,* p. 3.

Hesiod (Hesiodos). *Theogony and Works and Days.* Translated with an introduction and notes by M. L. West. New York: Oxford University Press, 1988.

Hippocrates. Translated and introduced by W. H. S. Jones. Loeb Classical Library. Cambridge: Harvard University Press, 1995.

Hippocrates of Cos. "Ancient medicine." In *Hippocrates.* Volume I, pp. 1–64.

_____. *The Book of Prognostics* (400 B.C). Translated by Francis Adams. Internet Classic Archive. http://classics.mit.edu.

_____. *Epidemics.* Books I and III. In *Hippocrates.* Volume I, pp. 139–287.

_____. "Precepts." In *Hippocrates.* Volume I, pp. 305–33.

"HIV. How [it] causes AIDS." National Institute of Allergy and Infectious Disease. National Institutes of Health. United States Department of Health and Human Services. October 2001. http://www.niaid.nih.gov.

Hodges, Nathaniel. *Loimologia: or, An Historical Account of the Plague in London in 1665: with precautionary Directions against the like Contagion.* Translated by John Quincy. (1720.) Appendix to *The Historical Sources of De Foe's Journal of the Plague Year* by Watson Nicholson. Port Washington, NY: Kennikat, 1920. Pp. 101–115.

Holmes, Oliver Wendell. "Border lines in medical science: An introductory lecture delivered before the Medical Class of Harvard University." November 6, 1861. Volume 9 of *The Works of Oliver Wendell Holmes.* (1861.) New York: Houghton-Mifflin,1892.

_____. "Contagiousness of puerperal fever." *Classics of Medicine and Surgery.* Edited by C. N. B. Camac. 1843 and 1855. New York: Dover, 1909. Pp. 399–435.

The Holy Bible. Containing the Old and New Testaments and the Apocrypha. Authorized King James Version. New York: Oxford University Press, n.d.

Homer. *The Iliad.* Translated with an introduction by Richard Lattimore. (1951.) Chicago: University of Chicago Press, 1967.

Homer, Frederic D, *Primo Levi and the Politics of Survival.* Columbia: University of Missouri Press, 2001.

Howard, Sidney Coe. Letter to Albert E. Truby. December 7, 1931. *Philip S. Hench Walter Reed Yellow Fever Collection.* http://etext.lib.virginia.edu.

_____. Letter to Albert E. Truby. December 19, 1931. *Philip S. Hench Walter Reed Yellow Fever Collection.* http://etext.lib.virginia.edu.

_____. Letter to John J. Moran. December 22, 1931. *Philip S. Hench Walter Reed Yellow Fever Collection.* http://etext.lib.virginia.edu.

_____. Letter to John J. Moran. January 12, 1932. *Philip S. Hench Walter Reed Yellow Fever Collection.* http://etext.lib.virginia.edu.

_____. Letter to John J. Moran. January 12, 1933. *Philip S. Hench Walter Reed Yellow Fever Collection.* http://etext.lib.virginia.edu.

_____. Letter to John J. Moran. March 6, 1934. *Philip S. Hench Walter Reed Yellow Fever Collection.* http://etext.lib.virginia.edu.

_____, in collaboration with Paul de Kruif. *Yellow Jack: A History.* New York: Harcourt. Brace, 1933.

Hug, p. L. "History, theology of." *New Catholic Encyclopedia.* Volume 7. Edited by William J. McDonald et al. New York: McGraw-Hill, 1967. Pp. 26–31.

Ingliss, T. J. J. "Legionellosis." *www.etiology.com.*

The Interpreter's Bible: The Holy Scriptures in the King James and Revised Standard Versions with General Articles and Introduction, Exegesis, Exposition for Each Book of the Bible. Edited by Arthur Buttrick et al. 12 volumes. (1953.) New York and Nashville: Abingdon, 1954.

The Interpreter's Dictionary of the Bible: An Illustrated Encyclopedia. Edited by George Arthur Buttrick et al. 4 volumes and supplement. 19th edition. Nashville: Abingdon, 1962.

Jenner, Edward. *The Origin of the Vaccine Inoculation.* London: D. M. Shury, 1801.

_____. *Vaccination against Smallpox.* Amherst, NY: Prometheus, 1996.

Jernigan, D.B., et al. "Outbreak of Legionnaires' disease among cruise ship passengers exposed to a contaminated whirlpool spa." *The Lancet,* 347.9000 (February 24, 1996): 494–9.

Johnson, Samuel. *Dictionary of the English Language.* Edited by Alexander Chalmers. (1843.) London: Studio Editions, 1994.

Kitasato, S[hibasaburo]. "The bacillus of bubonic plague." *The Lancet* 2 (August 25, 1894): 428–430.

Koch, Robert. "The aetiology of tuberculosis." Translated by Dr. and Mrs. Max Pinner. *Source Book of Medical History,* pp. 392–406

_____. "The etiology of anthrax, based on the life history of *Bacillus anthracis*" (1876). In Brock, *Milestones in Microbiology,* pp. 89–95.

_____. "The etiology of tuberculosis" [March 24, 1882]. In Brock, *Milestones in Microbiology,* pp. 109–115.

_____. "The etiology of tuberculosis" [Koch's Postulates] (1884). In Brock, *Milestones in Microbiology,* pp. 116–18.

_____. "On the anthrax inoculation [1872]." Translated by K. Codell Carter. Site by David V. Cohen. http://www.foundersofscience.

Kohn, George Childs, editor. *Encyclopedia of Plague and Pestilence from Ancient Times to the Present.* Foreword by Mary-Louise Scully. (Revised edition, 1995.) New York: Checkmark, 2001.

Kolata, Gina. *Flu: The Story of the Great Influenza Pandemic of 1918 and the Search for the Virus That Caused It.* 1999. New York: Simon and Schuster, 2001.

Koob, Derry D., and William E. Boggs. *The Nature of Life.* Reading, MA: Addison-Wesley, 1972.

Kuhn, Thomas S. "Anomaly and the emergence of scientific discoveries." In *The Structure of Scientific Revolutions.* 2nd edition. Volume 2.2. International Encyclopedia of Unified Science. Editor-in-chief Otto Neurath. Associate editors Rudolf Carnap and Charles Morris. (1962.) Chicago: University of Chicago Press, 1970. Pp. 52–65.

_____. "The historical structure of scientific discovery." In Conley et al., *Fields of Writing: Readings Across the Disciplines,* pp. 721–37.

Lederberg, Joshua. "Emerging infections: an evolutionary perspective." *Emerging Infectious Diseases* 4.3 (July–September 1998). *http://www.cdc.gov.*

_____. "Infectious disease as an evolutionary paradigm." *Emerging Infectious Diseases* 3.4 (October-December 1997): 417–23.

_____. "Infectious disease as an example of evolution." In De Salle, *Epidemic! The World of Infectious Disease*, pp. 13–17.

_____. "Infectious history" (2000). http://www.univie.ac.at/hygieneaktuell/lederberg.htm.

Lee, Bradford A. "Arms race." *Reader's Companion to Military History*. http://college.hm co.com.

"*Legionellosis*: Legionnaires' disease (LD) and Pontiac fever." Centers for Disease Control. Division of Bacterial and Mycotic Diseases. Disease Information. December 23, 2003. www.cdc.gov.

Levi, Primo. *Survival in Auschwitz: The Nazi Assault on Humanity*. Translated by Stuart Woolf. New York: Touchstone, 1958.

Lewis, Sinclair. *Arrowsmith*. (1924.) New York: Signet, 1998.

Liebig, Justis. "Concerning the phenomenon of fermentation, putrefaction and decay, and their causes" (1839). In Brock, *Milestones in Microbiology*, pp. 24–7.

Litsios, Socrates. *Plague Legends: From the Miasmas of Hippocrates to the Microbes of Pasteur*. Chesterfield, MO: Science and Humanities, 2001.

Livy, Titus (Livius). *The Early History of Rome*. Books I-V of *The History of Rome from its Foundation*. Translated by Aubrey de Sèlincourt with an Introduction by R. M. Ogilvie.(Reprinted 1960.) Harmondsworth, Middlesex, England: Penguin, 1971.

Lloyd, G. E. R. *Early Greek Science: Thales to Aristotle. Ancient Culture and Society*. Edited by M. I. Finley. New York: W. W. Norton, 1971.

Löffler, Friedrich, and Paul Frosch. "Report of the commission for research on the foot-and-mouth disease" (1898). In Brock, *Milestones in Microbiology*, pp. 149–53.

London, Jack. *The Cruise of the Snark*. (1919.) New York: Dover, 2000.

Lord, Alexandra M. "A brief history of anthrax." lhncbc.nlm-gov/apdb/phsHistory-/resources/printed_mat.html.

Lucretius (Titus Lucretius Carus). *On the Nature of the Universe*. Translated by Ronald Melville. Introduction by Don and Peta Fowler. New York: Oxford University Press, 1999.

Marks, Geoffrey, and William K. Beatty. *Epidemics: The Story of Mankind's Most Lethal and Elusive Enemies — From Ancient Times to the Present*. New York: Charles Scribner's Sons, 1976.

Mausner, Judith S., Anita K. Bahn, Sira Kramer, et al. *Epidemiology: An Introductory Text*. 2nd edition. Philadelphia: W. B. Saunders, 1985.

May, Arthur. *Europe Since 1939*. New York: Holt, Rhinehart, and Winston, 1966.

Mayr, Ernst. *The Growth of Biological Thought: Diversity, Evolution, and Inheritance*. Cambridge: The Belknap Press of Harvard University Press, 1982.

McDade, J.E. "The ecology of outbreaks: discovery of *Legionella pneumophila*." In De Salle, *Epidemic! The World of Infectious Disease*, pp. 135–38.

McDade, J. E., et al. "Legionnaires' disease: isolation of a bacterium and demonstration of its role in other respiratory disease." *The New England Journal of Medicine* 297.22 (December 1, 1977): 1197–1203.

McElroy, John. *This Was Andersonville*. Edited with an introduction by Roy Meredith. (1879.) New York: Bonanza, 1957.

McGinn, Bernard. *Anti-Christ: Two Thousand Years of the Human Fascination with Evil*. New York: HarperCollins, 1996.

McGovern, Thomas W., and Arthur M. Friedlander. "Plague." *Medical Aspects of Chemical and Biological Warfare*. http://www.cbwinfo.-com/History/History.html

McNeill, William H. *Plagues and Peoples*. New York: Anchor, 1976.

Medawar, Peter Brian. "Can scientific discovery be premeditated?" In Conley et al., *Fields of Writing: Readings Across the Disciplines*, pp. 731–37.

Messadié, Gerald. "Genetic Recombination." In Messadié, *Great Scientific Discoveries*, pp. 79–81.

_____. *Great Scientific Discoveries*. New York: W. R. Chambers, 1991.

_____. "Vaccination." In Messadié, *Great Scientific Discoveries*, pp. 209–10.

Mihelic, J. L., and G. E. Wright. "Plagues in Exodus." *The Interpreter's Dictionary of the Bible*. Vol. 3, K-Q, pp. 822–24.

Mollaret, H. H. "Paul-Louis Simond's discovery of the flea's role as vector of plague." *Journal of the Pasteur Institute*. In honor of Paul-Louis Simond. Reprinted from *Rev. Prat*, Paris 41 (1991): 1947–1951.

Montagu, Lady Mary Wortley. "Smallpox vaccination in Turkey." *Modern History Sourcebook*. http://www.fordham.edu.

Moran, John J. Letter to Howard A. Kelley. February 15, 1907. *Philip S. Hench Walter Reed Yellow Fever Collection*. http://etext.lib.virginia.edu.

_____. "Memoirs of a human guinea pig (19[49])." *Philip S. Hench Walter Reed Yellow Fever Collection*. http://etext.lib./virginia./edu

Murray, Oswyn. "Greek historians." *The Oxford History of Greece and the Hellenistic World*. Edited by John Boardman, Jasper Griffin, and Oswyn Murray. New York: Oxford University Press, 1991. Pp. 214–39.

Muscetta, Carlo. *Giovanni Boccaccio*. 2d edition. Bari: Laterza, 1974.

The New Cassell's German Dictionary: German-English / English-German. Edited by Karl Breul. Revised and re-edited by Harold T. Betteridge, with a foreword by Gerhard Cordes. (1958.) New York: Funk and Wagnalls, 1971.

The New Merriam-Webster Dictionary. Edited by Frederick C. Mish et al. Springfield, MA: Merriam-Webster, 1989.

"New York City reassures public on plague." November 8, 2002. CBS.com.

Nicholson, Watson. *The Historical Sources of De Foe's* Journal of the Plague Year. *Illustrated by Extracts from the Original Documents in the Burney Collection and Manuscript Room in the British Museum*. Port Washington, NY: Kennikat, 1920.

Nicolle, Charles. "Investigations on typhus." Presentation speech." The Nobel Prize in Physiology or Medicine 1928. http://www.nobel.se/medicine/laureates/-1928/nicolle-lectur.html.

Nuland, Sherwin B. *Childbed Fever, and the Strange Story of Ignaz Semmelweis*. New York: W. W. Norton, 2004.

Ogata, Masanori. " 'One should pay close attention to insects....': bubonic plague hits San Francisco, 1900–1907." *A Science Odyssey: People and Discoveries*. pbs.org/wgbh.

_____. "Über die Pestepidemie in Formosa." *Zentralbl Bakteriol Parasitkenkd Infekionskr* 21 (1897): 769–777.

Oldstone, Michael B. A. *Viruses, Plagues, and History*. New York: Oxford University Press, 2000.

Osterholm, M. T., et al. "A 1957 outbreak of Legionnaires' disease associated with a meat packing plant." *American Journal of Epidemiology* 17.1 (1987): 60–7.

Ovid (Publius Ovidius Naso). *Metamorphoses*. Translated by A. D. Melville. Introduction and notes by E. J. Kenney. Volume 7. New York: Oxford University Press, 1986. Pp. 523–613.

Owen, H. P. "Eschatology." *Interpreter's Dictionary of the Bible*. Volume 3, K-Q, pp. 48–9.

The Oxford English Dictionary. 21 volumes and Supplement (1933). Oxford: Clarendon, 1971.

Parish, H. J. *A History of Immunization*. Edinburgh: E. and S. Livingstone, 1965.

Pasteur, Louis. "Animal infusoria living in the absence of free oxygen, and the fermentations they bring about" (1861). In Brock, *Milestones in Microbiology*, pp. 39–41.

_____. "The anthrax vaccination: reply of M. Pasteur to a paper of M. Koch." Translated by Evelyn T. and David V. Cohen. Revised 30 March 2001. extract from the *Scientific Review*, Paris. 20 Jan.1883. http://www.foundersofscience.net/p's-Reply.htm

_____. "The attenuation of the causal agent of fowl cholera" (1880). In Brock, *Milestones in Microbiology*, pp. 126–31.

_____. *The Germ Theory and Its Applications to Medicine and Surgery* (1878). Translated by H. C. Ernst. Revised edition. Amherst, NY: Prometheus, 1996, pp. 110–17.

_____. "On a vaccine for fowl cholera and anthrax" (1881). In Brock, *Milestones in Microbiology*, pp. 131–32.

_____. "On the extension of the germ theory to the etiology of certain common diseases" (1880). In Pasteur, *The Germ Theory and Its Applications to Medicine and Surgery* (1878), pp. 118–30.

_____. "On the organized bodies which exist in the atmosphere; examinaton of the doctrine of spontaneous generation" (1861). In Brock, *Milestones in Microbiology*, pp. 43–8.

_____. "Prevention of rabies: a method by which the development of rabies after a bite may be prevented." Translated by D. Berger. In *The Founders of Modern Medicine: Pasteur, Koch, Lister*, edited by Elie Metchnikoff. New York: Walden, 1939. Pp. 379–87.

_____, and Louis Thuillier. *The Correspondence Concerning Anthrax and Swine Fever Vaccinations* (September 16, 1881–June 26, 1887). Translated and edited with an introduction by Robert M. Frank and Denise Wrotnowska, preface by Pasteur Vallery-Radot. University: University of Alabama Press, 1968.

_____, et al. "Summary report of the experiments conducted at Pouilly-le-Fort, near Melun, on the anthrax vaccination." Translated by Tina Dasgupsta. *Classics of Biology and Medicine* 22 (2002), pp. 59–62; reprinted from *Comptes Rendus de l'Academie des Sciences* 92 (June 13, 1881): 1378–1383.

Paul the Deacon. *History of the Langobards*. Translated by William Dudley Foulke. Philadelphia: University of Pennsylvania Press, 1907.

"Pediculosis: head lice infestation." Centers for Disease Control. http://www.cdc.gov.

"Pistoia: ordinances for sanitation in a time of mortality." *Plague and Public Health in Renaissance Europe*. http://jefferson.village.virginia.edu.

"Plague." In Chin, *Control of Communicable Diseases Manual*, pp. 381–87.

"Plague, information on." Centers for Disease Control. Division of Vector-Borne Infectious Diseases. www.cdc.gov.

Porter, Roy. *The Greatest Benefit to Mankind: A Medical History of Humanity*. New York: W. W. Norton, 1997.

Powell, J. H. *Bring Out Your Dead: The Great Plague of Yellow Fever in Philadelphia in 1793*. Philadelphia: University of Pennsylvania Press, 1949.

Preston, Richard. *The Demon in the Freezer: A True Story*. New York: Random House, 2002.

Procopius of Caesarea. *History of the Wars*. Books I–II. Translated by H. B. DeWing. Loeb Classical Library. Cambridge: Harvard University Press, 1992.

"Rabies." National Center for Infectious Disease. http://www.cdc.gov.

The Random House College Dictionary. Revised edition. Edited by Jess Stein, Leonore C. Hauck, and P. Y. Su. New York: Random House,1973.

Random House Webster's Dictionary of Scientists. Edited by Sara Jenkins-Jones et al. New York: Random House, 1997.

Reed, Walter. Letter to George Miller Sternberg. July 24, 1900. *Philip S. Hench Walter Reed Yellow Fever Collection*. http://etext.lib.virginia.edu.

_____. Letter to James Carroll. September 24, 1900. *Philip S. Hench Walter Reed Yellow Fever Collection*. http://etext.lib.virginia.edu.

_____. "Yellow Fever." *Source Book of Medical History*, pp. 479–84.

Reichenbach, Hans. *The Rise of Scientific Philosophy*. (1951.) Berkeley and Los Angeles: University of California Press, 1966.

Ricketts, H. T., and Russell M. Wilder. "The etiology of the typhus fever (tabardillo) of Mexico City." In Hahon, *Selected Papers on the Pathogenic Rickettsiae*, pp. 41–6.

Rosenthal, Elisabeth. "Girl is first to survive rabies without a shot." *The New York Times*, November 25, 2004, p. A28.

Roueché, Bernard. "A man named Hoffman." In Berton Roueché, *The Medical Detectives*. (1965.) New York: Truman Talley, 1988. Pp. 179–99.

Ryan, Kenneth J. "Childbed fever." In *Sherris Medical Microbiology: An Introduction to Infectious Disease*. Edited by Kenneth J. Ryan, C. George Ray, et al. New York: McGraw-Hill. 2004, pp. 915–16.

Semmelweis, Ignaz. "Lecture on the genesis of puerperal fever (childbed fever)" (1850). In Brock, *Milestones in Microbiology*, pp. 80–2.

Seneca, Lucius Annaeus. *Oedipus*. In *Seneca: Tragedies*. Translated by Frank Justus Miller. Loeb Classical Library. Cambridge, MA: Harvard University Press, 1917. Pp. 425–523.

"Shigellosis (bacillary dysentery)." In Chin, *Control of Communicable Diseases Manual*, pp. 451–55.

Simond, Paul-Louis. "Comment fut mis en évidence le rôle de la puce dans transmission de la peste." *Rev. Hyg.* 58 (1936): 1–17.

_____. "La propagation de la peste." *Annals of the Pasteur Institute* 12 (1898): 626–86.

Excerpts quoted in "La découverte par Paul-Louis Simond du role de la puce dans la transmission de la peste" by H. H. Mollaret. Reprinted in *Rev. Prat* Paris 41 (1991): 1947–1951.

Sinnigen, William G., and Arthur E. R. Boak. *A History of Rome to* A.D. *565.* 6th edition. New York: Macmillan, 1977.

"Smallpox." In *Handbook of Infectious Disease.* Edited by H. Nancy Holmes et al. Foreword by David L. Longworth. Springhouse, PA: Springhouse, 2002. Pp. 329–330.

"Smallpox overview." Public Health Emergency Preparedness and Response. Centers for Disease Control. http://www.bt.cdc.gov.

Smith, M. S. "The diagnosis and treatment of scurvy: an historical perspective." *J. R. Nav. Med. Serv.* 72.2 (Summer 1986): 104–06.

Snodgrass, Mary Ellen. *World Epidemics: A Cultural Chronology of Disease from Prehistory to the Era of SARS.* Jefferson, NC: McFarland, 2003.

Snow, John. "Cholera and the water supply in the South Districts of London, 1854." http://www.ph.ucla.edu.

_____. *On the Mode of Communication of Cholera.* London: John Churchill, 1855. http://www.ph.ucla.edu.

Sontag, Susan. *Illness as Metaphor and AIDS and Its Metaphors.* New York: AnchorDoubleday, 1990.

Sophocles. *Oedipus Rex.* Translated by Albert Cook. In *Ten Greek Plays in Contemporary Translations.* Edited by Gordon N. Ray. Boston: Houghton Mifflin, 1957. Pp. 117–153.

Source Book of Medical History. Compiled with notes by Logan Clendening. New York: Henry Schuman; New York: Dover, 1942.

Spielman, Andrew. "The emergence of new diseases." In De Salle, *Epidemic! The World of Infectious Disease,* pp. 19–22.

Stanley, Wendell M., and Evans G. Valens. *Viruses and the Nature of Life.* New York: Dutton, 1965.

Stent, Gunther S. *Molecular Biology of Bacterial Viruses.* San Francisco: W. H. Freeman, 1963. Pp. 1–22.

_____. "Reproduction and mutation." In Stanley and Valens, *Viruses and the Nature of Life,* pp. 72–87.

Sternberg, George M. Letter to Walter Reed. January 19, 1894. *Philip S. Hench Walter Reed Yellow Fever Collection.* http://etext.lib.virginia.edu.

Stinespring, W. F. "Ashdod." *The Interpreter's Dictionary of the Bible.* Volume 1, A–D, pp. 248–49.

_____. "Ekron." *The Interpreter's Dictionary of the Bible.* Volume 2, E–J, p. 69.

Stolley, Paul D., and Tamar Lasky. *Investigating Disease Patterns: The Science of Epidemiology.* New York: Scientific American Library, 1998.

Sulakvelidze, Alexander, et al. "Bacteriophage therapy: minireview." *Antimicrobial Agents and Chemotherapy* 45.3 (March 2001): 649–59. http://aac.asm.org.

Summers, William C. "Bacteriophage therapy." (Abstract.) *Annual Review of Microbiology* 55 (October 2001): 437–51.

_____. *Felix D'Hérelle and the Origins of Molecular Biology.* New Haven: Yale University Press, 1999.

Swiderski, Richard M. *Anthrax: A History.* Jefferson, NC: McFarland, 2004.

Szikszai, S. "Samuel I and II." *The Interpreter's Dictionary of the Bible.* Volume 4, R–Z, pp. 201–02.

Tebb, William. *The Recrudescence of Leprosy and Its Causation.* 1893. http://www.whale. to /vaccine/tebb.html.

Thomas, Rolla L. "Typhus fever." *The Eclectic Practice of Medicine.* 1907. http://www.ibiblio.org/herbmed/eclectic/thomas/typhus.html.

Thomson, Ian. *Primo Levi: A Life.* New York: Henry Holt, 2003.

Thrall, William Flint, Addison Hibbard, and Hugh Holman. *A Handbook to Literature.* (Revised and enlarged edition, 1936.) New York: Odyssey, 1960.

Thucydides. *The Complete Writings.* Translated by Richard Crawley. Introduction by John H. Finley, Jr. New York: Modern Library, 1951.

_____. *The Peloponnesian War.* Translated by Thomas Hobbes. Introduction and notes by

David Grene. (1959.) Chicago: University of Chicago Press, 1989.

Trawick, Buckner. B. *The Bible as Literature: The Old Testament and the Apocrypha.* 1963. New York: Barnes and Noble, 1970. Pp. 95–110.

Tsevat, M. "Samuel I and II." *Interpreter's Dictionary of the Bible.* Supplementary volume, pp. 777–81.

Tucker, Jonathan B. *Scourge: The Once and Future Threat of Smallpox.* New York: Grove, 2001.

"Two cases of travel-associated bubonic plague in New York City." Health Alert #36. The City of New York Department of Health and Mental Hygiene. November 6, 2002. www.nyc.gov.

Twort, F. W. "An investigation of the nature of ultra-microscopic viruses." (1915.) In *Selected Papers on Virology.* Edited by Nicholas Hahon. Englewood Cliffs, NJ: Prentice Hall, 1964, pp. 97–102.

"Typhus." In Chin, *Control of Communicable Diseases Manual,* pp. 541–558.

Virgil. "Polydore." In *The Georgics.* Translated with an introduction and notes by L. P. Wilkinson. Harmondsworth, Middlesex, England: Penguin, 1982.

Voltaire, François Marie Arouet de. "Inoculation." *The English Letters* in *The Portable-Voltaire.* Edited and translated by Ben Ray Redman. (1949.) New York: Penguin, 1977, pp. 524–30.

The Wanderer: Anglo-Saxon Poetry. Selected and translated with an introduction by R. K. Gordon. 1926. New York: Dutton; London: Dent, 1976. Pp. 73–75.

Watts, Sheldon. *Epidemics and History: Disease, Power and Imperialism.* (1997.) New Haven: Yale University Press, 1999.

Wilkinson, Lise. "Anthrax." *The Cambridge World History of Human Disease.* Cambridge: Cambridge University Press, 1993. Pp. 582–84.

Wills, Christopher. *Yellow Fever, Black Goddess: The Coevolution of People and Plagues.* Cambridge, MA: Perseus, 1996.

Winslow, Charles-Edward Amory. *The Conquest of Epidemic Disease: A Chapter in the History of Ideas.* (1943.) Madison: University of Wisconsin Press, 1980.

"Yellow fever." Fact Sheet 100. Revised December 2001. World Health Organization. http://www.who.int/int-fs/en/fact100.html

"Yellow fever / Reed Commission Exhibit." University of Virginia Health Sciences Library Historical Collection. http://www.med.virginia.edu.

Yersin, Alexandre. "La peste bubonique à Hong-Kong." (Translated by Charles De Paolo for use in this study.) *Archives of Naval Medicine* 62 (1894): 256–61.

Ziegler, Philip. *The Black Death.* New York: Harper and Row, 1969.

Zinsser, Hans. *Rats, Lice, and History.* Boston: Little, Brown, 1924.

INDEX